Lung Cancer, Part II: Surgery and Adjuvant Therapies

Editors

JEAN DESLAURIERS
F. GRIFFITH PEARSON
FARID M. SHAMJI

THORACIC SURGERY CLINICS

www.thoracic.theclinics.com

Consulting Editor
M. BLAIR MARSHALL

August 2013 • Volume 23 • Number 3

ELSEVIER

1600 John F. Kennedy Boulevard • Suite 1800 • Philadelphia, Pennsylvania, 19103-2899

http://www.theclinics.com

THORACIC SURGERY CLINICS Volume 23, Number 3
August 2013 ISSN 1547-4127, ISBN-13: 978-0-323-18617-9

Editor: Jessica McCool

Thoracic Surgery Clinics (ISSN 1547-4127) is published quarterly by Elsevier Inc., 360 Park Avenue South, New York, NY 10010-1710. Months of publication are February, May, August, and November. Business and editorial offices: 1600 John F. Kennedy Boulevard, Suite 1800, Philadelphia, PA 19103-2899. Periodicals postage paid at New York, NY, and additional mailing offices. Subscription prices are $335.00 per year (US individuals), $433.00 per year (US institutions), $159.00 per year (US Students), $416.00 per year (Canadian individuals), $547.00 per year (Canadian institutions), $216.00 per year (Canadian and foreign students), $443.00 per year (foreign individuals), and $547.00 per year (foreign institutions). Foreign air speed delivery is included in all Clinics' subscription prices. All prices are subject to change without notice. **POSTMASTER:** Send address changes to Thoracic Surgery Clinics, Elsevier Health Sciences Division, Subscription Customer Service, 3251 Riverport Lane, Maryland Heights, MO 63043. **Customer Service (orders, claims, online, change of address): Telephone: 1-800-654-2452 (U.S. and Canada); 314-447-8871 (outside U.S. and Canada). Fax: 314-447-8029. Email: journalscustomerservice-usa@elsevier.com (for print support); journalsonlinesupport-usa@elsevier.com (for online support).**

Reprints. For copies of 100 or more, of articles in this publication, please contact Commercial Rights Department, Elsevier Inc., 360 Park Avenue South, New York, NY 10010-1710. Tel: (212) 633-3812; Fax: (212) 462-1935; E-mail: reprints@elsevier.com.

Thoracic Surgery Clinics is covered in *MEDLINE/PubMed (Index Medicus)* and *EMBASE/Excerpta Medica*.

Printed and bound by CPI Group (UK) Ltd, Croydon, CR0 4YY

Transferred to digital print 2013

Contributors

CONSULTING EDITOR

M. BLAIR MARSHALL
Associate Professor of Surgery, Georgetown University School of Medicine; Chief, Division of Thoracic Surgery, Department of Surgery, Georgetown University Medical Center, Washington, DC

EDITORS

JEAN DESLAURIERS, MD, FRCS(C)
Professor of Surgery, Division of Thoracic Surgery, Institut Universitaire de Cardiologie et de Pneumologie de Québec (IUCPQ), Quebec City; Professor of Surgery, Laval University, Quebec, Canada

F. GRIFFITH PEARSON, MD, Bsc Med, FRCS(Can), FACS
Professor of Surgery Emeritus, Division of Thoracic Surgery, Department of Surgery, University Health Network – Toronto General Hospital, University of Toronto, Toronto, Ontario, Canada

FARID M. SHAMJI, MD, MBBS, FRCS(C), FACS
Professor of Surgery, Division of Thoracic Surgery, Ottawa Hospital – General Campus; Professor of Surgery, University of Ottawa, Ottawa, Ontario, Canada

AUTHORS

AYESHA S. BRYANT, MD, MSPH
Assistant Professor, Division of Cardiothoracic Surgery, University of Alabama at Birmingham, Birmingham, Alabama

ROBERT J. CERFOLIO, MD, FACS, FCCP
Professor of Surgery, Chief, Section of Thoracic Surgery, JH Estes Family Endowed Chair for Lung Cancer Research, Division of Cardiothoracic Surgery, University of Alabama at Birmingham, Birmingham, Alabama

JOE Y. CHANG, MD, PhD
Professor, Department of Radiation Oncology, The University of Texas MD Anderson Cancer Center, Houston, Texas

SARAH DANSON, BMedSci, BMBS, MSc, PhD, FRCP
Academic Unit of Clinical Oncology, Weston Park Hospital, Sheffield, United Kingdom

GAIL E. DARLING, MD, FRCS
Professor, Thoracic Surgery, Kress Family Chair in Esophageal Cancer, University of Toronto; Director of Clinical Research in Thoracic Surgery, Toronto General Hospital University Health Network, Toronto, Ontario, Canada

JEAN DESLAURIERS, MD, FRCS(C)
Professor of Surgery, Division of Thoracic Surgery, Institut Universitaire de Cardiologie et de Pneumologie de Québec (IUCPQ), Quebec City; Professor of Surgery, Laval University, Quebec, Canada

MARK K. FERGUSON, MD
Professor, Department of Surgery, The University of Chicago Medicine, The University of Chicago, Chicago, Illinois

DALILAH FORTIN, MD, FRCS(C)
Department of Thoracic Surgery, Schulich School of Medicine & Dentistry, London Health Science Centre, Critical Care Trauma Centre, Victoria Hospital, Western University, London, Ontario, Canada

SABHA GANAI, MD, PhD
Surgical Oncology Fellow, Department of Surgery, The University of Chicago Medicine, The University of Chicago, Chicago, Illinois

MOHSEN IBRAHIM, MD, PhD
Department of Thoracic Surgery, Sant'Andrea Hospital, Sapienza University of Rome, Rome, Italy

CELINE MASCAUX, MD, PhD
Princess Margaret Cancer Centre, University of Health Network, University of Toronto, Toronto, Ontario, Canada

GIULIO MAURIZI, MD
Department of Thoracic Surgery, Sant'Andrea Hospital, Sapienza University of Rome, Rome, Italy

REZA MEHRAN, MD
Professor of Surgery, Department of Thoracic and Cardiovascular Surgery, MD Anderson Cancer Center, Houston, Texas

SHINICHIRO MIYOSHI, MD, PhD
Professor and Chairman, Department of General Thoracic Surgery and Breast and Endocrinological Surgery (Surgery II), Okayama University Graduate School of Medicine, Dentistry and Pharmaceutical Sciences, Kitaku, Okayama, Japan

BILL NELEMS, MD, FRCSC, MEd
Professor Emeritus, University of British Columbia, British Columbia, Canada

MORIHITO OKADA, MD, PhD
Chair and Professor, Department of Surgical Oncology, Research Institute for Radiation Biology and Medicine, Hiroshima University, Minami-ku, Hiroshima City, Hiroshima, Japan

ERINO ANGELO RENDINA, MD
Department of Thoracic Surgery, Sant'Andrea Hospital, Sapienza University of Rome; Spencer-Cenci Lorillard Foundation, Rome, Italy

R. TAYLOR RIPLEY, MD
Fellow, Thoracic Service, Department of Surgery, Memorial Sloan-Kettering Cancer Center, New York, New York

JACK A. ROTH, MD, FACS
Professor and Bud Johnson Clinical Distinguished Chair, Department of Thoracic and Cardiovascular Surgery; Professor of Molecular and Cellular Oncology; Director, W.M. Keck Center for Innovative Cancer Therapies; Chief, Section of Thoracic Molecular Oncology Clinic, The University of Texas MD Anderson Cancer Center, Houston, Texas

VALERIE W. RUSCH, MD
Chief, Thoracic Service, Department of Surgery, Memorial Sloan-Kettering Cancer Center, New York, New York

FARID M. SHAMJI, MD, MBBS, FRCS(C), FACS
Professor of Surgery, Division of Thoracic Surgery, Ottawa Hospital – General Campus; Professor of Surgery, University of Ottawa, Ottawa, Ontario, Canada

FRANCES A. SHEPHERD, MD, FRCPC
Princess Margaret Cancer Centre, University of Health Network, University of Toronto, Toronto, Ontario, Canada

SHERVIN M. SHIRVANI, MD, MPH
Fellow, Department of Radiation Oncology, The University of Texas MD Anderson Cancer Center, Houston, Texas

SHOBHA SILVA, MBBS, MRCP
Department of Oncology, Weston Park Hospital, Sheffield, United Kingdom

LISE TREMBLAY, MD, FRCPC
Multidisciplinary Department of Pulmonology and Thoracic Surgery, Institut Universitaire de Cardiologie et de Pneumologie de Québec (IUCPQ), Quebec City, Quebec, Canada

FRANÇOIS TRONC, MD
Thoracic Surgeon, Department of Thoracic Surgery, Hôpital Louis-Pradel, Lyon, Cedex, France

FEDERICO VENUTA, MD
Department of Thoracic Surgery, Policlinico Umberto I, Sapienza University of Rome; Spencer-Cenci Lorillard Foundation, Rome, Italy

DENNIS A. WIGLE, MD, PhD
Thoracic Surgery, Mayo Clinic, Rochester, Minnesota

Contents

Management of Tumors Involving the Chest Wall Including Pancoast Tumors and Tumors Invading the Spine 313

Jean Deslauriers, François Tronc, and Dalilah Fortin

Bronchogenic carcinomas involving the chest wall include tumors invading the ribs and spine, as well as Pancoast tumors. In the past, such neoplasms were considered to be incurable, but with new multimodality regimens, including induction chemoradiation followed by surgery, they can now be completely resected and patients can benefit from prolonged survival. The most important prognostic factors are the completeness of resection and the pathologic nodal status.

The Role of Surgery in Patients with Clinical N2 Disease 327

Reza Mehran

Patients with N2 non–small cell lung carcinoma have ipsilateral mediastinal adenopathy with stage IIIA disease. Most of these patients are still staged solely using imaging techniques, which causes a significant error in staging if not combined with some form of surgical staging of the mediastinum. N2 disease forms a spectrum of disease ranging from occult microscopic disease to bulky multistation adenopathy. Proper understanding of the prognosis and treatment implications for each form of mediastinal lymph node metastases has led to the selective use of surgery to treat these patients. This article reviews the role of surgery in the management of patients with N2 mediastinal involvement.

Reconstruction of the Bronchus and Pulmonary Artery 337

Mohsen Ibrahim, Giulio Maurizi, Federico Venuta, and Erino Angelo Rendina

Sleeve lobectomy (SL) (lobectomy associated with resection and reconstruction of the bronchus, the pulmonary artery, or both) has proved to be a suitable choice for the treatment of centrally sited non–small cell lung cancer. SL for lung cancer is indicated when a tumor or an N1 lymph node infiltrates the origin of a lobar bronchus, the origin of the lobar branches of the pulmonary artery, or both but not to the extent that a pneumonectomy is required. SL can be performed safely and effectively, even after induction therapy, without an increased complication rate.

Current Status of Mediastinal Lymph Node Dissection Versus Sampling in Non-small Cell Lung Cancer 349

Gail E. Darling

This article addresses the appropriate use of lymph node sampling versus dissection, recommendations for minimum sampling for staging, and the role of lymph node dissection in improving survival.

Intraoperative Nodal Staging: Role of Sentinel Node Technology 357

Shinichiro Miyoshi

In cases of superficial malignancies such as melanoma or breast cancer, intraoperative lymph node mapping with a sentinel lymph node (SLN) biopsy is an effective and minimally invasive alternative to inguinal or axillary lymph node dissection for early-stage tumors. For primary lung cancer, although much effort has been made to investigate a variety of tracers, such as dyes, radioisotopes, magnetite, and iopamidol, for discerning SLNs, an appropriate agent that produces high identification and accuracy rates has yet to be developed. Further studies are needed to find an ideal tracer for practical use in patients with non–small cell lung cancer.

Can Stereotactic Ablative Radiotherapy in Early Stage Lung Cancers Produce Comparable Success as Surgery? 369

Shervin M. Shirvani, Joe Y. Chang, and Jack A. Roth

Early stage non–small cell lung cancer is a potentially curable manifestation of a disease that is typically associated with a grim prognosis. Therapies directed at early stage disease can be challenging to deliver because patients tend to be elderly with multiple comorbidities. Surgery, the standard of care, has been validated with long-term follow-up. However, the risk of perioperative mortality and morbidity can limit the feasibility of an operation for many high-risk patients. Stereotactic ablative radiotherapy uses highly focused, ablative doses of radiation to treat tumors and has emerged as an alternative to surgery.

Surgeon's View: Is Palliative Resection of Lung Cancer Ever Justified? 383

Farid M. Shamji and Jean Deslauriers

Thoracic surgeons are often asked to see patients with locally advanced primary lung cancer in whom the goal of treatment is palliation for relief of disabling symptoms. The last four decades have brought great changes in the care of patients with primary lung cancer. The goals of the treatment must be well-defined by the interdisciplinary team. The thoracic surgeon has to make the final decision on whether to consider an operation for palliation and what is the expectation of the recommended treatment.

Current Status of Systemic Therapies

Adjuvant Chemotherapy After Pulmonary Resection for Lung Cancer 401

Celine Mascaux and Frances A. Shepherd

Adjuvant chemotherapy using a cisplatin-based regimen is currently recommended for patients with stage II and III non–small cell lung cancer (NSCLC) after complete tumor resection and may be considered for patients with stage IB NSCLC. Although adjuvant chemotherapy after complete resection of localized NSCLC is associated with an absolute survival advantage of approximately 5% at 5 years, there is still a relatively high risk of relapse even for early-stage NSCLC. Efforts are ongoing to identify new treatments in the adjuvant setting and to select patients for individualized treatment based on biomarkers.

Targeted Therapy and New Anticancer Drugs in Advanced Disease 411

Shobha Silva and Sarah Danson

The development of targeted therapies in lung cancer (mainly non–small cell lung cancer) has led to improvement in clinical outcomes and a more personalized approach to the management of these patients. This article discusses the main categories of novel targeted agents and the evidence behind their use.

Biologic Approaches to Drug Selection and Targeted Therapy: Hype or Clinical Reality? 421

Dennis A. Wigle

Oncology remains at the forefront of the application of individualized or genomics-driven approaches to cancer care. This approach acknowledges cancer as a genetic disease, driven by alterations in oncogenes and tumor suppressors, with the strategy of using this information to guide therapy based on therapeutics capable of targeting specific alterations. Recent advances suggest a changing landscape in how management decisions are approached for the patient with non–small cell lung cancer. An expanding and functionally useful toolbox of novel targeted agents and biomarkers to drive therapeutic choices is beginning to impact patient care. This article reviews key advances, with commentary and perspective for the practicing thoracic surgical oncologist.

Follow-up After Surgery and Palliative Care

What is the Most Practical, Optimal, and Cost Effective Method for Performing Follow-up After Lung Cancer Surgery, and by Whom Should It be Done? **429**

Lise Tremblay and Jean Deslauriers

Surgery is the treatment of choice for early stage non-small cell lung cancer. In this context, postoperative follow-up is important to diagnose late postoperative complications, as well as to detect recurring cancer or new primaries as early as possible. There is, however, no high-quality evidence regarding the benefits of monitoring programs on survival and quality of life. Most studies recommend clinical and radiological follow-up (radiograph or chest computed tomography) performed more intensively during the first two years and annually thereafter. The physician doing the follow-up can be the thoracic surgeon, the diagnosing physician, or the family physician.

Quality of Life After Pulmonary Resections **437**

Robert J. Cerfolio and Ayesha S. Bryant

Quality of life (QOL) is an important component of the conversation between any physician and patient. It is especially important between a surgeon and an operative candidate when considering treatment of lung cancer. Patients want reassurance that after removal of part of their lung that not only will they be cancer-free but also that they will be able to breathe well even when active. They do not want to be left physically or mentally handicapped. Recent studies have also shown the correlation between QOL and survival after resection. In this article the literature concerning QOL after pulmonary resection is reviewed.

Palliative Care Principles for Thoracic Surgery **443**

Bill Nelems

Palliative care medicine is embedded within thoracic surgery due to its heavy oncological bias. Many thoracic procedures are entirely palliative in nature, designed to alleviate symptoms and to relieve suffering. At a global level, access to palliative care services is dismal, necessitating awareness and advocacy. Early identification of palliative needs improves patient quality and reduces cost.

Index **447**

THORACIC SURGERY CLINICS

FORTHCOMING ISSUES

November 2013
Evolving Therapies in Esophageal Carcinoma
Wayne L. Hofstetter, MD, *Editor*

February 2014
Tracheal Surgery
Erich Hecker, MD and
Frank Detterbeck, MD, *Editors*

May 2014
Robotic Surgery
Bernard Park, MD, *Editor*

RECENT ISSUES

May 2013
Lung Cancer, Part I: Screening, Diagnosis, and Staging
Jean Deslauriers, MD, F. Griffith Pearson, MD, and Farid M. Shamji, MD, *Editors*

February 2013
Management of Benign and Malignant Pleural Effusions
Cliff K.C. Choong, MBBS, FRCS, FRACS, *Editor*

November 2012
Patient Perspectives in Pulmonary Surgery
Alessandro Brunelli, MD, *Editor*

RELATED INTEREST

Surgical Oncology Clinics of North America, Volume 22, Issue 2 (April 2013)
Multidisciplinary Care of the Cancer Patient
Gregory A. Masters, MD, *Editor*
Available at http://www.surgonc.theclinics.com/

Preface

Recent Advances in the Surgery and Adjuvant Treatment of Lung Cancer: Tribute to Robert J. Ginsberg

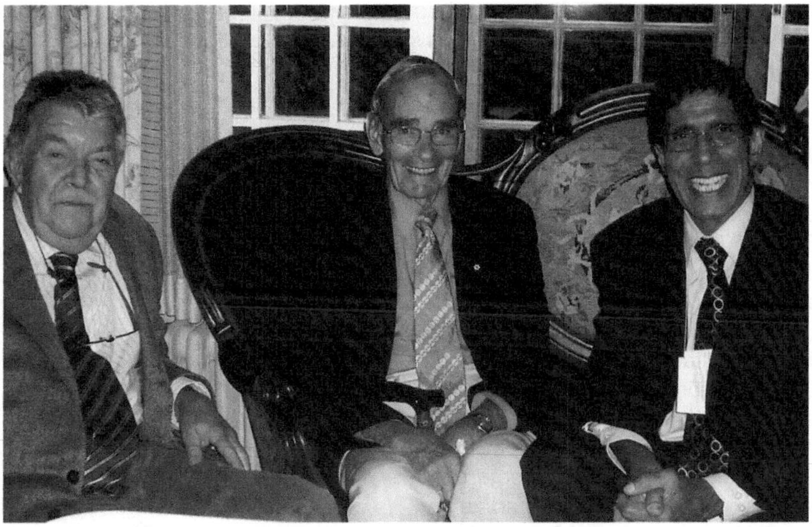

Jean Deslauriers, MD, FRCS(C), F. Griffith Pearson, MD, Bsc Med, FRCS(Can), FACS, and Farid M. Shamji, MD, MBBS, FRCS(C), FACS
Editors

On March 1, 2003, the Thoracic Surgical Community lost a valued member when Dr Robert Jason Ginsberg died of the very disease that he spent a lifetime studying. He was a leader in the field of Thoracic Surgical Oncology and had a profound impact on the career and life of many of the authors of this issue of *Thoracic Surgery Clinics* on surgery for lung cancer. Indeed, most articles presented in this issue have been written by thoracic surgeons and medical oncologists who were friends or trainees of Dr Ginsberg.

From our perspective as thoracic surgeons, we have elected to discuss in this issue those aspects of lung cancer surgery that are still intriguing and challenging to us. In 1982, one of us (F. Griffith Pearson) reported a series of 141 consecutive N_2 patients who had had cervical mediastinoscopy and subsequently had undergone surgical resection. In that series, the absolute 5-year survival was a disappointing 9% when mediastinoscopy had been positive, but when N_2 disease had only been identified at thoracotomy, a 24% overall 5-year survival was observed. This early report showed that pulmonary resection was clearly indicated in some patients with N_2 disease, but the current challenges are to determine which subset of patients should have surgery, who is likely to benefit from multimodality regimens, and should chemotherapy be administered as induction before the operation or as an adjuvant postoperatively.

Over the years, controversy has persisted about the indications for extended resections, although most surgeons will adopt an aggressive surgical approach if a complete resection appears possible. What is challenging is how much can be safely resected, especially if the tumor invades important extrapulmonary structures, such as the brachial plexus, the subclavian blood vessels, and the vertebral column, and should these patients receive induction chemoradiation therapy to downstage the tumor and possibly facilitate complete resection. Sleeve lobectomies are now used electively rather than being forced by

Thorac Surg Clin 23 (2013) xiii–xiv
http://dx.doi.org/10.1016/j.thorsurg.2013.04.008
1547-4127/13/$ – see front matter

impaired pulmonary function, but the issues of sleeve segmentectomies for patients with small diameter tumors or of sleeve resection of the pulmonary artery are most intriguing and will be addressed in this issue by Drs Okada and Rendina, respectively.

The issue of routine radical mediastinal lymphadenectomy versus mediastinal node sampling is still debated the world over, although the results of the ACOSOG randomized trial, as presented by Dr Gail Darling, have shown that it may not be necessary in patients with surgical N_0 disease. In this context, Dr Myoshi will describe sentinel node mapping techniques and their role in contemporary surgery for lung cancer.

Segmental resection of the lung was first reported by Churchill and Belsey in 1939 at a time when Mr Belsey was working as a fellow with Churchill in Boston. This early experience was in patients with bronchiectasis, which frequently involved selectively the lingula. In patients with lung cancer, Dr Ginsberg and the Lung Cancer Study Group have established that lobectomy should be the operation of choice in uncompromised patients, although, as discussed by Dr Okada, several recent studies, mostly from Japan, have shown that radical segmentectomies with nodal dissection should be considered as an alternative for a T_1N_0 lung cancer of 2 cm or less, even in low-risk patients.

Obviously some real progress has been made in the surgery of lung cancer since its beginning in the 1950s, but major challenges remain and it will be exciting to anticipate the changes in the understanding and management of lung cancer, which are likely to unfold during this early part of the 21st century.

Jean Deslauriers, MD, FRCS(C)
Division of Thoracic Surgery
Institut Universitaire de Cardiologie et de Pneumologie de Québec
2725 Chemin Sainte-Foy
Quebec City, Quebec G1V 4G5, Canada

F. Griffith Pearson, MD, Bsc Med, FRCS(Can), FACS
RR # 1
Mansfield, Ontario L0N 1M0, Canada

Farid M. Shamji, MD, MBBS, FRCS(C), FACS
Division of Thoracic Surgery
General Campus
The Ottawa Hospital
501 Smyth Road
Room 6362, Box 708
Ottawa, Ontario K1H 8L6, Canada

E-mail addresses:
jean.deslauriers@chg.ulaval.ca (J. Deslauriers)
fgpearson@hotmail.com (F.G. Pearson)
fshamji@ottawahospital.on.ca (F.M. Shamji)

Dedication

Tribute to Robert Jason Ginsberg (1940–2003)

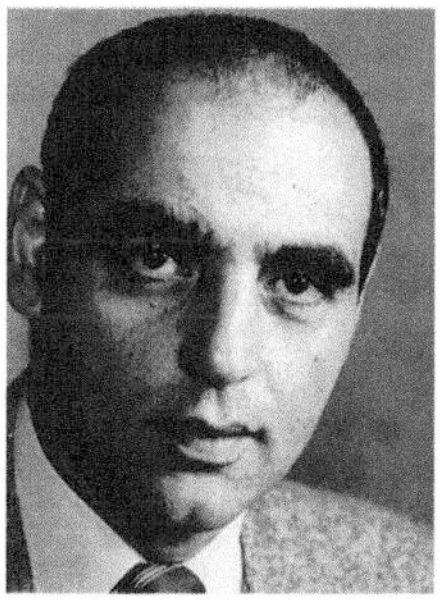

Robert Jason Ginsberg

To Robert Jason Ginsberg, surgery was an art, as well as a science, and he practiced it well because he recognized the most important ingredient necessary—the human relations between surgeon and patient. He reminded the young surgical residents that while cure may happen sometimes, and suffering alleviated frequently, being compassionate at all times was essential.

Postgraduate surgical education was important to Bob and he believed that the surgical residents must acquire knowledge on the Scientific Basis of Surgery and not to be merely a craftsman. His presentation in *The Coventry Conference on Trauma of the Chest* in 1977 on "The Management of Post-traumatic Pulmonary Insufficiency" was a reflection of what he wanted—that the surgeon must have knowledge on surgical physiology, chemical pathology and biochemistry, bacteriology, and metabolism.

Bob was not a textbook surgeon. He loved to be innovative and "innovation" was his favorite word during ward rounds and academic rounds and in the operating room. His enthusiasm was infectious. He carried the spirit of innovation to the time he spent in animal experiments during his surgical residency at the University of Toronto. Bob Ginsberg, Mel Goldberg, and Bob Stone, under the guidance of Griff Pearson, undertook an animal experiment on bronchial arterial circulation and published it in the *Surgery Forum* in 1966. This increased understanding of bronchial arterial circulation was applied to canine lung autotransplantation and many years later to clinical lung transplantation. Dr Joel Cooper, rightly regarded as the surgeon who finally made clinical single-lung transplantation a reality in 1982, used the knowledge gained on earlier experimental work on bronchial artery circulation to support healing of bronchial anastomosis with omentopexy, published in *Annals of Thoracic Surgery* in 1982 and 1984.

Bob had particular fascination with resection of Pancoast tumor, likely because of the time that he spent in Dallas, Texas with Dr Harold C. Urschel Jr and Dr Donald L. Paulson. It was because of Bob that a lasting friendship of the Toronto Thoracic Surgeons began with the two Texan surgeons. Bob wanted to make a video of the Paulson technique of the Posterior Surgical Approach for resection of Pancoast tumor in 1982. Bob told Farid Shamji to perform the operation without his surgical assistance, knowing very well that Farid had never seen one, let alone done one, while Bob stood on the platform making the movie for the entire 5 hours that it took to complete the operation. This is the type of confidence that Bob would impart to his residents. The movie is now in the *Society of Thoracic Surgeons* Video Library Section. Later, Bob published on Pancoast tumor in the *Annals of Thoracic Surgery* in 1994, in *Chest Surgery Clinics of North America* in 1995, *Journal of Thoracic and Cardiovascular Surgery* in 2000 with Dr Valerie Rusch, and in *Comprehensive Textbook of Thoracic Oncology* in 1996 with Dr David Payne and Dr Farid Shamji, all worth reading.

Bob loved to teach on the management of esophageal perforation and it was wonderful to listen to

Thorac Surg Clin 23 (2013) xv–xix
http://dx.doi.org/10.1016/j.thorsurg.2013.05.006
1547-4127/13/$ – see front matter

his words of practical wisdom conveyed so precisely in the *General Surgery and Emergency Medicine Specialist Programs* audiocassette produced by *Medifacts Limited* in 1986. He continued to write on this subject years later in the *Annals of Thoracic Surgery* in 2001.

Bob was a no-nonsense surgeon and an intelligent doctor. He was blessed with surgical intuition and this was clearly evident at the bedside of the patient imparting words of wisdom that patient care was based on rational thinking and not just on tests; he deplored premature and excessive use of diagnostic tests over organized thought process. Bob was very careful in his deliberation and delivery, and he was very fair. He spoke his mind when it was obvious to him that an error of judgment both outside and inside the operating room had occurred that had serious impact on the patient. Some examples include unsuccessful delayed distal tracheal resection after mediastinal sepsis complicating esophageal injury during cervical mediastinoscopy at another institution; unsuccessful distal tracheal resection for squamous cell cancer of trachea in a very elderly patient; inadvertent left subclavian artery injury during difficult decortication for empyema. Bob could speak his mind and everyone would listen to his rational approach to such surgical complications so as not to be repeated. Bob hated surgical complications with a passion. Training under the guiding hands of Bob was an absolute joy for Farid Shamji, whose attempts to emulate him were painful and met with precious little success.

The leadership and the enthusiasm that Bob displayed in clinical research became immediately recognized in the Lung Cancer Study Group, which conducted major clinical trials across North America and Canada between 1977 and 1989, a span of just 12 years, and with lasting success that is still as much remembered now as before on the methodology of conducting good clinical trials. A collective publication of these trials can be found in *Chest* 1994:106(6) Supplement.

One very important outcome of the clinical trials was the seminal article, often quoted, that Bob wrote in the *Journal of Cardiovascular and Thoracic Surgery* on "Modern Thirty-day Operative Mortality for Surgical Resections in Lung Cancer" in 1983. This publication set the bar for acceptable mortality in pulmonary resections against which future pulmonary resections have been measured.

Bob was very persistent when he believed that something that he thought was important should be carried to completion. This of course was on the role of surgical staging of mediastinum, which Griff Pearson was instrumental in advancing in the management of lung cancer reporting in 1965, 1968, and 1972. Bob insisted that Griff write on this subject again many years later after cervical mediastinoscopy had become routine in the staging of lung cancer. The first time Griff wrote on this subject was in 1965. At Bob's insistence, Griff revisited this subject as tribute to the work of the Division of Thoracic Surgery at the Toronto General Hospital after accumulating large experience. It was published in the *Journal of Thoracic and Cardiovascular Thoracic Surgery* in 1982. Griff did not have the heart to say "not now" to Bob. Such was the relationship between the master and the former student.

Bob was extremely popular at various national and international thoracic surgical meetings because he always spoke his mind, yet was courteous in his convincing delivery. Bob loved going to restaurants at meetings and the best one was in Atlanta, where he sat at the head of the long table, surrounded as always by many. On this particular occasion, he put on a bib and had a picture taken, where he was holding up two giant lobsters. He then went on to devour both with oil dripping from the corners of his mouth. It was a sight to remember.

He cherished the word "innovative" and believed that you had to think and use your mind without preconceived ideas. This was aptly reflected when he introduced his residents to the technique of one-lung anesthesia using an endobronchial blocker published in the *Journal of Cardiovascular and Thoracic Surgery* in 1981. It was about extended cervical mediastinoscopy as a single staging procedure for bronchogenic carcinoma of the left upper lobe, published in the same journal in 1987 and in *Chest Surgery Clinics of North America* in 1996. He taught surgical residents how to biopsy a scalene lymph node through the same little incision for cervical mediastinoscopy; he said it could be done and you just had to be careful.

Bob had particular interest in the surgical management of small-cell lung cancer. Together with the medical oncologists, Dr Frances Shepherd, Dr William Evans, and Dr Ronald Feld, a clinical trial was conducted by the University of Toronto Lung Oncology Group. Publications are in the *Journal of Thoracic and Cardiovascular Surgery* 1989 and 1991, *Seminars Radiation Oncology* in 1995, and in the *Annals of Thoracic Surgery* in 1990. Bob was an oncologist at heart and could converse easily with medical and radiation oncologists when it came to discussing induction and adjuvant chemotherapy and radiation therapy, not only for locally advanced lung cancer but also for malignant mesothelioma, chest wall sarcoma, esophageal cancer, and malignant mediastinal tumors. He was endowed with surgical intuition and his breadth of knowledge in cancer biology allowed him to converse easily and convincingly.

Thoracic surgery was his passion, not only as a gifted surgeon, but also as an educator, clinical investigator, and mentor.

The four conditions necessary for the surgeon that Guy De Chauliac described in 1300-1370 personifies Bob in all respects:

First, he should be learned and for this it is required that the surgeon should know not only the principles of surgery but also those of medicine in theory and practice.

Second, he should be expert, meaning that he should have seen others operate.

Third, he must be ingenious, of good judgment and memory to recognize conditions.

And fourth, he should be able to adapt and accommodate himself to circumstances.

When it came to leadership, Bob was second to none and he believed that everyone had a job to do and that each member of the Division of Thoracic Surgery at the Toronto General Hospital was a member of a team. The success of the Division of Thoracic Surgery was a team effort, under the leadership of Dr Joel Cooper, and was recognized when it performed the first successful single-lung transplantation in 1983. At this moment in time, while Dr Griff Pearson was responsible for performing lung extraction from the donor and Dr Joel Cooper was responsible for lung implantation in the recipient, Bob was the go-between, ensuring that it was well coordinated with a prepared captain's log book of sequences in the conduct of the operation. At this juncture, it is important to go back in time to 5 years earlier in 1977 and give credit to Dr Bill Nelems. Clinical lung transplantation at the Toronto General Hospital began with him suggesting that it was time to do it. He was the first clinical lung transplant coordinator during the first lung transplantation at the Toronto General Hospital. Unfortunately, the patient succumbed to rejection 18 days later. When Dr Bill Nelems left for British Columbia, Dr Joel Cooper became the lung transplant coordinator. Under the leadership of Dr Joel Cooper, important basic science research was conducted in animal lung transplantation to make it a successful reality 5 years later.

Going back in time to the days of residency training in General Thoracic Surgery in Canada as a specialty in itself, Dr Robert Ginsberg was the first chief resident and Dr Bill Nelems was his junior resident in the Toronto Training Program. An incident is fondly recalled by Dr Griff Pearson, who had brought back with him Dr Carlens' mediastinoscopy instrument from his visit to Karolinska Institute in Sweden. Bob suggested that they should do a study in 100 consecutive cases comparing chest tomograms and cervical mediastinoscopy in the assessment of mediastinal lymph nodes. Bob in his usual manner took responsibility of preparing thoughtful slides, which Griff presented at a meeting in Raleigh, North Carolina. Organized by Dr Gordon Murray and Ben Wilcox, Earl Wilkins and Dr Nael Martini were in attendance. The slide pictures were in a booklet prepared by Gordon Murray.

In closing, it is important to honor Dr Griff Pearson as the true giant on whose shoulders a group of Thoracic Surgeons at the Toronto General Hospital have looked beyond with enduring success. Across Canada, all thoracic surgeons can claim to have been taught directly or indirectly, through his trainees, by Griff Pearson. And many of us in the 1980s can make similar claims of having been taught as well by Bob Ginsberg and Joel Cooper. It was Griff who introduced endoscopy and mediastinoscopy in thoracic surgery at the Toronto General Hospital, recognizing that the need would be increased as the incidence of lung cancer increased. It was at this time of specialization that Dr Frederick Kergin, then Surgeon-in-Chief (1957-1966), approved creating a separate division of thoracic surgery with 2 representative surgeons—Dr F. Griffith Pearson, who did 100% thoracic surgery, and Dr Norman Delarue, who was part-time in thoracic surgery, having more interest in breast diseases. Dr F. Griffith Pearson was a disciple of Dr F. Kergin. There were 3 surgical wards and Thoracic Surgery began as a subspecialty of General Surgery on Ward "C." In 1966, Dr F. Kergin, then Associated Dean, and Dr William Drucker, new Surgeon-in-Chief (1966-1972), announced the formation of the first Division of Thoracic Surgery at the University of Toronto. They gave approval for redistribution of surgical beds and allowed 2 junior surgical residents to rotate on thoracic surgery service. Dr F. Griffith Pearson became the first Head of the Division of Thoracic Surgery at the Toronto General Hospital. Bob Ginsberg was influenced by Griff as much as Griff was influenced by Bob and they enjoyed mutual respect for each other that was to last the lifetime of Bob.

Today, largely due to the initiative of the Lung Cancer Study Group of the past, the standard of care expected in the education and practice of thoracic surgeons is based on certain guiding principles taught in the school of Dr F. Griffith Pearson and the late Dr Robert J. Ginsberg.

INFLUENCE OF THE LUNG CANCER STUDY GROUP IN STANDARDIZING TREATMENT FOR LUNG CANCER—LCSG

LCSG began in 1977 as a multicenter initiative at the advice of the National Cancer Institute to study lung cancer in a systematic manner to understand the pathology, staging, biology, and surgical and multimodality management of lung cancer. In the short lifespan of just 12 years, conducting clinical trials worthy of note and winding down in 1989 due to abrupt halting of funding, LCSG established the gold standard of excellence for future clinical studies in this disease.

Lung cancer continues to have the worldwide implications for mortality and is notorious for being the most lethal form of cancer in both men and women. There is an annual incidence of 1.3 million new cases of lung cancer and an annual incidence of death in 1.13 million. Tobacco smoking is the single most important causative agent in the destruction of human life, being responsible for 90% of all types of lung cancer. This is essentially a preventable disease in 90%, if only tobacco smoking were banned immediately. It was this disease that took the life of the late Dr Robert J. Ginsberg, the principal investigator with Dr F. Griffith Pearson in LCSG and the chairman of the LCSG surgery committee, to whom this issue on Lung Cancer is published as a tribute.

The Lung Cancer Study Group in 1977 recognized that there were issues of surgical importance in lung cancer treatment that required attention. These were studied in carefully conducted clinical trials:

Q1: Could a disparate group of surgeons produce reliable and uniform surgical results?
To look at the issues related to surgical treatment.
Q2: Does regional immune stimulation with BCG improve survival in stage I lung cancer?
To look at issues related to tumor immunity.
Q3: Can adjunctive chemotherapy improve survival in surgically resected lung cancer?
To look at postoperative chemotherapy.
Q4: What is the proper role of adjunctive radiation therapy in the management of locally advanced, resectable lung cancer?
To look at postoperative chemotherapy combined with radiotherapy.
Q5: Are smaller operations appropriate for smaller cancers?
To look at limited resection of small cancers.
Q6: Is neoadjuvant or induction therapy using chemotherapy and irradiation in a humane and rational treatment program justifiable to any critical reviewer of treatment policy?
To look at issues related to neoadjuvant treatment.

The Thoracic Surgical Community in Canada, United States, and other far-reaching countries will forever remain indebted to Bob in many ways. He was collegial, a good advisor, a friend indeed, and an excellent surgeon.

Farid M. Shamji, MBBS, FRCS(C), FACS
Division of Thoracic Surgery
General Campus
The Ottawa Hospital
501 Smyth Road, Room 6362
Box 708
Ottawa, Ontario K1H 8L6, Canada

Jean Deslauriers, MD, FRCS(C)
Division of Thoracic Surgery
Laval University
Institut Universitaire de Cardiologie et de Pneumologie de Québec
2725 Chemin Sainte-Foy
Quebec City, Quebec G1V 4G5, Canada

F. Griffith Pearson, MD, Bsc Med, FRCS(Can), FACS
Division of Thoracic Surgery
Department of Surgery
University Health Network–Toronto General Hospital
University of Toronto, 200 Elizabeth Street
Toronto, Ontario M5G 2C4, Canada

E-mail addresses:
fshamji@ottawahospital.on.ca (F.M. Shamji)
jean.deslauriers@chg.ulaval.ca (J. Deslauriers)
fgpearson@hotmail.com (F.G. Pearson)

SUGGESTED READINGS

Ginsberg RJ. Esophageal perforations. Issues of interest—general surgery and emergency medicine. Medifacts 1986.

Ginsberg RJ. Enbloc resection of a superior sulcus tumor. The Society of Thoracic Surgeons Video Library 312-644-6610.

Ginsberg RJ, Payne DG, Shamji FM. Superior sulcus tumors. Comprehensive Textbook of Thoracic Oncology. Williams & Wilkins - A Waverly Company; 1996. p. 357–87.

Ginsberg RJ, Rubinstein L. The comparison of limited resection to lobectomy for T1N0 non-small cell lung cancer: LCSG 821. Chest 1994;106:318S–9S.

Ginsberg RJ, Hill LD, Eagan RT, et al. Modern 30-day operative mortality after surgical resections in lung cancer. J Thorac Cardiovasc Surg 1983;86: 654–8.

Jones WG, Ginsberg RJ. Esophageal perforations: a continuing challenge. Ann Thorac Surg 1992;53: 534–43.

Ginsberg RJ. Extended cervical mediastinoscopy. Chest Surg Clin N Am 1996;6:21–30.

Lee JD, Ginsberg RJ. Lung cancer staging: the value of ipsilateral scalene lymph node biopsy performed at mediastinoscopy. Ann Thorac Surg 1996; 62:338–41.

Stone RM, Ginsberg RJ, Colapinto RF, et al. Bronchial artery regeneration after radical hilar stripping. Surg Forum 1966;17:109–10.

Ginsberg RJ. New technique for one-lung anesthesia using an endobronchial blocker. J Thorac Cardiovasc Surg 1981;82:542–6.

Ginsberg RJ. Operation for small cell lung cancer—where we are? Ann Thorac Surg 1990;49:692–3.

Shepherd FA, Ginsberg RJ, Feld R, et al. Surgical treatment for limited small-cell lung cancer. J Thorac Cardiovasc Surg 1991;101:385–93.

Role of Induction Therapies

Role of Induction Therapy

Surgical Resection of Non–Small Cell Lung Cancer After Induction Therapy

R. Taylor Ripley, MD, Valerie W. Rusch, MD*

KEYWORDS

• Induction therapy • Surgery • Stage III lung cancer

KEY POINTS

- Treatment of Stage III non–small cell lung cancer (NSCLC) can be subdivided according to whether a patient has N2 disease or a T3/T4N0 tumor.
- Induction therapy plus surgery is a standard treatment for Stage IIIA (N2) NSCLC, but should only be offered to patients who are medically fit for lung resection.
- Definitive chemoradiation is a standard treatment for patients with Stage IIIA (N2) disease whose performance status or lung functions preclude surgery.
- Induction chemoradiotherapy plus surgery is a standard treatment for NSCLC involving the superior sulcus or spine.

INTRODUCTION

Induction therapy was developed to overcome the dismal outcomes of patients with locally advanced non–small cell lung cancer (NSCLC) managed by surgery or radiotherapy alone. Despite many clinical trials, the use of induction therapy and surgery for locally advanced NSCLC remains controversial. This topic is most easily understood by considering the management of stage IIIA (N2) disease and T3-4 N0-1 tumors separately. In addition, an experience with induction therapy for earlier-stage NSCLC has begun to emerge.

Induction therapy has potential benefits in comparison with postoperative adjuvant therapy, including the assessment of systemic therapy in vivo, improved delivery of drugs to the tumor, earlier treatment of micrometastatic disease, an increased likelihood of patients receiving the planned regimen, and downstaging of disease before local therapy. Some of these, such as better drug delivery, are well accepted, whereas others, such as improved resectability, remain unproven.

OUTCOMES AFTER INDUCTION THERAPY

Induction Therapy for Stage III N2 Disease

Based on a large international database, Goldstraw and colleagues[1] reported that the 5-year survival after resection of stage IIIA (N2) disease was 24%. These results are similar to those reported by Martini and Flehinger[2] in 1987, with 5-year survivals of 30% and 5% after resection of stage IIIA (N2) NSCLC with single and multiple N2 station disease. Poor outcomes after surgical resection alone provided the rationale to study multimodality therapy for N2 disease. Both chemotherapy (**Table 1**) and chemoradiotherapy have been studied in the preoperative setting.

In a single-arm phase II trial, Martini and colleagues[3] reported a 41% 3-year survival in patients with N2 disease treated with 3 cycles of induction mitomycin, vinblastine, and cisplatin

Thoracic Service, Department of Surgery, Memorial Sloan-Kettering Cancer Center, 1275 York Avenue, New York, NY 10065, USA
* Corresponding author.
E-mail address: ruschv@mskcc.org

Thorac Surg Clin 23 (2013) 273–285
http://dx.doi.org/10.1016/j.thorsurg.2013.04.004

Table 1
Studies of induction chemotherapy and surgical resection for stage III (N2) disease

Authors,[Ref.] Year	Phase	Disease	Patients (N)	Resected (n)	Resected (%)	pCR (%)	5-y Survival (%)	N2 Downstaging
Burkes et al,[77] 1992	II	IIIA-N2	39	22	56	5	26 (3-y)	36
Sugarbaker et al,[8] 1995	II	IIIA-N2	74	46	62	NS	23 (3-y)	22
Rosell et al,[6,78] 1994, 1999	III	44/60 (N2)	60	23/27	85	3	17 (induction), 0 (no induction)	32
Roth et al,[4,5] 1994, 1998	III	IIIA	60	17/28	61	4	36 (induction), 15 (no induction)	NS
Van Zandwijk et al (EORTC),[79] 2000	II	IIIA-N2	47 (17 surgery)	16/17	94 (induction)	6 (1/17)	NS for surgical group	53
Betticher et al,[80] 2003	II	IIIA-N2	90	75	83	NS	34 (3-y)	61
Nagai et al,[81] 2003	III	IIIA-N2	62	20/31	65 (induction)	0 (0/31)	22 (induction), 10 (no Induction)	NS
O'Brien et al (EORTC),[82] 2003	II	IIIA-N2	52 (15 surgery)	12/15	80 (induction)	2	NS for surgical group	17
Garrido et al,[83] 2007	II	IIIA (N2)-B (T4N0–1)	69 (N2)	46 (N2)	67	2 (N2)	32 (N2 resected)	27

Abbreviations: EORTC, European Organization for Research and Treatment of Cancer; NS, not stated; pCR, complete pathologic response.

chemotherapy. Induction therapy was also tested in phase III trials. In 1998, Roth and colleagues[4,5] reported 5-year survivals of 36% for patients treated with perioperative chemotherapy (cyclophosphamide, etoposide, and cisplatin) versus 15% with surgery alone. Patients undergoing complete resection had a 5-year survival of 53% with combined modality therapy versus 24% after surgical resection alone, but the survivals were only 9% and 0%, respectively, after incomplete resection. Rosell and colleagues[6] reported a phase III study of induction chemotherapy plus surgery versus surgery alone with 5-year survivals of 17% versus 0%. In 2010, a meta-analysis of 13 randomized controlled trials testing neoadjuvant chemotherapy found a hazard ratio of 0.84 (95% confidence interval 0.77–0.92) in favor of induction therapy.[7] Platinum-based chemotherapy was the key component of effective preoperative treatment.

Additional trials tested the use of preoperative chemoradiotherapy (**Table 2**). In 1995, the Cancer and Leukemia Group B (CALGB) reported a phase II study of preoperative chemotherapy with cisplatin and vinblastine followed by resection, then adjuvant chemoradiotherapy.[8] This study had 5% treatment-related mortality and 3% postoperative mortality. Again, the importance of complete resection was noted; the 3-year survival for complete versus incomplete resections was 46% versus 21%. In a phase II study, the Southwest Oncology Group (SWOG 8805) showed the feasibility of induction chemotherapy (2 cycles of cisplatin and etoposide) with concurrent radiotherapy (45 Gy) for stage IIIA and selected IIIB NSCLC.[9] Among 126 eligible patients, the treatment-related mortality was 10% (13 patients) and postoperative mortality 6% (8 patients). The resectability rate was 85% and 3-year survival 27% for patients with N2 disease. The strongest prognostic factor was mediastinal downstaging (3-year survival of 44% for pN0 vs 18% for pN2 disease). This study also showed a poor survival for patients with stage IIIB (N3) disease, leading to the exclusion of such patients from subsequent trials of combined-modality therapy with surgery. The results of SWOG 8805 led to an intergroup phase III trial (Intergroup Trail 0139) to determine whether surgery improved survival over definitive chemoradiotherapy alone.

In 2009, Albain and colleagues[10] reported the mature results of the Intergroup Trial 0139 (Radiation Therapy Oncology Group 9309) comparing chemoradiotherapy followed by surgery versus definitive radiotherapy without surgery in patients with pathologically proven N2 disease. Two cycles of cisplatin and etoposide were delivered concurrently with 45 Gy of radiotherapy. Patients with responding or stable disease were then randomized to surgical resection or to continuation of radiotherapy to 61 Gy. Progression-free survival was 22% versus 11% at 5 years, significantly in favor of the surgical arm, but overall survival was not significantly different in the surgical versus the nonsurgical group (27% vs 20% at 5 years). A high operative mortality after pneumonectomy prompted an exploratory analysis excluding these patients. Patients who underwent lobectomy were compared with a matched cohort treated with definitive chemoradiotherapy, and were found to have a significantly better 5-year survival (36% vs 18%). These trial results highlighted the potential risks of pneumonectomy after induction therapy, established definitive chemoradiotherapy as a standard treatment option for stage IIIA (N2) NSCLC, and suggested a benefit for adding resection (via lobectomy) in selected patients.

Table 2
Select studies of induction chemoradiotherapy and surgery for stage III NSCLC

Authors,[Ref.] Year	Phase	Disease	Patients (N)	Resected (n)	pCR (%)	5-y Survival (%)	N2 Downstaging
Albain et al (SWOG 8805),[9] 1995	II	IIIA-N2	75 (N2 patients)	57	21	27 (3-y; N2)	51
Mathisen et al,[84] 1996	II	IIIA-N2	40	35	6	43	40
Katayama et al,[85] 2004	II	IIIA-B	22	19	23	66 (3-y)	NS
Albain et al (INT 0139),[10] 2009	III	IIIA	429	155/202	14	27 (induction), 20 (no induction)	41% (N0)
Steger et al,[86] 2009	II	III-N2/3	55	55	35	49	69

Abbreviations: INT, Intergroup Trial; NS, not stated; pCR, complete pathologic response; SWOG, Southwest Oncology Group.

The European Organization for Research and Treatment of Cancer (EORTC) compared surgery with radiation after induction chemotherapy.[11] Unlike Intergroup Trial 0139, the induction regimen did not include radiotherapy, so patients received either radiation or surgery. Moreover, only patients with response to induction chemotherapy were randomized, and the outcomes of the nonrandomized patients are unknown. No significant difference was noted for progression-free or overall survival, but better local control was observed in the surgical arm. In addition, patients who underwent an R0 resection experienced a 27% 5-year survival, which was significantly better than the 14% in the radiation group and 7% in the incomplete resection group. Similar to the Intergroup Trial 0139, an unplanned subgroup analysis revealed a significantly better survival for patients who underwent lobectomy rather than pneumonectomy.

Unsuspected N2 Disease Discovered at Surgery

A specific circumstance is the discovery of unsuspected N2 disease at surgery. This situation usually occurs when micrometastatic disease is present in the mediastinal lymph nodes, but is not enlarged or fluorodeoxyglucose-avid on positron emission tomography (PET). These patients have been shown in several randomized trials to benefit significantly from adjuvant chemotherapy,[12–16] although further detail is beyond the scope of this article.

Patterns of Relapse

In the SWOG 8805 trial only 11% of recurrences were locoregional, whereas the remaining 89% occurred in distant or both local and distant sites. Brain was the most common single site of relapse.[9] The Intergroup 0139 trial confirmed this pattern of relapse and showed that local-only relapses were uncommon in the surgery arm of the study (2% vs 14%).[10] In the EORTC trial, locoregional recurrences were more common in the radiotherapy group than in the surgical arm of the study (55% vs 32%).[11] These trials indicate that surgical resection leads to a low risk of local recurrence, and that survival is linked to the risk of distant metastases.

Induction Chemotherapy Versus Chemoradiotherapy for Stage IIIA (N2) NSCLC

The use of induction chemotherapy versus chemoradiotherapy for stage IIIA (N2) disease remains controversial. Chemoradiotherapy is associated with a higher rate of complete pathologic response (pCR) than chemotherapy alone (approximately 20% vs 5%), but overall survival is determined primarily by distant metastatic disease, which is similar between the 2 approaches. In addition, adding radiotherapy as adjuvant postoperative treatment allows the use of higher doses delivered to smaller fields.

Several studies have addressed this issue. Thomas and colleagues[17] evaluated whether the addition of chemoradiotherapy to induction chemotherapy improved survival in patients with stage III NSCLC. Only 37% and 32% of the intent-to-treat population underwent complete resection. Although chemoradiotherapy led to a higher pathologic response (60% vs 20%), no differences in progression-free survival, rate of complete resection, or overall survival were observed. Treatment-related mortality was 14% and 6% in patients who received and did not receive radiotherapy, respectively. Higgins and colleagues[18] performed a retrospective review of patients who received preoperative chemotherapy versus chemoradiotherapy. The mediastinal pathologic complete response was greater with radiotherapy (65% vs 35%). Radiotherapy was associated with improved disease-free survival and local control, but these findings did not translate into an overall survival benefit. In a meta-analysis of studies comparing induction chemotherapy with chemoradiotherapy, Shah and colleagues[19] found that although well-designed trials are lacking, no evidence of benefit to the addition of induction radiotherapy was noted. On balance, it seems that induction chemoradiotherapy is more appropriate in situations where the extent of the primary tumor requires maximal local control to allow for complete resection (eg, superior sulcus carcinomas; see later discussion). Stage IIIA (N2) is generally managed with induction chemotherapy alone, with radiotherapy administered postoperatively to reduce the risk of recurrence in the mediastinum.

Assessment of Response to Induction Therapy

Response to induction therapy is a key prognostic factor in long-term survival. Some investigators believe that surgical resection should only be offered to patients whose mediastinal nodal disease has been eradicated by the induction therapy. This criterion is controversial because patients with persistent N2 disease after induction therapy have a lower but distinct chance of 5-year survival if a complete resection can be performed. Nonetheless, great attention has been given to the best way to assess response after induction therapy.

Candela and Detterbeck[20] conducted a review of methods of restaging after induction therapy, and found only a 57% rate of pCR in patients with radiographic complete response by computed tomography (CT) scan. False negatives ranged from 0% to 100%, indicating that CT does not reliably predict pCR. In this review, PET scans had a false-negative rate of 30%, but if the standardized uptake value dropped by more than 80%, this decrease was associated with low false-positive and false-negative rates. Most PET studies focus on changes in imaging the primary tumor, whereas response in the mediastinal nodes is the most relevant information in patients with N2 disease. Minimal data exist for CT, but PET scans have a false-negative rate of 26% and a false-positive rate of 34% in evaluating mediastinal nodal disease after induction therapy. Rebollo-Aguirre and colleagues[21] reviewed trials that reported N2 restaging after induction therapy and found a sensitivity and specificity of 64% and 85%, respectively. These studies show that both CT and PET scans are poor in assessing mediastinal downstaging.

Pathologic evaluation of the mediastinum after induction therapy has also been studied. Repeat mediastinoscopy can often be performed even if it had been performed before induction therapy. Surprisingly, even if all involved stations were rebiopsied, the rate of false negatives was 22%.[20] Although data are limited, the false-negative rate of endobronchial ultrasonography (EBUS) is estimated to be 14%.[22–26] Given that 4 of these series reported 25 or fewer patients and that the false-negative rate for the largest series of 124 was an outlier,[25] the true incidence of false negativity is unclear. False-positive results are rare with EBUS or mediastinoscopy. Increasingly, repeat mediastinoscopy is being replaced by either EBUS before and after induction therapy, or EBUS before and mediastinoscopy after induction therapy. Conversely, in the absence of disease progression it is also acceptable to proceed directly to thoracotomy to determine whether a complete resection can be performed. No uniform standard currently exists with respect to mediastinal restaging.

Is Pneumonectomy Appropriate After Induction Therapy?

Mortality was higher than expected after pneumonectomy in cooperative group trials.[27] In Intergroup Trial 0139, 155 resections were performed with 54 (35%) pneumonectomies and 98 (63%) lobectomies.[10] Sixteen patients (8%) in the surgical group died, but 14 of these deaths were after pneumonectomy, giving a 26% mortality after pneumonectomy. Forty-five percent of patients with pT0N0 disease were treated with pneumonectomy, suggesting a lack of selectivity toward pneumonectomies in this multicenter study performed during an early time frame (1994–2001). Several subsequent reports show a lower mortality after pneumonectomy.[28–34] Barnett and colleagues[28] reported a recent series from Memorial Sloan-Kettering Cancer Center showing a decline in rates of both morbidity and mortality after pneumonectomy. Pneumonectomy was performed in 13% of patients with a 4% mortality, an improvement over the 11% mortality in a previous report from the same institution.[35] In another large contemporary series, Weder and colleagues[29] reported a 90-day mortality of 3% for 176 patients after pneumonectomy. Barnett and colleagues[28] reported that underlying pulmonary comorbidities were significantly associated with pulmonary complications. Grade 3 or higher adverse events were increased in patients who had a diffusion capacity (DLCO) of 58% or less of predicted. The explanation for the lower mortality in these single-institutional series compared with earlier cooperative group trials is likely multifactorial, and related to more careful patient selection, an increase in adenocarcinomas (relative to more centrally located squamous cell carcinomas), evolution in chemotherapy regimens, and greater attention to preoperative pulmonary evaluation.

Evans and colleagues[36] reviewed the Society of Thoracic Surgeons General Thoracic Surgical Database, and noted that only half of patients with stage IIIA N2 disease were treated with induction therapy. These differences in practice patterns may be driven by concerns of postoperative complications after induction therapy. Kim and colleagues[37] performed a meta-analysis of mortality after induction therapy and pneumonectomy, and found 30-day mortalities of 11% and 5% for right and left pneumonectomies.[34,35,37–43] It is clear that care must be exercised in selecting patients for pneumonectomy after induction therapy, but attention to pulmonary function, especially DLCO, permits pneumonectomy when necessary to achieve complete resection.

Surgical Management

As noted, the 2 most important factors for survival after surgical resection are complete (R0) resection and downstaging of mediastinal nodal disease. As discussed, mediastinal downstaging cannot be reliably assessed by imaging studies; therefore, surgical exploration is the only reliable method of assessment in the absence of progressive disease. Even for patients with persistent N2 disease, a small but real chance of long-term survival exists if complete resection can be obtained. This survival contrasts with a uniformly dismal prognosis among patients who do not undergo resection. In addition, surgical resection results in an improved local control, which is important given the morbidity of mediastinal disease.

The assessment of complete resection is the operative goal. This assessment begins with preoperative assessment of tolerability by pulmonary function testing, with particular attention to the DLCO. Quantitative ventilation, perfusion scanning, and exercise testing are used as clinically necessary. Intraoperatively, the assessment of resectability begins with the mediastinal lymph nodes. On the right, complete paratracheal lymphadenectomy with division of the azygous is critical. In addition, multiple frozen-section specimens to assess negative margins are appropriate. If the nodes are deemed resectable, attention is directed to the resectability of the primary tumor. Once both are assessed, every effort should be made to perform a complete resection. A lobectomy is preferable to pneumonectomy even if a sleeve resection is required, but given contemporary outcomes a pneumonectomy is acceptable for patients with adequate lung function. For patients who are unresectable, the operation should be terminated without an attempt to perform a partial resection. For unresectable patients, definitive radiotherapy can be administered postoperatively.

INDUCTION THERAPY FOR LOCALLY ADVANCED T3 AND T4 DISEASE

Induction Therapy for Superior Sulcus Tumors (Pancoast Tumors)

Superior sulcus tumors represent a rare subset of NSCLC invading the apex of the chest and potentially involving the brachial plexus, spine, or subclavian vessels. For purposes of treatment planning, patients with locally advanced paraspinal T3-4 disease that is not at the apex of the chest can also be included in this category. Historically these tumors were all stage III, but with the revised seventh edition of TNM lung cancer staging, this subset of T3N0 tumors are classified Stage IIB.

When first described by Pancoast[44] in 1932, these tumors were considered unresectable. In the 1950s Paulson and Shaw introduced the use of induction radiotherapy followed by en bloc resection.[45,46] This treatment remained standard until the 1990s. Rusch and colleagues[47] retrospectively reviewed the outcomes of patients with superior sulcus tumors, and found that complete resection was achieved in only 64% of patients with T3 and 39% of patients with T4 disease. The 5-year survival for patients with N2 disease was 0%. These results highlighted the need for better treatment. Innovative surgical approaches reported by Dartevelle and colleagues[48] improved local control, but better systemic therapy was still needed. The success of combined-modality therapy in Stage IIIA (N2) NSCLC led to a North American trial testing this approach in superior sulcus NSCLC.

Intergroup Trial 0160 (SWOG 9416) was a phase II study of induction chemoradiotherapy followed by resection.[49,50] Patients with clinical T3-4, N0-1 (N2 disease excluded by mediastinoscopy) received 2 cycles of cisplatin and etoposide with 45 Gy of concurrent radiotherapy. Patients without progressive disease then underwent thoracotomy. Complete resection was achieved in 91% and 87% of patients with T3 and T4 tumors, respectively. One-third of patients had a pCR, one-third minimal microscopic disease, and one-third grossly viable tumor within the resected specimen. Pathologic complete response was the main predictor of overall survival. The median survival was 94 months for patients with complete resections, compared with 33 months for all eligible patients. Postoperative mortality was 2.3%. This study showed that complete responses can be achieved with induction chemoradiotherapy, the morbidity of trimodality therapy is low, and complete resection is achievable in most patients. Complete resectability and overall survival were markedly better than in all previously reported series using preoperative radiation alone and, thus, this approach to treatment has become standard management for superior sulcus NSCLC. In contrast to stage IIIA (N2) disease, this experience is a good example of how the synergism of concurrent induction chemoradiotherapy can lead to improved outcomes for some T3 and T4 tumors. Several additional retrospective series and prospective clinical trials (**Table 3**) corroborate the results of this North American intergroup trial.

Surgical Management of Stage IIB/III (T3, T4) NSCLC

The approach to resection of superior sulcus and paravertebral tumors depends on the specific tumor locations. Both posterior and anterior approaches may be used.[51]

In the posterior Paulson approach, a posterolateral thoracotomy is performed to determine whether the pleural space is free of disease. The incision is then extended to the seventh cervical vertebra and the serratus anterior detached from

Table 3
Series reporting the results of induction therapy and surgical resection of superior sulcus NSCLC

Authors,[Ref.] Year	Patients (N)	Treatment	Complete Resection (%)	Local Recurrence Rate (%)	5-y Survival (%)
Paulson,[87] 1975	61	RT	NS	NS	26
Attar et al,[88] 1979	73	RT	48	NS	NS
Ginsberg et al,[89] 1994	124	RT	56	72	26
Maggi et al,[90] 1994	60	RT	60	15	17
Hagan et al,[91] 1999	34	RT	NS	20	33
Komaki et al,[92] 2000	62	RT, RT/CT	53	NS	38
Rusch et al,[47] 2000	225	RT, RT/CT	56	40	29
Martinod et al,[93] 2002	139	None, RT	81	31	35
Kwong et al,[31] 2005	36	RT/CT	97	14	50
Marra et al,[94] 2007	31	CT, RT/CT	94	6	46
Rusch et al,[50] 2007	88	RT/CT, CT	76	11	44
Pourel et al,[95] 2008	72	RT/CT	98	34	51 (3-y)
Kunitoh et al,[96] 2008	57	RT/CT	68	33	56

Abbreviations: CT, chemotherapy; NS, not stated; RT, radiotherapy.

its insertion to expose the upper chest wall. An alternative incision with an extension anteriorly to the midclavicular line was described by the groups of Masaoka and Niwa.[52,53] The scalene muscles are detached to expose the first rib. The chest-wall resection is performed anteriorly, obtaining 4-cm margins. The erector spinae muscles are elevated to expose the transverse processes, which are then resected en bloc with the heads of the involved ribs. This step of the operation is generally performed in collaboration with a spine neurosurgeon and is critical to obtaining an adequate margin posteriorly. The intercostal nerve roots are clipped to prevent cerebrospinal fluid leak. Intraoperative nerve monitoring helps define whether it is safe to resect the T1 nerve root, which can sometimes affect motor function to the hand. Division of the C8 nerve root usually results in severe loss of motor function to the hand and arm, and involvement of this root defines nonresectability. Frozen section should be liberally used because abnormal tissue often is the result of scar without viable tumor from induction therapy. After chest-wall resection, standard lobectomy and mediastinal lymph node dissection are performed.

Dartevelle and colleagues[48] popularized the anterior approach for tumors with involvement of the subclavian vessels, describing an incision along the anterior border of the sternocleidomastoid muscle extended through the sternoclavicular joint into a horizontal incision in the second intercostal space. A variation on this uses an L-shaped incision through the manubrium, allowing it to be elevated along with the clavicle and facilitating subsequent closure.[54] The scalene muscles are detached from the first and second ribs, preserving the phrenic nerve. The subclavian vein is resected, exposing the subclavian artery, which is resected and reconstructed. The tumor is mobilized from the brachial plexus. An additional posterolateral thoracotomy may be needed to complete the resection, depending on the extent of the tumor and the patient's body habitus.

With induction chemoradiotherapy, NSCLC with vertebral body involvement can also be cured with resection. When only the transverse process is invaded, a posterolateral thoracotomy is adequate. True vertebral body involvement requires a combined posterior and anterior approach. The posterior part of the operation is performed by a spine neurosurgeon with the patient in the prone position. After vertebral body resection and internal rod fixation, the patient is rotated to the lateral decubitus position, and the remainder of the chest wall and lung resection is performed via a posterolateral thoracotomy.[55]

Regardless of the technical approach to resection, the most critical aspect of management of these locally advanced NSCLCs is complete resection with histologically negative margins. The use of induction chemoradiotherapy has facilitated in achieving this goal.

Patterns of Relapse

Induction chemoradiotherapy followed by complete resection has decreased the local failure rates in superior sulcus tumors. In the Intergroup Trial 0160 locoregional recurrences occurred in 23% of the patients, whereas distant-only relapse occurred in 66% of the patients.[49] The brain was the most common single site of recurrence.[31,50]

SPECIAL SITUATIONS RELATED TO INDUCTION THERAPY

Elderly Patients

Another concern is whether operative risk is higher in elderly patients after induction therapy. Seventy percent of all cancer-related deaths and more than 50% of all lung cancers occur in patients older than 65 years.[56,57] However, the elderly are underrepresented in clinical trials, and trial results may not be generalizable to older patients.[58–63] The benefit of induction therapy is primarily based on extrapolation from younger cohorts.[64–67] Some trials show that the elderly experience the same responses as younger patients when they receive the same treatment, but the likelihood of experiencing toxicity and discontinuing treatment or reducing the dose is higher in the elderly. In a case-control study, Rivera and colleagues[68] found that patients older than 75 years experienced an increase in the incidence and severity of postoperative morbidity and length of stay even though mortality was similar to that in younger patients. Induction therapy should be offered to the elderly for the same indications as for younger patients, but chemotherapy dose modifications and extra vigilance in perioperative care may be needed.

Induction Therapy for Early-Stage NSCLC

Experience with induction therapy for early-stage NSCLC is more limited than for stage III disease. Although stage I and II NSCLC is considered a curable disease with resection, the 5-year survival of pathologically staged IA and IB tumors is 50% and 43%, respectively.[1] Therefore, strategies to improve outcomes are needed. Several randomized trials have tested induction therapy for early-stage NSCLC.

In SWOG Trial S9900, patients with clinically staged IB-IIIA disease were randomized to surgery or 3 cycles of paclitaxel and carboplatin chemotherapy followed by surgery.[69] Patients with N2 disease or superior sulcus tumors were excluded. Five-year survival was 50% in the induction therapy versus 41% in the surgery-alone groups. Though not statistically significant, the absolute improvement in 5-year survival was 9%. The Chemotherapy in Early Stages NSCLC Trial (ChEST) reported a difference in 3-year progression-free survival of 2.9 years for surgery versus 4.0 years for induction chemotherapy and surgery.[70] A subgroup analysis suggested that only patients with IIB or IIIA disease benefited from therapy. These results differed from those of the S9900 trial, which showed no difference in outcomes for stages IB/IIA versus IIB/IIIA NSCLC.

The MRC-LU 22/NVALTs/EORTC 08012 multicenter randomized trial reported the results of neoadjuvant therapy with resectable NSCLC.[71] Although stage IIIA patients were included, they accounted for only 7% of all cases. There was no difference in morbidity or mortality, procedures performed, progression-free survival, or overall survival. The 5-year survivals were 44% versus 45% for induction therapy versus surgery alone. The investigators suggest that because more than 60% of tumors were stage I and the survival of the surgery-alone arm was better than expected, a difference still may exist despite this trial failing to show a statistically significant benefit.

The NATCH (Neoadjuvant/Adjuvant Taxol/Carboplatin Hope) 3-arm phase III trial compared disease-free survival in patients treated with surgery alone, induction therapy, and adjuvant therapy.[72] Patients enrolled in this study had stage IA (greater than 2 cm in size), IB, II, or T3N1 disease. The 5-year disease-free survivals were 25%, 37%, and 31% in the surgery-alone, induction, and adjuvant groups, respectively, and overall survivals were 44%, 47%, and 46% for the same groups. No statistically significant survival benefit was found, but subgroup analysis suggested that patients with T3N1 disease benefited from the addition of chemotherapy. An important finding from this trial was that 90% of patients completed induction therapy whereas only 61% completed adjuvant therapy, suggesting that induction therapy is better tolerated than adjuvant therapy. Similar to the S9900 and ChEST trials, a trend toward an improved survival with combined-modality therapy was observed but failed to meet statistical significance. This finding could be related to these trials being underpowered.

Future Directions: Targeted Therapies

The development of therapy with small-molecule tyrosine kinase inhibitors or monoclonal antibodies targeted to epidermal growth factor (gefitinib and erlotinib), vascular endothelial growth factor (bevacizumab), and EML4-ALK (crizotinib) has introduced new options for patients with lung cancer. These therapies have primarily been studied in the metastatic setting, and the toxicities are typically less severe than with cytotoxic chemotherapy. Because these drugs are not curative, treatment with induction therapy followed by surgical resection may be a reasonable approach.[73,74] In patients with early-stage NSCLC, Rizvi and colleagues[75] reported that preoperative gefitinib correlated with radiologic response in patients with sensitizing mutations of epidermal growth factor receptor. Schaake and colleagues[76] reported a phase II of induction erlotinib in patients with early-stage NSCLC, and reported greater than 25% reduction in PET avidity in 27% of patients. After surgery, 5% had greater than 95% necrosis and 25% had greater than 50% necrosis. No unexpected postoperative complications occurred. These studies show the feasibility of using targeted therapy for induction treatment of tumors with specific molecular abnormalities. Phase III trials are needed to show the efficacy and survival benefit of this approach.

SUMMARY

Multimodality therapy with induction therapy for NSCLC is accepted as optimal management for stage III disease. For superior sulcus and locally advanced paravertebral tumors, induction chemoradiotherapy and surgery provide the best treatment. Surgically, complete resection of these locally advanced NSCLCs is key to achieving long-term survival.

Multimodality therapy is standard for N2 disease, although the optimal regimens remain controversial. Definitive chemoradiotherapy can be used, but complete resection after induction chemotherapy remains appropriate for selected patients. Careful evaluation of preoperative pulmonary function with particular attention to the DLCO is critical to assessing the patient's ability to tolerate the planned procedure. Again, complete resection of both the mediastinal disease and the primary tumor play a pivotal role in long-term survival. A lobectomy is preferable, but if a pneumonectomy is required technically, it can be performed in carefully selected patients. Inclusion of radiotherapy in the induction regimen remains controversial. Current evidence does not support chemoradiotherapy over chemotherapy alone, and radiotherapy is usually given postoperatively to reduce the risk of mediastinal recurrence. For all patients with locally advanced NSCLC, well-coordinated multidisciplinary care is key to a successful outcome.

REFERENCES

1. Goldstraw P, Crowley J, Chansky K, et al. The IASLC Lung Cancer Staging Project: proposals for the revision of the TNM stage groupings in the forthcoming (seventh) edition of the TNM classification of malignant tumours. J Thorac Oncol 2007;2:706–14.
2. Martini N, Flehinger BJ. The role of surgery in N2 lung cancer. Surg Clin North Am 1987;67:1037–49.
3. Martini N, Kris MG, Flehinger BJ, et al. Preoperative chemotherapy for stage IIIa (N2) lung cancer: the Sloan-Kettering experience with 136 patients. Ann Thorac Surg 1993;55:1365–74.
4. Roth JA, Atkinson EN, Fossella F, et al. Long-term follow-up of patients enrolled in a randomized trial comparing perioperative chemotherapy and surgery with surgery alone in resectable stage IIIA non-small cell lung cancer. Lung Cancer 1998;21:1–6.
5. Roth JA, Fossella F, Komaki R, et al. A randomized trial comparing perioperative chemotherapy and surgery with surgery alone in resectable stage IIIA non-small-cell lung cancer. J Natl Cancer Inst 1994;86:673–80.
6. Rosell R, Gómez-Codina J, Camps C, et al. A randomized trial comparing preoperative chemotherapy plus surgery with surgery alone in patients with non-small-cell lung cancer. N Engl J Med 1994;330:153–8.
7. Song WA, Zhou NK, Wang W, et al. Survival benefit of neoadjuvant chemotherapy in non-small cell lung cancer: an updated meta-analysis of 13 randomized control trials. J Thorac Oncol 2010;5(4): 510–6.
8. Sugarbaker DJ, Herndon J, Kohman LJ, et al. The Cancer and Leukemia Group B Thoracic Surgery Group. Results of Cancer and Leukemia Group B protocol 8935. A multiinstitutional phase II trimodality trial for stage IIIA (N2) non-small-cell lung cancer. J Thorac Cardiovasc Surg 1995;109:473–85.
9. Albain KS, Rusch VW, Crowley JJ, et al. Concurrent cisplatin/etoposide plus chest radiotherapy followed by surgery for stages IIIA (N2) and IIIB non-small cell lung cancer: mature results of Southwest Oncology Group Phase II study 8805. J Clin Oncol 1995;13:1880–92.
10. Albain KS, Swann RS, Rusch VW, et al. Radiotherapy plus chemotherapy with or without surgical resection for stage III non-small cell lung cancer: a phase III randomised controlled trial. Lancet 2009; 374:379–86.
11. Van Meerbeeck JP, Kramer GW, Van Schil PE, et al. Randomized controlled trial of resection versus radiotherapy after induction chemotherapy in Stage IIIA-N2 non-small cell lung cancer. J Natl Cancer Inst 2007;99:442–50.
12. Arriagada R, Dunant A, Pignon JP, et al. Long-term results of the International Adjuvant Lung Cancer Trial evaluating adjuvant cisplatin-based chemotherapy in resected lung cancer. J Clin Oncol 2010;28(1):35–42.
13. Pignon JP, Tribodet H, Scagliotti GV, et al. Lung adjuvant cisplatin evaluation: a pooled analysis by the LACE Collaborative Group. J Clin Oncol 2008;26(21):3552–9.

14. Douillard JY, Rosell R, De Lena M, et al. Adjuvant vinorelbine plus cisplatin versus observation in patients with completely resected stage IB-IIIA non-small cell lung cancer (Adjuvant Navelbine International Trialist Association [ANITA]): a randomised controlled trial. Lancet Oncol 2006;7:719–27.
15. Winton T, Livingston R, Johnson D, et al. Vinorelbine plus cisplatin vs. observation in resected non-small cell lung cancer. N Engl J Med 2005; 352:2589–97.
16. Strauss GM, Herndon JE II, Maddaus MA, et al. Adjuvant paclitaxel plus carboplatin compared with observation in Stage IB non-small cell lung cancer: CALGB 9633 with the Cancer and Leukemia Group B, Radiation Therapy Oncology Group, and North Central Cancer Treatment Group Study Groups. J Clin Oncol 2008;26(31):5043–51.
17. Thomas M, Rübe C, Hoffknecht P, et al. Effect of preoperative chemoradiation in addition to preoperative chemotherapy: a randomised trial in stage III non-small cell lung cancer. Lancet Oncol 2008; 9(7):636–48.
18. Higgins K, Chino JP, Marks LB, et al. Preoperative chemotherapy versus preoperative chemoradiotherapy for stage III (N2) non-small cell lung cancer. Int J Radiat Oncol Biol Phys 2009;75(5): 1462–7.
19. Shah AA, Berry MF, Tzao C, et al. Induction chemoradiation is not superior to induction chemotherapy alone in stage IIIA lung cancer. Ann Thorac Surg 2012;93(6):1807–12.
20. de Cabanves Candela S, Detterbeck FC. A systematic review of restaging after induction therapy for stage IIIA lung cancer: prediction of pathologic stage. J Thorac Oncol 2010;5(3):389–98.
21. Rebollo-Aguirre AC, Ramos-Font C, Villegas Portero R, et al. Is FDG-PET suitable for evaluating neoadjuvant therapy in non-small cell lung cancer? Evidence with systematic review of the literature. J Surg Oncol 2010;101(6):486–94.
22. Stigt JA, Oostdjik AH, Timmer PR, et al. Comparison of EUS-guided fine needle aspiration and integrated PET-CT in restaging after treatment for locally advanced non-small cell lung cancer. Lung Cancer 2009;66(2):198–204.
23. Kunst PW, Lee P, Paul MA, et al. Restaging of mediastinal nodes with transbronchial needle aspiration after induction chemoradiation for locally advanced non-small cell lung cancer. J Thorac Oncol 2007; 2(10):912–5.
24. Annema JT, Veseliç M, Versteegh MI, et al. Mediastinal restaging: EUS-FNA offers a new perspective. Lung Cancer 2003;42:311–8.
25. Herth FJ, Annema JT, Eberhardt R, et al. Endobronchial ultrasound with transbronchial needle aspiration for restaging the mediastinum in lung cancer. J Clin Oncol 2008;26(20):3346–50.
26. Varadarajulu S, Eloubeidi M. Can endoscopic ultrasonography-guided fine-needle aspiration predict response to chemoradiation in non-small cell lung cancer? A pilot study. Respiration 2006; 73(2):213–20.
27. Van Schil P, van Meerbeeck J, Kramer G, et al. Morbidity and mortality in the surgery arm of EORTC 08941 trial. Eur Respir J 2005;26:1–6.
28. Barnett SA, Rusch VW, Zheng J, et al. Contemporary results of surgical resection of non-small cell lung cancer after induction therapy: a review of 549 consecutive cases. J Thorac Oncol 2011; 6(9):1530–6.
29. Weder W, Collaud S, Eberhardt WE, et al. Pneumonectomy is a valuable treatment option after neoadjuvant therapy for stage III non-small cell lung cancer. J Thorac Cardiovasc Surg 2010;139: 1424–30.
30. Cerfolio RJ, Bryant AS, Spencer SA, et al. Pulmonary resection after high-dose and low-dose chest irradiation. Ann Thorac Surg 2005;80:1224–30.
31. Kwong KF, Edelman MJ, Suntharalingam M, et al. High-dose radiotherapy in trimodality treatment of Pancoast tumors results in high pathologic complete response rates and excellent long-term survival. J Thorac Cardiovasc Surg 2005; 129:1250–7.
32. Daly BD, Fernando HC, Ketchedjian A, et al. Pneumonectomy after high-dose radiation and concurrent chemotherapy for nonsmall cell lung cancer. Ann Thorac Surg 2006;82:227–31.
33. Edelman MJ, Suntharalingam M, Burrows W, et al. Phase I/II trial of hyperfractionated radiation and chemotherapy followed by surgery in Stage III lung cancer. Ann Thorac Surg 2008;86:903–11.
34. Krasna MJ, Gamliel Z, Burrows WM, et al. Pneumonectomy for lung cancer after preoperative concurrent chemotherapy and high-dose radiation. Ann Thorac Surg 2010;89(1):200–6.
35. Martin J, Ginsberg RJ, Abolhoda A, et al. Morbidity and mortality after neoadjuvant therapy for lung cancer: the risks of right pneumonectomy. Ann Thorac Surg 2001;72:1149–54.
36. Evans NR 3rd, Li S, Wright CD, et al. The impact of induction therapy on morbidity and operative mortality after resection of primary lung cancer. J Thorac Cardiovasc Surg 2010;139(4):991–6.
37. Kim AW, Boffa DJ, Wang Z, et al. An analysis, systematic review, and meta-analysis of the perioperative mortality after neoadjuvant therapy and penumonectomy for non-small cell lung cancer. J Thorac Cardiovasc Surg 2012;143(1):55–63.
38. Doddoli C, Barlesi F, Trousse D, et al. One hundred consecutive pneumonectomies after induction therapy for non-small cell lung cancer: an uncertain balance between risks and benefits. J Thorac Cardiovasc Surg 2005;130:416–25.

39. Martin J, Ginsberg RJ, Venkatraman ES, et al. Long term results of combined modality therapy in resectable non-small cell lung cancer. J Clin Oncol 2002;20(8):1989–95.
40. Kim AW, Faber LP, Warren WH, et al. Pneumonectomy after chemoradiation therapy for non-small cell lung cancer: does "side" really matter? Ann Thorac Surg 2009;88:937–44.
41. Allen AM, Mentzer SJ, Yeap BY, et al. Pneumonectomy after chemoradiation: the Dana-Farber Cancer Institute/Brigham and Women's Hospital experience. Cancer 2008;112(5):1106–13.
42. Mansour Z, Kochetkova EA, Ducrocq X, et al. Induction chemotherapy does not increase the operative risk of pneumonectomy! Eur J Cardiothorac Surg 2007;31:181–5.
43. Doddoli C, Thomas P, Thirion X, et al. Postoperative complications in relation with induction therapy for lung cancer. Eur J Cardiothorac Surg 2001;20: 385–90.
44. Pancoast HK. Superior pulmonary sulcus tumor. J Am Med Assoc 1932;99:1391–6.
45. Chardack WM, MacCallum JD. Pancoast tumor (five year survival without recurrence or metastases following radical resection and postoperative irradiation). J Thorac Surg 1956;31:535–42.
46. Shaw RR, Paulson DL, Kee JL Jr. Treatment of the superior sulcus tumor by irradiation followed by resection. Ann Surg 1961;154:29–40.
47. Rusch VW, Parekh KR, Leon L, et al. Factors determining outcome after surgical resection of T3 and T4 lung cancers of the superior sulcus. J Thorac Cardiovasc Surg 2000;119:1147–53.
48. Dartevelle PG, Chapelier AR, Macchiarini P, et al. Anterior transcervical-thoracic approach for radical resection of lung tumors invading the thoracic inlet. J Thorac Cardiovasc Surg 1993;105:1025–34.
49. Rusch VW, Giroux DJ, Kraut MJ, et al. Induction chemoradiation and surgical resection for non-small cell lung carcinomas of the superior sulcus: initial results of Southwest Oncology Group trial 9416 (Intergroup trial 0160). J Thorac Cardiovasc Surg 2001;121:472–83.
50. Rusch VW, Giroux DJ, Kraut MJ, et al. Induction chemoradiation and surgical resection for superior sulcus non-small cell lung carcinomas: long-term results of Southwest Oncology Group trial 9416 (Intergroup trial 0160). J Clin Oncol 2007;25:313–8.
51. Rusch VW. Management of Pancoast tumours. Lancet Oncol 2006;7(12):997–1005.
52. Masaoka A, Ito Y, Yasumitsu T. Anterior approach for tumor of the superior sulcus. J Thorac Cardiovasc Surg 1979;78:413–5.
53. Niwa H, Masaoka A, Yamakawa Y, et al. Surgical therapy for apical invasive lung cancer: different approaches according to tumor location. Lung Cancer 1993;10:63–71.
54. Grunenwald D, Spaggiari L. Transmanubrial osteomuscular sparing approach for apical chest tumors. Ann Thorac Surg 1997;63:563–6.
55. Bilsky MH, Vitaz TW, Boland PJ, et al. Surgical treatment of superior sulcus tumors with spinal and brachial plexus involvement. J Neurosurg 2002;97(Suppl 3):301–9.
56. Jemal A, Siegel R, Ward E, et al. Cancer statistics, 2009. CA Cancer J Clin 2009;59:225–49.
57. Rocha Lima CM, Herndon JE II, Kosty M, et al. Therapy choices among older patients with lung carcinoma: an evaluation of two trials in the Cancer and Leukemia Group B. Cancer 2002;94(1):181–7.
58. Peake MD, Thompson S, Lowe D, et al, Participating Centers. Ageism in the management of lung cancer. Age Ageing 2003;32(2):171–7.
59. Owonikoko TK, Ragin CC, Belani CP, et al. Lung cancer in elderly patients: an analysis of the surveillance, epidemiology, and end results database. J Clin Oncol 2007;25(35):5570–7.
60. Smith TJ, Penberthy L, Desch CE, et al. Differences in initial treatment patters and outcomes of lung cancer in the elderly. Lung Cancer 1995;13(3): 235–52.
61. Oxnard GR, Fidias P, Muzikansky A, et al. Non-small cell lung cancer in octogenarians: treatment practices and preferences. J Thorac Oncol 2007; 2(11):1029–35.
62. Cudennec T, Gendry T, Labrune S, et al. Use of a simplified geriatric evaluation in thoracic oncology. Lung Cancer 2010;67(2):232–6.
63. Girre V, Falcou MC, Gisselbrecht M, et al. Does a geriatric oncology consultation modify the cancer treatment plan for elderly patients? J Gerontol A Biol Sci Med Sci 2008;63(7):724–30.
64. Früh M, Rolland E, Pignon JP, et al. Pooled analysis of the effect of age on adjuvant cisplatin-based chemotherapy for completely resected non-small cell lung cancer. J Clin Oncol 2008; 26(21):3573–81.
65. Pepe C, Hasan B, Winton TL, et al. Adjuvant vinorelbine and cisplatin in elderly patients: National Cancer Institute of Canada and Intergroup Study JBR.10. J Clin Oncol 2007;25(12):1553–61.
66. Gridelli C, Maione P, Comunale D, et al. Adjuvant chemotherapy in elderly patients with non-small-cell lung cancer. Cancer Control 2007;14(1):57–62.
67. Gridelli C, Langer C, Maione P, et al. Lung cancer in the elderly. J Clin Oncol 2007;25(14):1898–907.
68. Rivera C, Jougon J, Dahan M, et al. Are postoperative consequences of neoadjuvant chemotherapy for non-small cell lung cancer more severe in elderly patients? Lung Cancer 2012;76(2):216–21.
69. Pisters KM, Vallières E, Crowley JJ, et al. Surgery with or without preoperative paclitaxel and carboplatin in early stage non-small cell lung cancer: Southwest Oncology Group trial S9900, an

intergroup, randomized, phase III trial. J Clin Oncol 2010;28(11):1843–9.
70. Scagliotti GV, Pastorino U, Vansteenkiste JF, et al. Randomized phase III study of surgery alone or surgery plus preoperative cisplatin and gemcitabine in stages IB to IIIA non-small cell lung cancer. J Clin Oncol 2012;30:172–8.
71. Gilligan D, Nicolson M, Smith I, et al. Preoperative chemotherapy in patients with resectable non-small cell lung cancer: results of the MRC LU22/NVALT 2/EORTC 08012 multicentre randomised trial and update of systematic review. Lancet 2007;369:1929–37.
72. Felip E, Rosell R, Maestre JA, et al. Preoperative chemotherapy plus surgery versus surgery plus adjuvant chemotherapy versus surgery alone in early-stage non-small cell lung cancer. J Clin Oncol 2010;28(19):3138–45.
73. Lynch TJ, Bell DW, Sordelia R, et al. Activating mutations in the epidermal growth factor receptor underlying responsiveness of non-small-cell lung cancer to gefitinib. N Engl J Med 2004;350(21):2129–39.
74. Reungwetwattana T, Weroha SJ, Molina JR. Oncogenic pathways, molecularly targeted therapies, and highlighted clinical trials in non-small cell lung cancer (NSCLC). Clin Lung Cancer 2012;13(4):252–66.
75. Rizvi NA, Rusch V, Pao W, et al. Molecular characteristics predict clinical outcomes: prospective trial correlating response to the EGFR tyrosine kinase inhibitor gefitinib with the presence of sensitizing mutations in the tyrosine binding domain of the EGFR gene. Clin Cancer Res 2011;17(10):3500–6.
76. Schaake EE, Kappers I, Codrington HE, et al. Tumor response and toxicity of neoadjuvant erlotinib in patients with early-stage non-small cell lung cancer. J Clin Oncol 2012;30(22):2731–8.
77. Burkes RL, Ginsberg RJ, Shepherd FA, et al. Induction chemotherapy with mitomycin, vindesine, and cisplatin for stage III unresectable non-small cell lung cancer: results of the Toronto phase II trial. J Clin Oncol 1992;10:580–6.
78. Rosell R, Gómez-Codina J, Camps C, et al. Preresectional chemotherapy in stage IIIA non-small cell lung cancer: a 7-year assessment of a randomized controlled trial. Lung Cancer 1999;47:7–14.
79. Van Zandwijk N, Smit EF, Kramer GW, et al. Gemcitabine and cisplatin as induction regimen for patients with biopsy-proven stage IIIA N2 non-small cell lung cancer: a phase II study of the European Organization for Research and Treatment of Cancer Lung Cancer Cooperative Group (EORTC 08955). J Clin Oncol 2000;18(14):2658–64.
80. Betticher DC, Hsu Schmitz SF, Tötsch M, et al. Mediastinal lymph node clearance after docetaxel-cisplatin neoadjuvant chemotherapy is prognostic of survival in patients with stage IIIA pN2 non-small cell lung cancer: a multicenter phase II trial. J Clin Oncol 2003;21:1752–9.
81. Nagai K, Tsuchiya R, Mori T, et al. A randomized trial of comparing induction chemotherapy followed by surgery with surgery alone for patients with stage IIIA N2 non-small cell lung cancer (JCOG 9209). J Thorac Cardiovasc Surg 2003;125:254–60.
82. O'Brien ME, Splinter T, Smit EF, et al. Carboplatin and paclitaxol (Taxol) as an induction regimen for patients with biopsy-proven stage IIIA N2 non-small cell lung cancer. An EORTC phase II study (EORTC 08958). Eur J Cancer 2003;39(10):1416–22.
83. Garrido P, González-Larriba JL, Insa A, et al. Long-term survival associated with complete resection after induction chemotherapy in stage IIIA (N2) and IIIB (T4N0-1) non-small cell lung cancer patients: the Spanish Lung Cancer Group trial 9901. J Clin Oncol 2007;25(30):4736–42.
84. Mathisen DJ, Wain JC, Wright C, et al. Assessment of preoperative accelerated radiotherapy and chemotherapy in stage IIIA (N2) non-small cell lung cancer. J Thorac Cardiovasc Surg 1996;111:123–33.
85. Katayama H, Ueoka H, Kiura K, et al. Preoperative concurrent chemoradiotherapy with cisplatin and docetaxel in patients with locally advanced non-small cell lung cancer. Br J Cancer 2004;90(5):979–84.
86. Steger V, Walles T, Kosan B, et al. Trimodal therapy for histologically proven N2/3 non-small cell lung cancer: mid-term results and indicators for survival. Ann Thorac Surg 2009;87(6):1676–83.
87. Paulson DL. Carcinomas in the superior pulmonary sulcus. J Thorac Cardiovasc Surg 1975;70:1095–104.
88. Attar S, Miller JE, Satterfield J, et al. Pancoast's tumor: irradiation or surgery? Ann Thorac Surg 1979;28:578–86.
89. Ginsberg RJ, Martini N, Zaman M, et al. Influence of surgical resection and brachytherapy in the management of superior sulcus tumor. Ann Thorac Surg 1994;57:1440–5.
90. Maggi G, Casadio C, Pischedda F, et al. Combined radiosurgical treatment of Pancoast tumor. Ann Thorac Surg 1994;57:198–202.
91. Hagan MP, Choi NC, Mathisen DJ, et al. Superior sulcus lung tumors: impact of local control on survival. J Thorac Cardiovasc Surg 1999;117:1086–94.
92. Komaki R, Roth JA, Walsh GL, et al. Outcome predictors for 143 patients with superior sulcus tumor treated by multidisciplinary approach at the University of Texas M.D. Anderson Cancer Center. Int J Radiat Oncol Biol Phys 2000;48:347–54.
93. Martinod E, D'Audiffret A, Thomas P, et al. Management of superior sulcus tumors: experience with

139 cases treated by surgical resection. Ann Thorac Surg 2002;73:1534–40.

94. Marra A, Eberhardt W, Pöttgen C, et al. Induction chemotherapy, concurrent chemoradiation and surgery for Pancoast tumour. Eur Respir J 2007; 29:117–27.
95. Pourel N, Santelmo N, Naafa N, et al. Concurrent cisplatin/etoposide plus 3D-conformal radiotherapy followed by surgery for stage IIB (superior sulcus T3N0)/III non-small cell lung cancer yields a high rate of pathological complete response. Eur J Cardiothorac Surg 2008;33:829–36.
96. Kunitoh H, Kato H, Tsuboi M, et al. Phase II trial of preoperative chemoradiotherapy followed by surgical resection in patients with superior sulcus non-small cell lung cancers: report of Japan Clinical Oncology Group Trial 9806. J Clin Oncol 2008;26:644–9.

Surgery for Lung Cancer

Can We Predict Morbidity and Mortality Before an Operation?

Sabha Ganai, MD, PhD[a], Mark K. Ferguson, MD[b,*]

KEYWORDS

• Prediction • Complications • Morbidity • Mortality • Thoracic • Lung resection

KEY POINTS

- Although risk assessment is often based on surrogate parameters of patient fitness, decisions regarding risk are typically made in the context of both patient and physician perceptions and expectations.
- Current predictive tools for morbidity and mortality are limited in usefulness by the quality of their data, the variables that are included in their models, and the degree of uncertainty provided in parameters and predicted outcomes.
- The rationale for predictive tools is not simply for internal audits and quality improvement purposes, but ideally to provide patients with a reasonable estimate of their risk within a range of uncertainty before undergoing an intervention.

It is exceedingly difficult to make predictions, particularly about the future.[1]

—*Neils Bohr*

In 1983, Professor Robert J. Ginsberg and the Lung Cancer Study Group published the first modern surgical series by a cooperative group examining operative mortality in patients with bronchogenic lung cancer.[2] After compiling data on patients who were resected with complete mediastinal lymph node staging across 7 treatment protocols, these investigators reported that among the 9 of 12 institutions that performed 10 or more lung resections per year (n = 1770), 30-day mortality was 6.2% for pneumonectomy, 2.9% for lobectomy, and 1.4% for sublobar resections. Mortality was noted to increase with age, ranging from 1.3% when younger than 60 years, 4.1% from 60 to 69 years, up to 7.1% for age 70 years and older. Major causes of death were attributed to postoperative pneumonia and respiratory failure (29%), bronchopleural fistula and empyema (26%), myocardial infarction (23%), and pulmonary embolus (13%). Only bronchopleural fistula and postoperative hemorrhage (3%) were interpreted as directly related to operative technique, with implications that recognizable preoperative risk factors may help determine outcome after resection.

Over the subsequent 30 years, despite progress in staging, decreases in pneumonectomy rates,[3] innovations in surgical technique and perioperative care, and concurrent improvements in morbidity and mortality from lung resection,[4] surgeons struggle with estimation of perioperative risk.[5] The understanding that most postoperative morbidity after lung resection is related to pulmonary complications has led to greater use of spirometry, measures of gas exchange, and assessments of exercise capacity to select for appropriate

The authors have nothing to disclose.
[a] Department of Surgery, The University of Chicago Medicine, The University of Chicago, 5841 South Maryland Avenue, MC 6040, Chicago, IL 60637, USA; [b] Department of Surgery, The University of Chicago Medicine, The University of Chicago, 5841 South Maryland Avenue, MC 5040, Chicago, IL 60637, USA
* Corresponding author.
E-mail address: mferguso@surgery.bsd.uchicago.edu

Thorac Surg Clin 23 (2013) 287–299
http://dx.doi.org/10.1016/j.thorsurg.2013.04.001
1547-4127/13/$ – see front matter

operative candidates, as well as further development of multivariate risk models using these and various other metrics. This article explores how clinical data have been used to infer relationships between patient-related factors and outcome, and discusses if it is ever possible to predict risk of morbidity and mortality after major lung resection.

UNCERTAINTY AND BIAS

Any rational discussion on prediction must begin with the knowledge that nothing can be understood with absolute precision or accuracy. The inherent error in measurement tools and the variables chosen or neglected to study become compounded with every iteration and attempt to create and validate relationships. Although cause and effect between variables and outcome is typically assumed, relationships may be nonlinear, stochastic, and probabilistic rather than deterministic. Assumptions are limited by current knowledge, and investigators may be led astray by their beliefs, focusing on noise rather than signal within a data set.[6] Data may be limited in its usefulness by the era in which it was collected, especially with dynamic innovations in staging, technique, and perioperative care over time. Prediction models may be applicable only to populations from which the data were derived and may never correlate with the outcomes of a single surgeon. Although many assumptions are based on bell-curve distributions, in reality, accurate predictions and forecasts may be limited by the presence of outliers, especially in highly complex and chaotic systems.[7]

Although risk assessment is often based on surrogate parameters of patient fitness, decisions regarding risk are typically made in the context of both patient and physician perceptions and expectations.[8] By underestimating uncertainty and overestimating what we as clinicians truly know, our ability to discuss the risks and benefits of a treatment plan in a way that is meaningful to decision making may be distorted.[6,7] Despite the rigor put into many prediction models, physicians tend to use objective data inconsistently and make decisions that are altered by experience, exposure, and internal biases.[9] Paradoxically, experts may enhance their capabilities at prediction by combining objective, measurable findings with subjective and qualitative data obtained through contextual relationships.[5,6] To complicate the issue further, although patient-related factors are often modeled as risk factors, systems-related factors (such as relationships between hospital volume, surgeon volume, and surgeon specialty on outcome)[10–13] may further confound the ability to generalize conclusions related to morbidity and mortality after pulmonary resection, whether derived from population-based or single-institutional databases. It can be argued that knowledge of one's personal surgical experience is the best way to gain understanding of the risks that a patient may be subject to, but that argument is still suspect to biases of selection and perhaps some self-deception. A limitation of human perception is that we interpret the data we are presented with in a way that is framed by our own expectations.[6]

PHYSIOLOGIC EVALUATION AND SELECTION

Current evidence-based clinical practice guidelines highlight the importance of objective preoperative physiologic assessment of perioperative risk to help identify patients who are at an increased risk of complications, disability, and mortality from lung resection using the least invasive tests possible.[14–16] Assessment of cardiovascular risk is generally performed as described by the American College of Cardiology (ACC) and American Heart Association (AHA) guidelines for noncardiac surgery,[17] which review major risk factors that should initiate further cardiologic evaluation, diagnostic testing, and use of prophylactic therapies (eg, perioperative β-blockade). Because pulmonary complications are more prevalent than cardiovascular complications after lung resection, further evaluation of fitness for thoracic surgery has focused on exploring the use of pulmonary function measures such as forced expiratory volume in 1 second (FEV_1), diffusion capacity of the lung for carbon monoxide (DLCO), and exercise testing for optimal patient selection.[8,18–20]

Although predicted postoperative (ppo) FEV_1 has been advocated as an important correlate for risk of complications after lung resection,[21] the importance of FEV_1 has been questioned in recent years.[8] The European Respiratory Society and European Society of Thoracic Surgeons (ESTS) clinical guidelines for evaluation of fitness in patients with lung cancer recommends that although ppo FEV_1 of 30% predicted is suggested as a high-risk threshold, it should not be used alone to select patients for surgery.[15] Their algorithm recommends routine measurement of DLCO in lung resection patients, and that a ppo DLCO of 30% predicted be used as a high-risk threshold for intervention, in addition to the use of exercise tests measuring oxygen consumption on patients with FEV_1 and DLCO lower than 80% of normal values. The British Thoracic Society (BTS) and the Society for Cardiothoracic Surgery in Great Britain and Ireland guidelines for lung resection recommend measurement of DLCO in all patients, regardless of spirometric values, as well as the selective use of exercise testing for evaluation of patients at high risk of postoperative dyspnea.[16] Although decreased DLCO has been associated with adverse outcomes after surgery, including morbidity, mortality, and impaired quality of life,[8,19,22] it has also been shown to be prognostic for long-term survival after resection for cancer.[23,24] Despite its importance as an independent predictor of risk, as well as recent changes in clinical practice guidelines to include it as an important part of risk assessment, it has not yet been well incorporated into clinical practice, possibly limiting the value of some of the predictive models discussed in this article.

MODELS FOR MORTALITY

In 1999, the Veterans Affairs National Surgical Quality Improvement Program (VA NSQIP) published the results of data obtained prospectively on 3516 consecutive patients who had undergone major lung resection across 123 medical centers over almost 4 years.[25] Each patient had 143 variables recorded with use of imputation techniques for missing data. Thirty-day morbidity and mortality were 25.7% and 11.5% for pneumonectomy, and 23.8% and 4.0% for lobectomy, respectively. Examining mortality with multivariable logistic regression, independent predictors of death were age, serum albumin, transfusion before operation of more than 4 units of red blood cells, disseminated cancer (clinical evidence of mediastinal lymph nodes with non–small cell lung cancer (NSCLC) or resection of a pulmonary metastasis), impaired sensorium, operation type (eg, pneumonectomy), intraoperative blood loss, and the presence of dyspnea (**Table 1**). Predictors of morbidity were also analyzed, as summarized in **Table 2**. Although the VA NSQIP group analyzed the largest data set of its time with the aim of creating a risk-adjusted model for selection of patients for lung resection, their data set lacked pulmonary function testing and was heavily biased toward a male population, leading to questions regarding its generalizability. The VA NSQIP group reported an approach for future outcome studies and emphasized the importance of consistency in prospective data collection across multiple centers.

The ESTS and the European Association of Cardiothoracic Surgeons modeled the risk of in-hospital death on patients entered in their database who underwent lung resection between 2001 and 2003.[26] Although ppo DLCO was a significant predictor of mortality in univariate analysis, data were missing from 77% of cases, so it was excluded from multivariate modeling. Using available data, the investigators created 2 models for in-hospital mortality: (1) the European Society Subjective Score (ESSS.01) and (2) the European Society Objective Score (ESOS.01). The ESSS.01 was developed using a training set of 2056 cases and validated in 1370 patients using a combination of dyspnea grade, American Society of Anesthesiologists (ASA) score, age, and procedure type to predict mortality. The ESOS.01 was developed in 1753 patients and validated in 1166 patients using a model that focused on age and ppo FEV_1. Although observed-to-predicted mortality plots were provided showing reliable prediction characteristics, receiver-operating characteristic (ROC) statistics were not reported. Recent validation in a small cohort of 290 patients showed that the ESOS.01 was reasonably accurate at predicting mortality, with area under ROC curve values of 0.8.[27] The ESOS.01 was also used to compare observed and predicted in-hospital mortality across 3 European thoracic surgery units and has been suggested as a methodology for performance of objective, risk-adjusted, multi-institutional audits on lung resection patients.[28]

The French Society of Thoracic and Cardiovascular Surgery used their national database from 2002 to 2005 to develop a risk model for in-hospital mortality after thoracic surgery called Thoracoscore.[29] Analyzing a selected group of more than 15,000 patients with more than 95% of completed data, these investigators developed a 9-variable risk model including gender, age, ASA score, performance status, dyspnea score, urgency of surgery, malignant diagnosis, type of resection, and number of comorbidities. Because DLCO was not regularly used in French practice,[30] it was not included in their initial training set. In an effort to better assess mortality risk, Thoracoscore has been incorporated as a global risk score for perioperative death as part of the BTS guidelines for tripartite risk assessment in patients with lung cancer[16] in combination with the ACC/AHA guidelines for cardiovascular risk evaluation,[17] and DLCO measurement for assessment of risk for respiratory morbidity. Performance of the prediction model was reasonable, with an ROC curve concordance (c)-statistic of 0.86 (95% confidence interval 0.83–0.89) and a Hosmer-Lemeshow goodness-of-fit P value of 0.92 when initially validated. However, there are several recent reports that Thoracoscore may fail in its predictive capacity when it has been applied to broader populations.[27,31,32] Although it can be argued that Thoracoscore is more cumbersome to use than a 2-variable risk model like ESOS.01, recent development of Web-based and smart phone applications[33,34] may influence its use by clinicians as a decision tool.

Table 1
Risk models for predicted perioperative mortality after major lung resection

	VA NSQIP[25]	ESSS.01[26]	ESOS.01[26]	Thoracoscore[29]	Norway[35]	SEER-Medicare[37]	STS[38]	Liverpool[32]
N	3516	3426	2822	15,183	1844	14,297	18,800	2574
Mortality (%)	5.2	1.9	2.0	2.2	4.4	4.6	2.2	2.3
Covariates included in prediction model	Preoperative transfusion >4 units PRBCs[a] DNR status Pneumonectomy[a] Impaired sensorium[a] Disseminated cancer[a] Dyspnea[a] Increased prothrombin time Age[a] Intraoperative blood loss[a] Albumin[a]	Dyspnea score[a] ASA score[a] Age[a] Procedure type[a]	Age[a] ppo FEV_1[a,b]	Malignancy[a] Pneumonectomy[a] Age[a] Dyspnea score[a] Comorbidities[a] Urgency of surgery[a] Performance status[a] ASA score[a] Gender[a]	Age[a] Charlson comorbidity index[a] Procedure[a] Pathologic stage[a] Histology[a] Laterality[a] Gender[a] VATS Tumor size Hospital volume	Acute MI[a] Severe ulcer[a] Procedure[a] Cerebrovascular disease[a] Complicated diabetes[a] Congestive heart failure[a] Laterality[a] Age[a] Tumor size[a] Pathologic stage[a] Histology[a] Gender[a]	Performance status[a] ASA score[a] Dialysis[a] Procedure[a] Creatinine >2 mg/dL[a] Induction chemoradiation therapy[a] Pathologic stage[a] Steroids[a] Age[a] Urgency[a] Gender[a] Hypertension Peripheral vascular disease BMI[a,b] VATS Diabetes FEV_1[a,b] Coronary artery disease Cerebrovascular disease Recent cigarette use Surgery year Induction chemotherapy alone Congestive heart failure Thoracic reoperation	Age[a] ppo FEV_1[a,b] Gender[a] Alcohol consumption[a] Renal failure[a] Emphysema[a] Tobacco pack-years Diabetes Resection margin BMI Tumor diameter

ROC c-statistic (95% CI)	0.75	NR	NR	0.86 (0.83–0.89)	NR	0.72	0.77	0.82 (0.80–0.84)
Hosmer-Lemeshow test (P)[c]	.58	NR	NR	.92	.93	.67	.17	.19

Abbreviations: ASA, American Society of Anesthesiologists; BMI, body mass index; CI, confidence interval; DNR, do not resuscitate; ESOS, European Society Objective Score; ESSS, European Society Subjective Score; MI, myocardial infarction; NR, not reported; PRBC, packed red blood cell; ROC c-statistic, receiver-operating characteristic concordance statistic; SEER, Surveillance Epidemiology and End Results; STS, Society of Thoracic Surgeons; VATS, video-assisted thoracoscopic surgery.

[a] $P<.05$.

[b] Inversely related.

[c] A larger *P* value indicates greater model reliability.

Table 2
Risk models for predicted perioperative morbidity after major lung resection

	VA NSQIP[25]	EVAD[46]	MSKCC[49]	ThRCRI[50]	STS[38]	STS-DLCO Subgroup[56]
N	3516	619	956	1696	18,800	7891
Morbidity (%)	24.1 (all)	13.9 (pulmonary), 32.0 (all)	12.7 (pulmonary)	3.3 (cardiac)	8.6 (all)	13.0 (pulmonary)
Covariates included in prediction model	Preoperative transfusion >4 units PRBCs[a] Hemiplegia[a] Weight loss >10%[a] COPD[a] Dyspnea[a] Smoking[a] Intraoperative blood transfusion Operative time Age[a] Albumin[a]	FEV_1[a,b] Age DLCO[a,b]	Preoperative chemotherapy[a] ppo DLCO[a,b]	Ischemic heart disease[a] Cerebrovascular disease[a] Pneumonectomy[a] Creatinine >2 mg/dL[a]	Performance status[a] ASA score[a] Procedure[a] Induction chemoradiation therapy[a] Dialysis[a] Creatinine >2 mg/dL[a] VATS[a] Steroids[a] Congestive heart failure[a] Recent cigarette use[a] Thoracic reoperation Age[a] Coronary artery disease[a] Pathologic stage Gender BMI[a,b] Hypertension Cerebrovascular disease FEV_1[a,b] Diabetes Urgency Peripheral vascular disease Surgery year Induction chemotherapy alone	Bilobectomy or sleeve lobectomy[a] Congestive heart failure[a] Performance status[a] Renal insufficiency[a] Preoperative chemotherapy or radiotherapy[a] Recent smoking history[a] ASA class[a] Diabetes Gender COPD DLCO[a,b] Coronary artery disease Abnormal spirometry (without COPD) Hypertension Pneumonectomy FVC FEV_1[a]

ROC c-statistic (95% CI)	0.65	0.65	0.63	0.72 (0.65–0.78)	0.69	NR
Hosmer-Lemeshow test (*P*)[c]	.39	NR	.43	NR	.46	NR

Abbreviations: ASA, American Society of Anesthesiologists; BMI, body mass index; CI, confidence interval; COPD, chronic obstructive pulmonary disease; EVAD, % FEV_1, age, and % DLCO score; FVC, forced vital capacity; NR, not reported; PRBC, packed red blood cell; ROC c-statistic, receiver-operating characteristic concordance statistic; STS, Society of Thoracic Surgeons; ThRCRI, Thoracic Revised Cardiac Risk Index; VATS, video-assisted thoracoscopic surgery.

[a] $P<.05$.

[b] Inversely related.

[c] A larger *P* value indicates greater model reliability.

Strand and colleagues[35] from the Cancer Registry of Norway reported predictors of 30-day mortality in more than 4000 patients undergoing surgical treatment of NSCLC between 1993 and 2005 (see **Table 1**). Although their model included hospital volume of more than 20 procedures per year as a covariate, this was not statistically significant in univariate or multivariate analysis as a predictor of mortality, a finding that is consistent with other data suggesting that hospital volume of lung cancer resections may not correlate with mortality risk.[36] More important relationships were related to risk of death from pneumonectomy, especially of the right lung, and in male patients older than 70 years. These investigators also noted general trends showing improvements in postoperative mortality and decreasing pneumonectomy rates over time.

Kates and colleagues[37] examined outcomes from the Surveillance Epidemiology and End Results Registry linked with Medicare claims (SEER-Medicare) in patients older than 65 years who underwent lung resection for NSCLC. Their analysis comprised more than 14,000 patients and included numerous variables specific to comorbidities, procedure, age, and tumor, as seen in **Table 1**. The investigators sought to validate the prediction rule developed by Strand and colleagues[35] by initially fitting similar and available covariates, but found improved predictive characteristics after including individual comorbidities rather than the Charlson comorbidity score. Although this model has strengths related to its development in a large population-based cancer registry, it is limited by a lack of pulmonary function data.

The Society of Thoracic Surgeons (STS) General Thoracic Surgery Database was used to develop models for mortality, morbidity, and a composite outcome measure that could be used to evaluate hospital performance for quality improvement purposes.[38] Investigators examined more than 18,000 patients who underwent resection for NSCLC between 2002 and 2008. Although imputation techniques were used for missing data, information on clinical staging and DLCO was missing in almost 40% of patient records, so these variables were excluded. Performance characteristics for their mortality and morbidity models (see **Tables 1** and **2**) suggest average predictive capacity, with limitations including the large number of covariates in their models. Although the STS has developed online decision-making software for cardiac procedures,[39] they have not yet expanded this to the general thoracic surgery population.

In an effort to improve on Thoracoscore, ESOS.01, and the STS risk models, Poullis and colleagues[32] presented a model for prediction of in-hospital mortality developed and validated from approximately 2500 lung resections at a single institution in the United Kingdom. These investigators included operative factors, including tumor size and bronchial margin, as well as patient factors such as alcohol consumption, renal disease, and ppo FEV_1 (see **Table 1**). DLCO was once again excluded because of missing data. The investigators found improved performance characteristics compared with the other models tested, with an ROC c-statistic of 0.82. Their use of a close resection margin as a covariate may be difficult to assess preoperatively, and although this was not statistically significant, it improved the predictive characteristics of the model. Other limitations of use of this model include development in a single institution and a lack of validation. Further examination of the methodological issues and biases limiting accurate prediction of risk of mortality is warranted, especially if these models are to be used for patient selection rather than quality-of-care purposes.

PREDICTING COMPLICATION RISK

A recent focus on improving the quality of health care delivery has led to systems-related approaches to addressing morbidity using objective outcomes data.[40] Challenges from interpreting institutional variability in the reporting of complications and their severity have led to further efforts to define and grade postoperative complications in a reproducible fashion.[41,42] Although studying operative mortality outcomes seems straightforward in definition (ie, patient death), there are still important differences in reporting in terms of scope and time frame, whether defining in-hospital, 30-day, or 90-day outcomes.[43] Reporting of complications is even more inconsistent, and details are often not captured by large databases. Although complication severity grading has been applied to esophagectomy, examining morbidity relationships with cost and length of stay,[44] it has been performed in only a limited fashion in lung resection patients.[45] In the general thoracic literature, most predictive models discussed for complications either focus on overall incidence in complications or specifically pulmonary or cardiac complications.

In 2003, Ferguson and Durkin[46] validated 3 algorithms for prediction of major postoperative complications in patients undergoing major lung resection: (1) the Cardiopulmonary Risk Index (CPRI),[47] (2) the Physiologic and Operative Severity Score for Enumeration of Mortality and Morbidity (POSSUM),[48] and (3) the % FEV_1, age, and % DLCO (EVAD) score.[46] The CPRI is a composite point score combining presence of cardiac variables (congestive heart failure, myocardial infarction, premature ventricular contractions, irregular preoperative electrocardiogram, age more than 70 years, aortic stenosis, and poor medical condition) with pulmonary variables (obesity, recent smoking history, productive cough, diffuse wheezing or rhonchi, FEV_1 less than 70%, and $Paco_2$ (partial pressure of carbon dioxide, arterial) greater than 45 mm Hg.[47] The POSSUM score is a risk-adjusted score that combines a 12-factor physiologic score with a 6-factor operative severity score.[48] Morbidity was compared between scoring systems across a variety of complication categories (eg, pulmonary, cardiovascular, infectious, total) and with specific definitions for complications within these categories. After developing the EVAD score, the investigators were able to predict risk of most types of complications with ROC analysis area under the curve of approximately 0.65, which although less than ideal, was better than the other methods validated.[46] The EVAD score has the added advantages of being a parsimonious, easy-to-use metric, with objective parameters that can be clearly defined preoperatively.

Amar and colleagues[49] at Memorial-Sloan Kettering Cancer Center reviewed outcomes of 956 patients who underwent lung resection between 1992 and 2003. Pulmonary complications occurred in 12.7% of patients, with oxygen needed on discharge in 2.5%. Patients with pulmonary complications were associated with an increased median length of stay (12 vs 6 days) and 30-day mortality (13.2% vs 0.7%). Important univariate associations included albumin, preoperative chemotherapy, DLCO, and ppo DLCO. FEV_1 was not significant. Multivariate analysis found that preoperative chemotherapy and decreased ppo DLCO were independent risk factors for pulmonary complications. These investigators developed a prediction model that assigned a point score of 2 for history of preoperative chemotherapy and a point score of 1 for each 5% decrement in ppo DLCO lower than 100%. By partitioning point scores to low-risk (0–10), intermediate-risk (11–13), and high-risk (14–19) groups, they were able to achieve adequate stratification of pulmonary complications at 9%, 14%, and 26%, respectively. Their model had an ROC c-statistic of 0.63, suggesting average predictive capacity with their simple and practical scoring system.

To develop a tool for cardiac risk stratification before lung resection, Brunelli and colleagues[50] modified the Revised Cardiac Risk Index (RCRI) to better fit a thoracic population.[51] They developed the Thoracic RCRI (ThRCRI) in a cohort of 1696 major lung resections, finding 4 independent predictors of cardiac complications (3% risk): (1) ischemic heart disease, (2) creatinine more than 2 mg/dL, (3) cerebrovascular disease, and (4) pneumonectomy. Risk of major cardiac complications ranged from 1.5% to 23% depending on ThRCRI score. ROC curve analysis c-statistic was 0.72 (95% confidence interval, 0.65–0.78), suggesting reasonable performance for this predictive metric specific to cardiac morbidity. The ThRCI was later externally validated as able to successfully stratify risk of cardiac complications in 2 separate cohorts of 2621 and 1255 patients, respectively.[52,53]

Brunelli and colleagues[54] later developed a combined outcome index score in an effort to create a composite, risk-adjusted outcome metric using 4 separate models for (1) 30-day mortality, (2) 30-day cardiopulmonary morbidity, (3) unplanned admission to the intensive care unit, and (4) prolonged hospital stay. Parameters used as covariates included age, ppo FEV_1, cardiac comorbidities, pneumonectomy, and performance status. Although it may be difficult for clinicians to assign value of a composite score relative to standard terms like morbidity and mortality, they may have value in defining global quality of care. Composite performance scores have been shown to be able to rank institutions distinctly compared with morbidity or mortality scores alone.[55] These metrics may not be as important to prediction as they are for evaluation of quality of care examining structure, processes, and outcomes, especially because they include a posteriori measures determined at preoperative, intraoperative, and postoperative time points.

Ferguson and colleagues[56] reviewed outcomes in 7891 patients included in the STS General Thoracic Database between 2002 and 2008 who had DLCO measurements recorded. This review comprised only 57% of available records during the time interval. Percent decrease in predicted DLCO was noted to be a significant predictor of pulmonary morbidity, independent of whether patients had preexisting chronic obstructive pulmonary disease. Further incorporation of DLCO into thoracic practice and development of databases that further highlight these objective parameters are necessary to improve predictive models.

Takamochi and colleagues[57] reviewed 1073 patients with NSCLC who underwent pulmonary resection between 1996 and 2009, comparing patients younger and older than 70 years. Although no significant difference in overall morbidity or 30-day mortality was seen between groups, these investigators found that arrhythmias and delirium were more common in the older cohort. On multivariate analysis, independent predictors of morbidity in the younger cohort were FEV_1 less than

70%, lobectomy or greater resection, and squamous cell histology. Independent risk factors for morbidity in the older cohort were a smoking history of more than 40 pack-years, hypertension, creatinine more than 1 mg/dL, and DLCO less than 60%. Although chronologic age is not necessarily a limiting factor for decision making around surgery, there may be relevant changes in global physiologic reserve related to age (ie, frailty) that may affect morbidity, mortality, and quality of life.[58] Important to this study is the knowledge that predictors of risk may be highly dependent on patient subgroup or population studied, requiring more complex algorithms for future analysis.

With recent improvements in computational power, fuzzy logic algorithms have been examined as a method to evaluate predictors of morbidity after lung resection.[59] Fuzzy logic is a form of multivalued logic that deals with reasoning that is approximate rather than exact and has value in representing areas in which precise description of processes is impossible, especially the complex feedback processes seen in medical decision making.[60] Fuzzy logic assigns a degree of uncertainty to each categorical parameter and propagates that uncertainty across each decision node.[61] For example, although our clinical definition of a term like elderly may be highly variable, most standard analyses use discrete binary cutoffs such as an age of 70 years. Instead, a fuzzy set may use overlapping definitions of terms, such as a range from 55 to 100 years for elderly patients and 15 to 70 years for younger patients. Turna and colleagues[59] examined 92 patients who underwent thoracotomy and used fuzzy logic for parameters including number of smoking pack-years, predicted FEV_1, $Pa{O_2}$ (partial pressure of oxygen, arterial), sedimentation rate, and leukocyte count to develop a tool for predicting risk of complications. Their model was able to stratify risk of complications into low-risk, intermediate-risk (unclassifiable), and high-risk groups with an ROC curve c-statistic of 0.76. Although this study was limited by number of patients studied and the types of parameters assessed, fuzzy logic may be an important methodology for future study, especially because it incorporates uncertainty into prediction rules.

Artificial neural networks are learning models that use numerous interconnected units with forward and backward feedback loops that work together to solve problems and model complex systems.[62] Neural networks are able to find subtle associations between parameters that are not obvious and learn by adaptation to improve their predictive capacity. Esteva and colleagues[63] examined the use of neural networks to estimate risk of morbidity and mortality after lung resection using 96 variables as parameters for 4 training models. These investigators developed models for estimating mortality and morbidity that had 100% specificity and sensitivity in classifying 28 cases. Santos-García and colleagues[64] examined neural networks to predict cardiopulmonary morbidity after pulmonary resection for NSCLC by using a training set of 348 patients and then validating this in 141 cases. Their neural network ensemble model combined 100 separate neural networks with different structures and parameters and showed a remarkably high predictive performance, with an ROC c-statistic of 0.98. Although promising, their model was developed using intraoperative and postoperative factors in addition to preoperative factors, which limits its use as an a priori predictive tool. Neural network models warrant further development and validation using larger, multi-institutional data sets before conclusions can be made on their usefulness.

SUMMARY

There are many challenges in the prediction of morbidity and mortality. Because of limited event rates, especially for mortality, large population-based or multi-institutional databases are ideal, although the overall quality of data collection may then become a concern. Missing data, such as that seen for DLCO in many of the described studies, limits the use and interpretation of several prediction models. Inaccurate reporting and manipulation of data can occur, such as presumed ASA score gaming described in development of the ESSS.01.[26] Overfitting, or the use of too many parameters relative to the number of observations, leads to a focus on random noise instead of signal within a data set and increases the instability and possibility of error from the model.[65] The simpler a model is to use, the more likely it is to be useful for busy clinicians. However, reporting of risk only as odds ratios and neglecting to indicate error limits or confidence intervals effectively limits the ability of clinicians to provide any useful information on individual prognosis with these tools. Ideally, these metrics should be designed to allow stratification of patients into groups at moderate and high risk of complications, as well as prohibitive risk of in-hospital mortality.[58]

By taking a skeptical viewpoint, it may seem that the accurate prediction of outcome after surgery is impossible, yet we still argue that thoughtful use of data using our current best evidence can help inform treatment decisions in accordance to patient preferences. The rationale for predictive tools is not just for internal audits, but ideally to provide patients with a reasonable estimate of their risk within a range of uncertainty before undergoing an intervention. Although many efforts at risk stratification have led to improved selection of operative candidates, by gaining an understanding of the risks of morbidity, mortality, and impaired functional outcomes from different treatment choices, we can also help inform decisions for patients who may be at high risk of surgical complications.[58] These discussions are a challenge for clinicians, who are as susceptible to framing biases as their patients[66] and may not be adequately trained to effectively communicate risk, despite the practical importance related to the process of informed consent.

Recommended strategies to assist patients in their understanding of risk and uncertainty include using visual decision aids for discussion of probabilities, presenting absolute numbers whenever possible rather than relative risks, and framing outcomes in both positive and negative forms (eg, likelihood of survival and of mortality).[67] Awareness that patients' assessments of risk are based more on emotion than on fact fundamentally requires fostering a doctor-patient relationship built on trust. Because recent pay-for-performance initiatives to incentivize high-quality surgical care may affect complication and failure-to-rescue rates after surgery by promoting a culture of safety,[40] it remains imperative to further gain an understanding of predictors of morbidity and mortality for specific procedures through feedback from high-quality data. Although it may not be possible to accurately forecast postoperative morbidity and mortality, with further scholarship greater understanding of the level of complexity surrounding prediction may be gained, new tools, processes of care, and interventions to avoid or select against complications may be developed, and patients may be provided with the data and contextual information that they need to help with evidence-based decision making.

REFERENCES

1. Petersson B. The perils of prediction, June 2nd [Letters to the editor]. The Economist 2007. Available at:. http://www.economist.com/blogs/theinbox/2007/07/the_perils_of_prediction_june. Accessed January 22, 2013.
2. Ginsberg RJ, Hill LD, Eagen RT, et al. Modern thirty-day operative mortality for surgical resections in lung cancer. J Thorac Cardiovasc Surg 1983;86:654–8.
3. Strand TE, Bartnes K, Rostad H. National trends in lung cancer surgery. Eur J Cardiothorac Surg 2012;42:355–8.
4. Ferguson MK, Vigneswaran WT. Changes in patient presentation and outcomes for major lung resection over three decades. Eur J Cardiothorac Surg 2008;33:496–500.
5. Ferguson MK, Stromberg JD, Celauro AD. Estimating lung resection risk: a pilot study of trainee and practicing surgeons. Ann Thorac Surg 2010;89:1037–43.
6. Silver N. The signal and the noise: why so many predictions fail–but some don't. New York: The Penguin Press; 2012.
7. Taleb NN. The black swan: the impact of the highly improbable. New York: Random House; 2010.
8. Brunelli A. Risk assessment for pulmonary resection. Semin Thorac Cardiovasc Surg 2010;22:2–13.
9. Brunelli A, Pompili C, Salati M. Patient selection for operation: the complex balance between information and intuition. J Thorac Dis 2013;5:8–11.
10. Bach PB, Cramer LD, Schrag D, et al. The influence of hospital volume on survival after resection for lung cancer. N Engl J Med 2001;345:181–8.
11. Birkmeyer JD, Siewers AE, Finlayson EV, et al. Hospital volume and surgical mortality in the United States. N Engl J Med 2002;346:1128–37.
12. Birkmeyer JD, Stukel TA, Siewers AE, et al. Surgeon volume and operative mortality in the United States. N Engl J Med 2003;349:2117–27.
13. Goodney PP, Lucas FL, Stukel TA, et al. Surgeon specialty and operative mortality with lung resection. Ann Surg 2005;241:179–84.
14. Colice GL, Shafazand S, Griffin JP, et al. Physiologic evaluation of the patient with lung cancer being considered for resectional surgery: ACCP evidenced-based clinical practice guidelines (2nd edition). Chest 2007;132:161S–77S.
15. Brunelli A, Charloux A, Bollinger CT, et al. ERS/ESTS clinical guidelines on fitness for radical therapy in lung cancer patients (surgery and chemoradiotherapy). Eur Respir J 2009;34:17–41.
16. Lim E, Baldwin D, Beckles M, et al. Guidelines on the radical management of patients with lung cancer. Thorax 2010;65:iii1–27.
17. Fleisher LA, Beckman JA, Brown KA, et al. ACC/AHA 2007 guidelines on perioperative cardiovascular evaluation and care for noncardiac surgery: a report of the American College of Cardiology/American Heart Association Task Force on Practice Guidelines. Circulation 2007;116:e418–99.
18. Ferguson MK. Preoperative assessment of pulmonary risk. Chest 1999;115:58S–63S.
19. Ferguson MK, Lehman AG, Bolliger CT, et al. The role of diffusing capacity and exercise tests. Thorac Surg Clin 2008;18:9–17.
20. Poonyagariyagorn H, Mazzone PJ. Lung cancer: preoperative pulmonary evaluation of the lung resection candidate. Semin Respir Crit Care Med 2008;29:271–84.

21. Kearney DJ, Lee TH, Reilly JJ, et al. Assessment of operative risk in patients undergoing lung resection: importance of predicted pulmonary function. Chest 1994;105:753–9.
22. Ferguson MK, Vigneswaran WT. Diffusing capacity predicts morbidity after lung resection in patients without obstructive lung disease. Ann Thorac Surg 2008;85:1158–64.
23. Liptay MJ, Basy S, Hoaglin MC, et al. Diffusion lung capacity for carbon monoxide (DLCO) is an independent prognostic factor for long-term survival after curative lung resection for cancer. J Surg Oncol 2009;100:703–7.
24. Ferguson MK, Dignam JJ, Siddique J, et al. Diffusing capacity predicts long-term survival after lung resection for cancer. Eur J Cardiothorac Surg 2012;41:e81–6.
25. Harpole DH Jr, DeCamp MM Jr, Daley J, et al. Prognostic models of thirty-day mortality and morbidity after pulmonary resection. J Thorac Cardiovasc Surg 1999;117:969–79.
26. Berrisford R, Brunelli A, Rocco G, et al. The European Thoracic Surgery Database project: modeling the risk of in-hospital death following lung resection. Eur J Cardiothorac Surg 2005;28: 306–11.
27. Barua A, Handagala SD, Socci L, et al. Accuracy of two scoring systems for risk stratification in thoracic surgery. Interact Cardiovasc Thorac Surg 2012;14:556–9.
28. Brunelli A, Varela G, Van Schil P, et al. Multicentric analysis of performance after major lung resections by using the European Society Objective Score (ESOS). Eur J Cardiothorac Surg 2008;33:284–8.
29. Falcoz PE, Conti M, Brouchet L, et al. The Thoracic Surgery Scoring System (Thoracoscore): risk model for in-hospital death in 15,183 patients requiring thoracic surgery. J Thorac Cardiovasc Surg 2007; 133:325–33.
30. Bernard A, Rivera C, Pages PB, et al. Risk model of in-hospital mortality after pulmonary resection for cancer: a national database of the French Society of Thoracic and Cardiovascular Surgery (Epithor). J Thorac Cardiovasc Surg 2011;141:449–58.
31. Bradley A, Marshall A, Abdelaziz M, et al. Thoracoscore fails to predict complications following elective lung resection. Eur Respir J 2012; 40:1496–501.
32. Poullis M, McShane J, Shaw M, et al. Prediction of in-hospital mortality following pulmonary resections: improving on current risk models. Eur J Cardiothorac Surg 2013 [Epub ahead of print], [PMID: 23345183].
33. Société Française de Cirurgie Thoracique et Cardio-Vasculaire. Epithor: Thoracoscore. Available at: http://sfctcv.fr/pages/epithor/thoracoscore_engl.php. Accessed February 6, 2013.
34. HEVA: health evaluation. Thoracoscore version 1.1. Available at: https://itunes.apple.com/us/app/thoracoscore/id452004201?mt=8. Accessed February 6, 2013.
35. Strand TE, Rostad H, Damhuis RA, et al. Risk factors for 30-day mortality after resection of lung cancer and prediction of their magnitude. Thorax 2007;62:991–7.
36. Kozower BD, Stukenborg GJ. The relationship between hospital lung cancer resection volume and patient mortality risk. Ann Surg 2011;254:1032–7.
37. Kates M, Perez X, Gribetz J, et al. Validation of a model to predict perioperative mortality from lung cancer resection in the elderly. Am J Respir Crit Care Med 2009;179:390–5.
38. Kozower BD, Sheng S, O'Brien SM, et al. STS database risk models: predictors of mortality and major morbidity for lung cancer resection. Ann Thorac Surg 2010;90:875–83.
39. STS Risk Calculator. Available at: http://riskcalc.sts.org/STSWebRiskCalc273/. Accessed February 6, 2013.
40. Birkmeyer JD. Progress and challenges in improving surgical outcomes. Br J Surg 2012;99: 1467–9.
41. Dindo D, Demartines N, Clavien PA. Classification of surgical complications: a new proposal with evaluation in a cohort of 6336 patients and results of a survey. Ann Surg 2004;240:205–13.
42. Strasberg SM, Linehan DC, Hawkins WG. The Accordian severity grading system of complications. Ann Surg 2009;250:177–86.
43. Bryant AS, Rudemiller K, Cerfolio RJ. The 30- versus 90-day operative mortality after pulmonary resection. Ann Thorac Surg 2010;89:1717–23.
44. Carrott PW, Markar SR, Kuppusamy MK, et al. Accordian severity grading system: assessment of relationship between costs, length of hospital stay, and survival in patients with complications after esophagectomy for cancer. J Am Coll Surg 2012;215:331–6.
45. Seely AJ, Ivanovic J, Threader H, et al. Systematic classification of morbidity and mortality after thoracic surgery. Ann Thorac Surg 2010;90: 936–42.
46. Ferguson MK, Durkin AE. A comparison of three scoring systems for predicting complications after major lung resection. Eur J Cardiothorac Surg 2003;23:35–42.
47. Epstein SK, Faling LJ, Daly BD, et al. Predicting complications after pulmonary resection. Preoperative exercise testing vs. a multifactorial cardiopulmonary risk index. Chest 1993;104:694–700.
48. Brunelli A, Fianchini A, Gesuita R, et al. POSSUM scoring system as an instrument of audit in lung resection surgery. Ann Thorac Surg 1999;67: 329–31.

49. Amar D, Munoz D, Shi W, et al. A clinical prediction rule for pulmonary complications after thoracic surgery for primary lung cancer. Anesth Analg 2010;110:1343–8.
50. Brunelli A, Varela G, Salati M, et al. Recalibration of the revised cardiac risk index in lung resection candidates. Ann Thorac Surg 2010;90:199–203.
51. Lee TH, Marcantonio ER, Mangione CM, et al. Derivation and prospective validation of a simple index for prediction of cardiac risk of major noncardiac surgery. Circulation 1999;100:1043–9.
52. Brunelli A, Cassivi SD, Fibla J, et al. External validation of the recalibrated thoracic revised cardiac risk index for predicting the risk of major cardiac complications after lung resection. Ann Thorac Surg 2011;92:445–58.
53. Ferguson MK, Celauro AD, Vigneswaran WT. Validation of a modified scoring system for cardiovascular risk associated with major lung resection. Eur J Cardiothorac Surg 2012;41:598–601.
54. Brunelli A, Refai M, Salati M, et al. Standardized combined outcome index as an instrument for monitoring performance after pulmonary resection. Ann Thorac Surg 2011;92:272–7.
55. Brunelli A, Berrisford RG, Rocco G, et al. The European Thoracic Database project: composite performance score to measure quality of care after major lung resection. Eur J Cardiothorac Surg 2009;35:769–74.
56. Ferguson MK, Gaissert HA, Grab JD, et al. Pulmonary complications after lung resection in the absence of chronic obstructive pulmonary disease: the predictive role of diffusing capacity. J Thorac Cardiovasc Surg 2009;138:1297–302.
57. Takamochi K, Oh S, Matsuoka J, et al. Risk factors for morbidity after pulmonary resection for lung cancer in younger and elderly patients. Interact Cardiovasc Thorac Surg 2011;12:739–43.
58. Ganai S, Ferguson MK. Quality of life in the high-risk candidate for lung resection. Thorac Surg Clin 2012;22:497–508.
59. Turna A, Mercan CA, Bedirhan A. Prediction of morbidity after lung resection in patients with lung cancer using fuzzy logic. Thorac Cardiovasc Surg 2005;53:368–74.
60. Hazelzet JA. Can fuzzy logic make things more clear? Crit Care 2009;13(1):116.
61. Vitez TS, Wada R, Macario A. Fuzzy logic: theory and medical applications. J Cardiothorac Vasc Anesth 1996;10(6):800–8.
62. Esteva H, Núñez TG, Rodríguez RO. Neural networks and artificial intelligence in thoracic surgery. Thorac Surg Clin 2007;17:359–67.
63. Esteva H, Marchevsky A, Núñez T, et al. Neural networks as a prognostic tool of surgical risk in lung resections. Ann Thorac Surg 2002;73:1576–81.
64. Santos-García G, Varela G, Novoa N, et al. Prediction of postoperative morbidity after lung resection using an artificial neural network ensemble. Artif Intell Med 2004;30:61–9.
65. Ranucci M, Castelvecchio S, Menicanti L, et al. Accuracy, calibration and clinical performance of the EuroSCORE: can we reduce the number of variables? Eur J Cardiothorac Surg 2010;37:724–9.
66. Perneger TV, Agoritsas T. Doctors and patients' susceptibility to framing bias: a randomized trial. J Gen Intern Med 2011;26:1411–7.
67. Paling J. Strategies to help patients understand risks. BMJ 2003;327:745–8.

Radical Sublobar Resection for Small-Diameter Lung Cancers

Morihito Okada, MD, PhD

KEYWORDS

• Segmentectomy • Wedge resection • Lobectomy • Adenocarcinoma

KEY POINTS

- From an oncological viewpoint, in sublobar resections, segmentectomy is superior to wedge resection as a cancer treatment.
- Radical (intentional) indication and compromised one for sublobar resection must be separately discussed.
- Sublobar resection could be considered an alternative for treating cT1N0 lung cancer of 2 cm or smaller, even in low-risk patients.
- Radical wedge resection should be confined to indolent tumors confirmed by imaging modalities such as high-resolution CT and positron emission tomography-CT.

INTRODUCTION

The treatment of choice for early-stage non-small cell lung cancer (NSCLC) is generally surgery. Lobectomy combined with systematic lymph node dissection, which can establish complete removal of the primary tumor and its lymphatic supply, has become the standard procedure even for tiny NSCLC over the past 5 decades. On the other hand, sublobar resection that comprises segmentectomy and wedge resection is considered inadequate as a curative procedure for NSCLC and it is applied only as a compromise for patients in whom lobectomy is contraindicated because of poor cardiopulmonary function.

Jensik and colleagues[1] comprehensively designated the role of segmentectomy for lung cancer in 1973, and demonstrated that it could be an acceptable procedure for early-stage NSCLC with the advantage of saving lung function. In the 1980s, several investigators reported that segmentectomy is feasible and effective for selected patients.[2–5] Preserving even a little healthy lung tissue can improve the postoperative quality of life, reduce operative morbidity, and provide more opportunities for additional resection. The incidence of developing a second primary lung cancer could be about 3% per year[6,7] and, accordingly, patients would face a significant cumulative risk of second cancers after a first resection. Removing large amounts of lung parenchyma for an early-stage NSCLC limits the choice of future surgical strategies. This is an important consideration because many such patients are likely to survive long enough to be at risk for a second, or even a third, NSCLC.

INTERPRETATION OF LUNG CANCER STUDY GROUP RESULTS

A shocking report released by the Lung Cancer Study Group (LCSG) in 1995 has remained very influential because it concerns the first and last randomized trial that examined whether sublobar resection is comparable to standard lobectomy for stage IA NSCLC.[8] The LCSG trial found a significantly higher incidence of local recurrence with a tendency toward poorer survival in subjects after sublobar resection, and concluded that lobectomy was the only choice for subjects with stage IA NSCLC. This report exerted a negative influence on the subsequent spread of sublobar

Department of Surgical Oncology, Research Institute for Radiation Biology and Medicine, Hiroshima University, 1-2-3-Kasumi, Minami-ku, Hiroshima City, Hiroshima 734-0037, Japan
E-mail address: morihito@hiroshima-u.ac.jp

Thorac Surg Clin 23 (2013) 301–311
http://dx.doi.org/10.1016/j.thorsurg.2013.04.003
1547-4127/13/$ – see front matter

resection, although more recent comparative studies of sublobar resection and lobectomy for stage IA NSCLC have revealed equivalent postoperative prognoses.[9–14]

The diagnostic capabilities of radiographic modalities have remarkably improved since the 1980s. The 1982 to 1988 LCSG study enrolled subjects with a clinical T1N0 peripheral tumor smaller than or equal to 3 cm in all dimensions on posteroanterior and lateral chest roentgenogram and, notably, not CT images. Patel and colleagues[15] highlighted several serious problems associated with the LCSG trial. Their detailed review of the data found a lower rate of perioperative lung morbidity, a similar cancer-related mortality rate, and better postoperative lung function in subjects after sublobar resection compared with lobectomy. One of the strongest criticisms of the LCSG trial was the inclusion of many subjects who underwent wedge resections. This is because segmentectomy is generally believed to be a much more effective procedure for cancer than wedge resection from the viewpoints of nodal assessment and surgical margin. The LCSG study demonstrated a high incidence of local recurrence after sublobar resection, whereas current Japanese studies did not despite progress in follow-up modalities that can easily identify local recurrence.[7,10,13,16] The high prevalence of wedge resection within the subjects who were treated by sublobar resection (32.8%) in the LCSG study is rather remarkable considering that the ratio is around 10% in most Japanese studies. In addition, the LCSG study included tumors up to 3 cm in diameter, whereas most Japanese studies analyzed tumors up to 2 cm. The predominance of wedge resection and the acceptance of larger tumors would undoubtedly have affected the frequency of local recurrence. The reasons for the lower rate of local recurrence in the Japanese studies might be associated with a preference for segmentectomy, which could improve the surgical margin.[9,10,13,14] Also, wedge resection might be related to less extensive intraoperative nodal surveillance, resulting in the potential understaging of disease, whereas the nodal status of the hilum can be assessed during segmentectomy. Nodal assessment is mandatory for even small tumors, except for noninvasive pure bronchioloalveolar carcinoma (BAC).

In the LCSG study, six subjects developed postoperative respiratory failure requiring ventilatory assistance for more than 24 hours after lobectomy, compared with none after sublobar resection. An earlier investigation of 2220 resections for lung cancer by LCSG uncovered the operative mortality rates of 6.2%, 2.9%, and 1.4% after pneumonectomy, lobectomy, and sublobar resection, respectively.[17] Preserving as much lung tissue as possible contributed to a lower occurrence of pulmonary complications and operative deaths, suggesting that postoperative morbidity and mortality rates would be improved with less resection. A noteworthy benefit missed in the conclusions of the LCSG trial is that of better lung function after sublobar resection. Among the subjects treated by sublobar resection, the forced volume capacity (FVC), 1-second forced expiratory volume (FEV_1), and maximal voluntary ventilation were all significantly better at 6 months after surgery, and FEV_1 remained significantly better even at 12 months thereafter.

SURGICAL RESULTS OF SUBLOBAR RESECTION FOLLOWING THE LCSG TRIAL

With the outstanding increase in the early detection of ever smaller lung cancers and BAC through the development of radiographic tools such as high-resolution CT (HR-CT) and widespread screening with low-dose helical CT,[18] several physicians, particularly in Japan, have expressed doubt that a uniform procedure comprising whole lobectomy is appropriate for small peripheral lesions. In practice, patients with smaller tumors have a better prognosis and a lower frequency of hematogenous and lymphatic metastases. Because biologic malignant behavior is more indolent (not only among smaller tumors but also those with a higher BAC component), consistently removing the entire lobe for such tiny peripheral lesions when sufficient surgical margins can be ensured by sublobar resection is questionable. **Table 1** summarized the outcomes of current comparisons of sublobar resection with lobectomy for small NSCLC.

In 2002, Yoshikawa and colleagues[14] published the final report on the 1992 Tsubota and colleagues[19] prospective Japanese multi-institutional trial of extended segmentectomy for NSCLC with a diameter smaller than or equal to 2 cm. The 5-year survival rate of 55 subjects was 92%, and local recurrence developed only in one, in whom the margins of resection were problematic at pathologic review. This initial prospective trial of radical sublobar resection for small NSCLC proceeded after thin-sliced CT was established as a tool for diagnosing lung cancer. Landreneau and colleagues[20] compared lobectomy with extended wedge resection, not with segmentectomy for T1N0 NSCLC, in a prospective nonrandomized multi-institute setting during 1997. They found that the 5-year survival and local recurrence rates were lower for subjects after wedge resection than after lobectomy (58% vs 70% and

Table 1
Survival and local recurrence rates of patients after sublobar resection or lobectomy to treat early-stage NSCLC

Study	Stage	Lobectomy Pts/Local Rec/5-YS	Sublobar Resection Pts/Local Rec/5-YS
1. LCSG,[8] 1995	T1N0	122/2.1/89.1	125/6.3/83.1
2. Landreneau et al,[20] 1997	T1N0	117/30/70	42[a]/24/58
3. Kodama et al,[9] 1997	T1N0[b]	46/N/A/93	77/N/A/88
4. Okada et al,[13] 2001	T1N0[b]	139/N/A/87.7	70/N/A/87.1
5. Koike et al,[10] 2003	T1N0[b]	159/1.3/90.1	74/2.7/89.1
6. Okada et al,[16] 2006	T1N0[b]	262/6.9/89.1	305/4.9/89.6

Sublobar resection comprised wedge resection in Study 2, segmentectomy in Study 4, and both in the other studies.
Abbreviations: 5-YS, 5-year survival (%); LCSG, Lung Cancer Study Group; Local Rec, Local recurrence (%); N/A, not available; Pts, Number of patients.
[a] Wedge resection.
[b] Tumor diameter ≤2 cm.

24% vs 30%, respectively) and that operative mortality, complications, and length of hospital stay were also significantly reduced. Kodama and colleagues[9] found that the 5-year survival rates of 77 and 46 subjects treated with sublobar resection and lobectomy, respectively, for NSCLC of smaller than or equal to 2 cm in the same year did not significantly differ (88% vs 93%).

Okada and colleagues[13] reported the consequences of a prospective comparison of radical segmentectomy and standard lobectomy for tumors of smaller than or equal to 2 cm in 2001. Radical segmentectomy, defined as removal of both the diseased segment and the adjacent segment or subsegment for sufficient surgical margins, with intraoperative lymph node assessment proceeded only when the surgical margins were sufficient. The procedure starts by isolating the veins, arteries, and bronchi connected to the affected segments, then exposing the intersegmental veins, which is a key process during anatomic segmentectomy (**Fig. 1**). Initially, the lobe is inflated with air and only the responsible segmental bronchus is tied to maintain air within the segments scheduled for removal and cut at the bronchial site proximal to the tie to deflate the preserved segments. An inflation-deflation

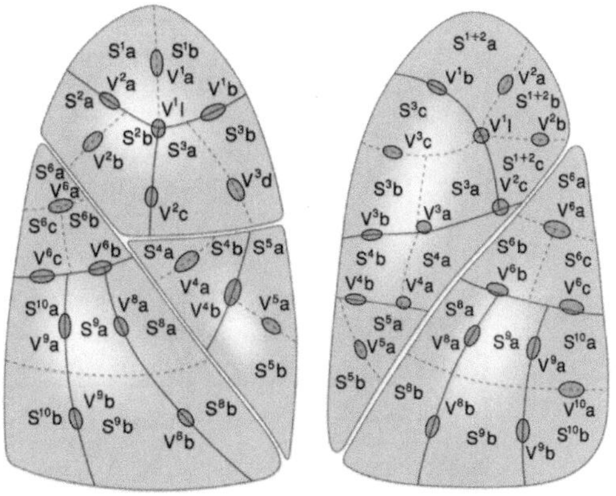

Fig. 1. External view for location of numbered segments and veins.

line that represents the anatomic intersegmental plane is consequently created for resection (**Fig. 2**). More recently, the Okada and colleagues[21] developed an original technique in which the intersegmental boundary is selectively identified using jet ventilation to the resected segments and cutting along the border using electrocautery without using mechanical staplers to fully expand adjacent preserved segments.[21] Subjects with an insufficient margin, intrapulmonary metastases, or nodal involvement judged intraoperative underwent lobectomy with complete nodal dissection instead. The 5-year survival rates of subjects treated by segmentectomy (n = 70) or lobectomy (n = 139) were 87.1% and 87.7%, respectively (*P* = .8008), indicating that radical segmentectomy could be an alternative to standard lobectomy for subjects with NSCLC of smaller than or equal to 2 cm.

In 2003, Koike and colleagues[10] retrospectively compared the outcomes of 159 and 74 subjects after lobectomy and sublobar resection, respectively, for T1N0 NSCLC of smaller than or equal to 2 cm. The 5-year survival rates did not significantly differ between the groups (90.1% vs 89.1%), although the ratios of local recurrence were 1.3% and 2.7%, respectively. In the following year, Keenan and colleagues[12] retrospectively analyzed the surgical outcomes of subjects treated with lobectomy (n = 147) or segmentectomy (n = 54) for stage I NSCLC between 1996 and 2001. Overall 4-year survival rates were 67% versus 62% (*P* = .406). They concluded that pulmonary function was better preserved after segmentectomy than after lobectomy and that survival was not compromised in subjects with stage I NSCLC.

Whether segmentectomy is superior to wedge resection as a cancer treatment strategy is

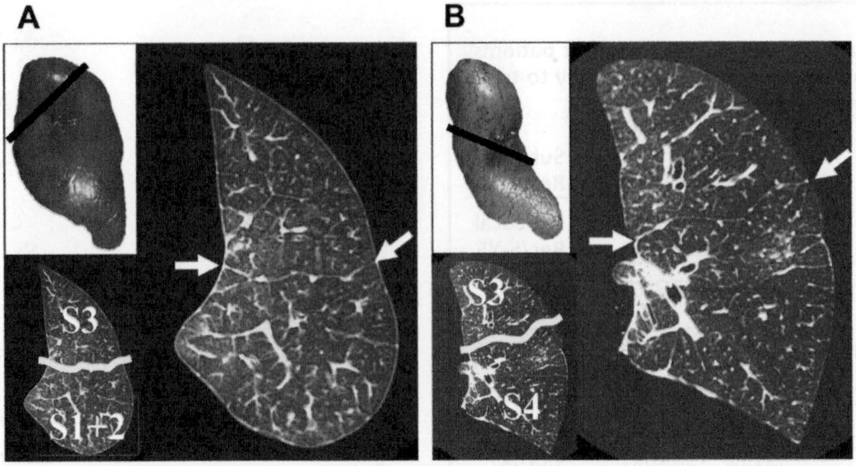

Fig. 2. Transaxial (*A*) and coronal (*B*) CT views of left upper lobe tissue specimen. (*A*) Anatomic intersegmental lines between S1+2 (apical and posterior segments) and S3 (anterior segment), and (*B*) between S3 and S4 (superior segment) are considered inflation-deflation lines (*arrows*). (*From* Okada M, Mimura T, Ikegaki J, et al. A novel video-assisted anatomic segmentectomy technique: selective segmental inflation via bronchofiberoptic jet followed by cautery cutting. J Thorac Cardiovasc Surg 2007;133:753–8; with permission.)

unknown, although several reports have suggested poorer surgical outcomes after wedge resection.[22–24] In 2005, Okada and colleagues[22] retrospectively examined surgical outcomes associated with tumor size and surgical procedure in 1272 consecutive subjects who underwent complete NSCLC resection. The subjects were stratified based on tumor sizes of smaller than or equal to 10 mm (n = 50), 11 to 20 mm (n = 273), 21 to 30 mm (n = 368), and larger than 30 mm (n = 581). The cancer-specific 5-year survival rates were 100%, 83.5%, 76.5% and 57.9%, respectively. For subjects with pathologic stage I (no nodal metastasis) disease, the rates were 100%, 92.6%, 84.1%, and 76.4%, respectively. The 5-year cancer-specific survival rates of subjects with pathologic stage I tumors smaller than or equal to 20 and 21 to 30 mm were 92.4% and 87.4% after lobectomy, 96.7% and 84.6% after segmentectomy, and 85.7% and 39.4% after wedge resection, respectively. In contrast, the survival rates for tumors greater than 30 mm were 81.3%, 62.9% and 0% after lobectomy, segmentectomy and wedge resection, respectively. These data revealed that tumor size is an important prognostic determinant for planning surgical strategies for patients with NSCLC.

In 2005, Martin-Ucar and colleagues[11] compared the long-term outcomes of lobectomy and segmentectomy in high-risk subjects with stage I disease defined by a predicted postoperative FEV_1 of less than 40%.[11] Seventeen subjects who underwent segmentectomy were matched with 17 others who underwent lobectomy. Hospital mortality, complications, hospital stay, overall 5-year survival (64% after lobectomy, 70% after segmentectomy), and local recurrence rates (18% in both groups) did not significantly differ between the groups, although pulmonary function was significantly better preserved after segmentectomy than lobectomy (P = .02). In the following year, Okada and colleagues[16] reported the long-term surgical outcomes of a multicenter study of subjects with peripheral cT1N0M0 NSCLC of smaller than or equal to 2 cm who could tolerate lobectomy. The prognosis was similar in both groups with 5-year disease-free and overall survival rates of 85.9% and 89.6% after sublobar resection (n = 305) and 83.4% and 89.1% after lobectomy (n = 262), respectively. However, postoperative lung function was significantly better in subjects who had undergone sublobar resection. Many more subjects were assessed in this study, which contributed not only to the furtherance of starting new randomized controlled trials (JCOG0802/WJOG4607L)[25] but also to the potential for remarkable changes occurring in current surgical approaches to treating lung cancer in the era of earlier detection.

In 2010, Wisnivesky and colleagues[26] compared the survivals of 1165 subjects with stage I lung cancer of smaller than or equal to 2 cm who were treated using lobectomy or sublobar resection and listed in the Surveillance, Epidemiology, and End Results registry linked to Medicare records. They found 196 (17%) subjects who underwent sublobar resection and that, overall, lung cancer-specific survival rates did not significantly differ between the two groups when stratified and matched by propensity scores.

Video-assisted thoracic surgery (VATS) during segmentectomy for lung cancer has recently become more popular.[27] The 2012 study by Okada and colleagues[28] analyzed the results of radical segmentectomy achieved through a hybrid VATS approach that used both direct vision and television monitor visualization at a median follow-up of over 5 years (**Fig. 3**). Hybrid VATS segmentectomy was applied to 102 consecutive subjects with clinical T1N0M0 NSCLC who could tolerate lobectomy. Electrocautery was used without a stapler to divide the intersegmental plane identified selectively by jet ventilation in addition to the path of the intersegmental veins. Curative resection was achieved in all subjects, and the median duration and blood loss during surgery were 129 minutes and 50 mL, respectively. The overall and disease-free 5-year survival rates were 89.8% and 84.7%, respectively, without any in-hospital deaths or 30-day mortality. These

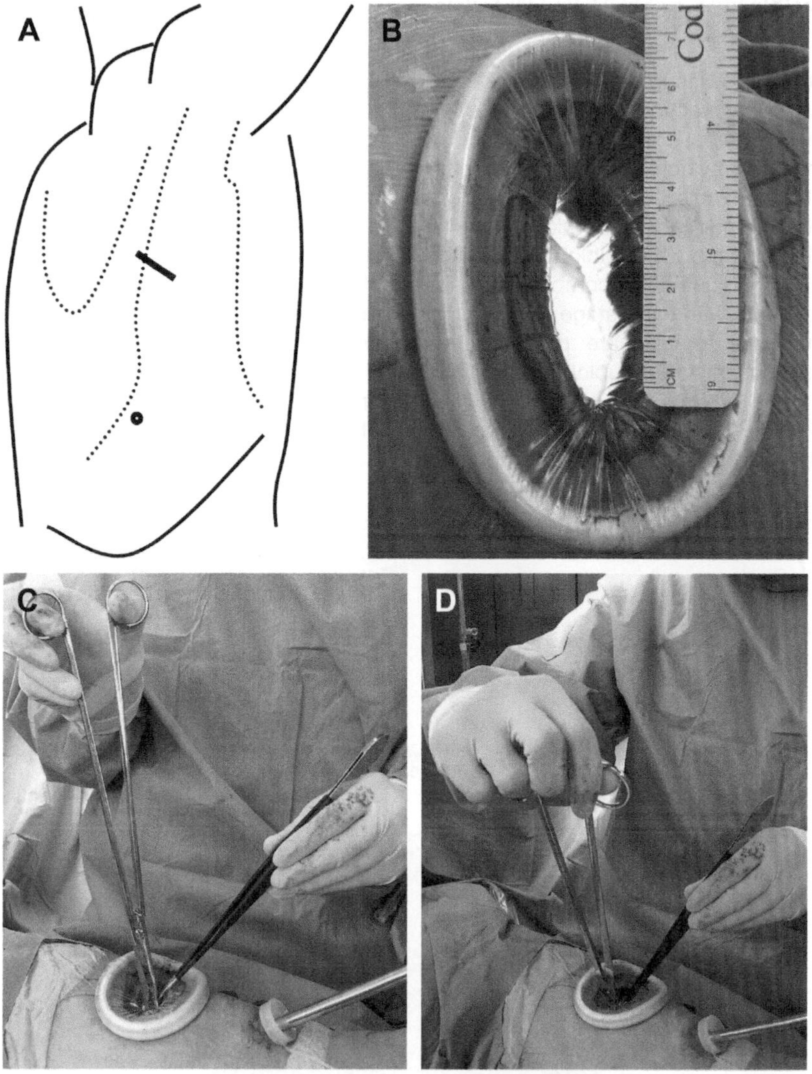

Fig. 3. Hybrid VATS approach. (*A*) Skin incisions for thoracoscopic (*circle*) access and for thoracotomy (*solid line*) are positioned over midaxillary line in fourth interspace for upper or middle lobe tumors. Lower lobe tumors are approached through auscultatory triangle in the fifth interspace. (*B*) Operative field is widened about 2-cm using wound retractor. Rib spreading is not required. (*C* and *D*) Sharp dissection in depths of directly visualized open thorax using upside-down grip on 30-cm scissors manipulated with thumb and index finger through loops and turning the wrist. Ulnar side of the hands rests comfortably alongside margins of the incision to avoid awkward elevation of the forearms or elbows. (*From* Okada M, Tsutani Y, Ikeda T, et al. Radical hybrid video-assisted thoracic segmentectomy: long-term results of minimally invasive anatomic sublobar resection for treating lung cancer. Interact Cardiovasc Thorac Surg 2012;14:5–11; with permission.)

data demonstrated that radical segmentectomy, including atypical resection of segment or subsegment via hybrid VATS, is a useful option for clinical stage-I NSCLC. Regarding the technical aspects of the procedure, understanding the anatomy of the intersegmental veins and precisely identifying the anatomic intersegmental plane followed by dissection using electrocautery is important from oncological and functional perspectives (**Figs. 4** and **5**).[28]

EFFECT OF SUBLOBAR RESECTION ON LUNG FUNCTION

The degree of resected lung volume directly affects the loss of pulmonary function; thus, less resection helps to preserve postoperative lung function. In theory, segmentectomy could save some lung tissue segments that would be removed by lobectomy and thus confer an anatomic functional advantage. The concept that sublobar resection might have oncologic outcomes comparable to lobectomy in patients with early-stage NSCLC has prompted surgeons to compare postoperative lung function in patients after sublobar resections versus lobectomy (**Table 2**).

The LCSG study[8] showed that pulmonary function tested at 6 months after surgery had improved in the sublobar resection group, and that lung function did not significantly differ between the two groups at 12 months after surgery. However, their data should be interpreted with caution because the investigators stated that the number of subjects undergoing pulmonary functional tests in either group was significantly decreased at the 12-month postoperative assessment due to a lack of funding for such tests beyond 6 months after surgery. In 2004, Keenan and colleagues[12] investigated pulmonary function after segmentectomy or lobectomy in 201 subjects with stage I NSCLC. The preoperative FEV_1 and FVC values were significantly lower after segmentectomy than after lobectomy, but overall survival between both groups was similar. At 1 year, FVC, FEV_1, maximum voluntary ventilation, and lung diffusing capacity for carbon monoxide (DLCO) significantly declined after lobectomy, whereas a decline in DLCO was the only significant change after segmentectomy. The investigators, therefore, concluded that pulmonary function was better preserved after segmentectomy than lobectomy with no influence on survival.

In 2005, a logistic regression analyses by Harada and colleagues[29] investigated whether the quantity of segments removed by segmentectomy or lobectomy correlated with a loss of pulmonary

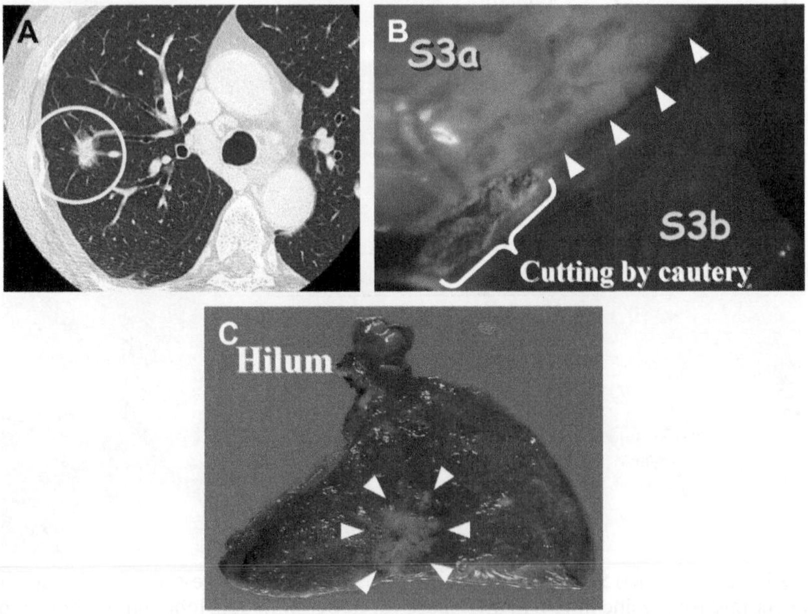

Fig. 4. Representative atypical segmentectomy: S2b (anterior subsegment of posterior segment) + S3a (posterior subsegment of anterior segment) resection of the right upper lobe. (*A*) HR-CT image shows tumor (*yellow circle*) located at S2b and S3a border. (*B*) Intraoperative findings show inflation-deflation line (*arrowheads*) between inflated (resected) S3a and deflated (preserved) S3b segments. (*C*) Resected surgical specimen shows tumor (*arrowheads*) with sufficient margin. (*From* Okada M, Mimura T, Ikegaki J, et al. A novel video-assisted anatomic segmentectomy technique: selective segmental inflation via bronchofiberoptic jet followed by cautery cutting. J Thorac Cardiovasc Surg 2007;133:753–8; with permission.)

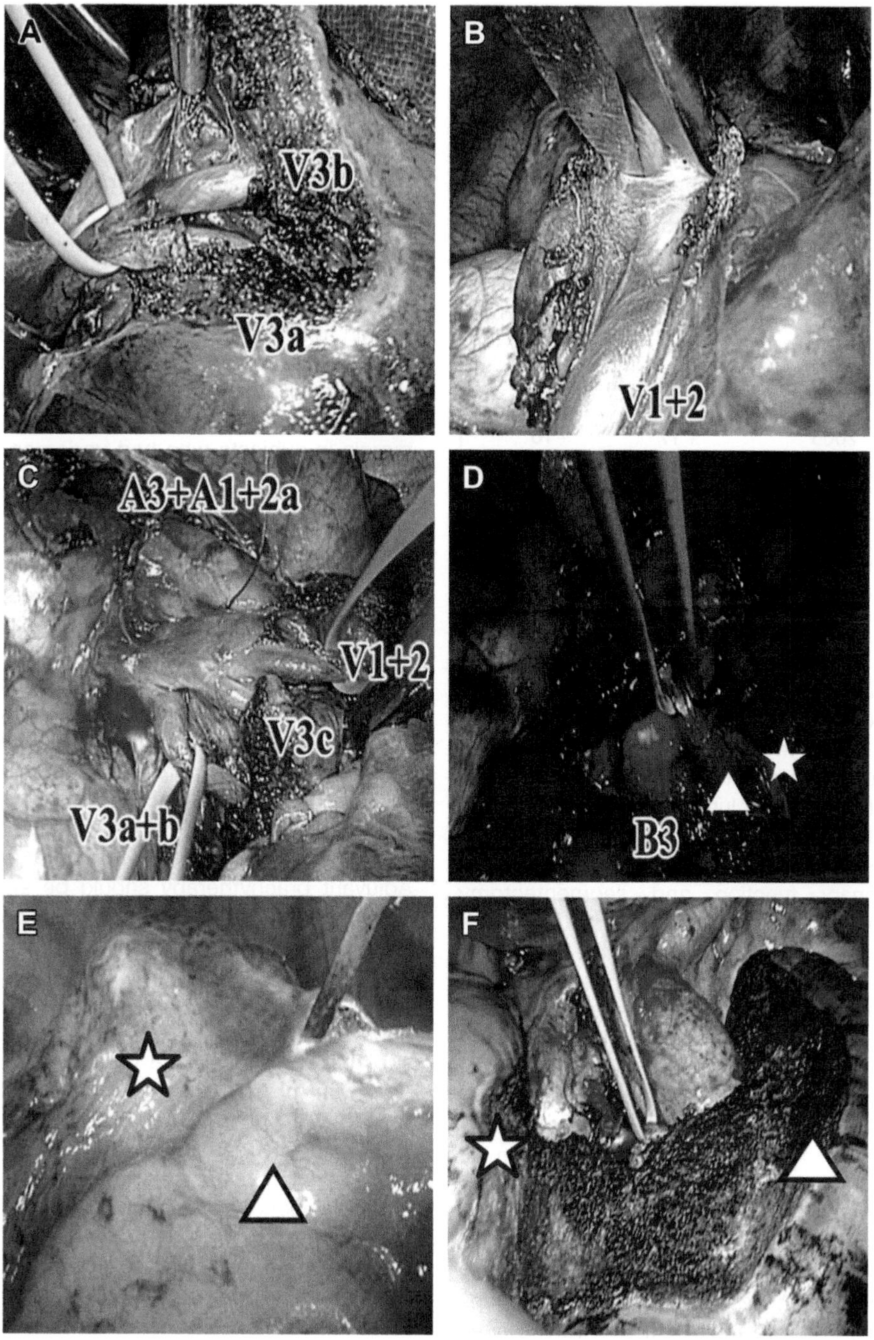

Fig. 5. Left S3 + S1+2a segmentectomy. (*A*) V3a and V3b branches of vein running between upper division and lingular segment are identified and exposed distally. (*B*) V1+2 vein branch is also exposed distally and V1+2a, V1+2b+c, and V1+2 superior branches are identified. V1+2a runs between S3c and S1+2a and V1+2b+c runs between S1+2a and S1+2b+c. (*C*) The first two branches of the artery (A3 and A1+2a) and vein (V1+2a, V1+2b+c, V3a, V3b, and V3c) are uncovered. V1+2b+c, V3b intersegmental branches of the vein are saved for venous return from preserved adjacent segments. (*D*) Bronchofiberscope inserted through a double-lumen tube into the orifice of a targeted segmental bronchus (B3) and B1+2a (*asterisk*), where high-frequency oscillation is applied. V1+2b+c (*triangle*) is preserved. (*E*) Inflation-deflation line between inflated (resected, *triangle*) S1+2a and deflated (preserved, *asterisk*) S1+2b+c subsegments, along which the anatomic inter-subsegmental plane is dissected with cautery. (*F*) Saved parenchyma of S1+2b+c (*triangle*) and S4 (*asterisk*) is fully inflated after S3 + S1+2a is removed. (*From* Okada M, Tsutani Y, Ikeda T, et al. Radical hybrid video-assisted thoracic segmentectomy: long-term results of minimally invasive anatomic sublobar resection for treating lung cancer. Interact Cardiovasc Thorac Surg 2012;14:5–11; with permission.)

Table 2
Postoperative pulmonary function in patients after sublobar resection and lobectomy for early-stage NSCLC

Study	Stage	Lobectomy Number/ FEV1[a]/FVC[a]	Sublobar Resection Number/ FEV1[a]/FVC[a]
1. LCSG,[8] 1995	T1N0	58/−11.1/ −5.7	71/−5.2/ 0.52
2. Keenan et al,[12] 2004	Stage I	147/−9.2/ −4.2	54/−3.2/ −2.7
3. Harada et al,[29] 2005	T1N0	45/−18/ −17	38[b]/−12/ −10
4. Okada et al,[16] 2006	T1N0	168/−16.8/ −16.0	168[b]/−9.1/ −10.4

Abbreviation: LCSG, Lung Cancer Study Group.
[a] Ratio (%) of change between postoperative and preoperative values.
[b] Segmentectomy only.

function. Correlations between the number of removed segments and the postoperative loss of FVC as well as FEV1 were positive and significant at both 2 and 6 months after surgery ($P<.0001$). Functional data correlated more closely with the extent of removed lung parenchyma at 6, compared with 2, months. The amount of anatomically resected lung directly affects long-term loss of pulmonary function and segmentectomy contributes to the better preservation of lung function than lobectomy. In addition, the anaerobic threshold, which expresses exercise capacity, was better maintained in the segmentectomy group. Moreover, Okada and colleagues[16] reported functional data from a multicenter study of radical sublobar and lobar resection to treat clinical stage IA NSCLC of smaller than or equal to 2 cm. The functional values before surgery were similar after wedge resection (n = 18), segmentectomy (n = 168), [16] and lobectomy (n = 168), indicating that the outcomes of sublobar resection and lobectomy were functionally equal. A direct comparison of functional changes among the three groups associated more resected lung tissue with reduced postoperative pulmonary function.

SUBLOBAR RESECTION WITH BRACHYTHERAPY

Postoperative local recurrence is a concern associated with compromise sublobar resection for high-risk patients with poor cardiopulmonary function. Several investigators, therefore, started to evaluate the effect of additional intraoperative brachytherapy on local tumor recurrence and patient survival after sublobar resection. In 2003, Santos and colleagues[30] reported the outcomes of 101 subjects after sublobar resection through the VATS approach with brachytherapy consisting of ^{125}I seed placement along the staple line, and demonstrated that brachytherapy reduced local recurrence compared with 102 historical controls (2% vs 18.6%, P = .0001). Although hospital stay, operative mortality, distant recurrence, or prognosis did not significantly differ, none of the subjects in the brachytherapy group developed radiation pneumonitis, implant migration, or decreased pulmonary function. In the same year, Lee and colleagues[31] found a low ratio of local recurrence after ^{125}I seed implantation along the margin in subjects who had undergone sublobar resection. The 5-year survival of subjects with T1N0 tumors was 67% with a cancer-specific survival of 77%, and a local recurrence rate of 10.5%, which was better than that of historical controls. In 2005, Fernando and colleagues[32] reported their findings of 124 subjects after sublobar resection for T1N0 NSCLC. Of these, 60 (48%) underwent brachytherapy with ^{125}I Vicryl suture implantation along the resection line. The data showed that local recurrence was significantly lower with brachytherapy compared with none (3.3% vs 17.2%, P = .012). The affect of brachytherapy on local recurrence seems encouraging, although the influence on overall survival remains unknown. Adjuvant brachytherapy should be applied after sublobar resection for compromised patients and not for those undergoing intentional radical sublobar resection.

The American College of Surgeons Oncology Group conducted a randomized comparison of sublobar resection alone versus sublobar resection with brachytherapy for high-risk subjects with NSCLC (Z4032) and permanently closed subject accrual in January 2010 at 224 subjects. Pulmonary function data currently available for 148 of the subjects indicates that adjuvant intraoperative brachytherapy together with sublobar resection does not significantly worsen pulmonary function or dyspnea at 3 months, and was is associated with increased perioperative pulmonary adverse events.[33] In addition, sublobar resection with brachytherapy can be safe for high-risk patients with NSCLC with low 30-day and 90-day mortality and acceptable morbidity.[34]

COMMENT

The detection rates of small lung cancers, especially adenocarcinoma, have recently increased and this trend will accelerate. The progress of radiographic modalities is mandatory for an understanding of their malignant aggressiveness, which is critical for the selection of suitable therapeutic strategies, such as sublobar resection. Fluorodeoxyglucose positron emission tomography (PET)-CT, as well as HR-CT findings, is important to determine the appropriateness of sublobar resection for treating clinical stage IA adenocarcinomas of the lung.[35–37] The maximum standardized uptake value on PET-CT and the size of solid tumors on HR-CT excluding ground-glass opacity (GGO) areas are notably useful predictors of high-grade malignancy and prognosis in small adenocarcinomas, whereas whole tumor size is not.[38] These determinants can also properly predict node-negative status criteria and might be helpful for avoiding lymphadenectomy and choosing optimal candidates for sublobar resection for clinical stage IA lung adenocarcinomas, even patients with T1b (2–3 cm) tumors.[39] On HR-CT, solid tumors exhibit behavior that is more malignant and have a poorer prognosis than mixed tumors that include a GGO component. However, differences in malignant behavior can be appropriately identified using maximum standardized uptake values on PET-CT.[40] The need for advanced radiographic diagnoses of small adenocarcinoma malignancy is increasing. In addition, similar to that of breast and prostate cancer, the role of clinical decision making for treating lung adenocarcinoma could be based on histologic subtyping, which is an important independent prognostic variable.[41]

Sublobar resection has conventionally been a type of parenchymal-sparing procedure for treating lung cancer in compromised patients with cardiopulmonary impairment who would otherwise be denied surgery.[1–5] However, current evidence indicates that sublobar resection can be a viable alternative to standard lobectomy in selected populations, including patients at low risk who could tolerate lobectomy. This could overthrow the established concept.[9,10,13,14,16,42] The frequency of local recurrence, which is one of the major disadvantages of radical sublobar resection, widely varies between Western and Japanese reports.[8,16] The lower amount in Japan might be linked to severe indications for the procedure and the predominance of segmentectomy favored by Japanese surgeons compared with wedge resection. Also, surgeons have to seek for an ideal segmentectomy technique to obtain postoperative function resulting from the full expansion of remaining segments or subsegments by trying to cut anatomic intersegmental planes using cautery and not staplers.[43]

The current information about sublobar resections can be summarized as follows. First, segmentectomy seems more useful than wedge resection from an oncological viewpoint. The lower rate of local recurrence after segmentectomy than after wedge resection results from the surgical margins. Also, segmentectomy can allow nodal dissection at the hilum, selection of the most appropriate procedure including conversion to lobectomy or not, and accurate pathologic staging. Thus, the higher ratio of wedge resection among sublobar resection categories in the Western literature could be involved in the higher ratio of local recurrence. Second, the indication for sublobar resection should be restricted only to small cancers. Surgical outcomes such as local recurrence and survival are comparable between segmentectomy and lobectomy for tumors smaller than or equal to 2 cm in diameter. Any suspicious lymph nodes must be intraoperatively diagnosed with direct tissue sampling, and sublobar resection should be converted to lobectomy when nodal involvement or an insufficient margin is detected or suspected. Third, radical and compromise indications for sublobar resection must be separately discussed. Radical sublobar resection is resolutely performed for low-risk patients who can tolerate lobectomy. Fourth, radical wedge resection should be confined to tumors identified as pure GGO on HR-CT images because lymph nodes are considered not to be involved. The temptation for surgeons to perform a technically simpler procedure, such as wedge resection, when planning radical sublobar resection, needs to be overcome. Because small cancers are becoming detectable, thoracic surgeons must learn to mater segmentectomy as a key technique.

The ongoing, multicenter phase III clinical trials of the propriety of radical segmentectomy in the United States (CALGB-140503) and Japan (JCOG0802/WJOG4607L) should be carefully watched.[25] Anatomic segmentectomy is more technically demanding than either lobectomy or wedge resection, thus incorrect outcomes in these clinical trials induced by procedural errors eg, recurrent resection lines or excessive loss of lung function) will be a concern. Surgeons must carefully avoid local failure at the margin and fully expand adjacent segments to maximize lung function after segmentectomy.[21] The acknowledgment of radical sublobar resection as a standard surgery for small cancers is eagerly anticipated.

REFERENCES

1. Jensik RJ, Faber LP, Milloy FJ, et al. Segmental resection for lung cancer. A fifteen-year experience. J Thorac Cardiovasc Surg 1973;66:563–72.

2. Bennett WF, Smith RA. Segmental resection for bronchogenic carcinoma: a surgical alternative for the compromised patient. Ann Thorac Surg 1979;27:169–72.
3. Errett LE, Wilson J, Chiu RC, et al. Wedge resection as an alternative procedure for peripheral bronchogenic carcinoma in poor-risk patients. J Thorac Cardiovasc Surg 1985;90:656–61.
4. Hoffmann TH, Ransdell HT. Comparison of lobectomy and wedge resection for carcinoma of the lung. J Thorac Cardiovasc Surg 1980;79:211–7.
5. Miller JI, Hatcher CR Jr. Limited resection of bronchogenic carcinoma in the patient with marked impairment of pulmonary function. Ann Thorac Surg 1987;44:340–3.
6. Gail MH, Eagan RT, Feld R, et al. Prognostic factors in patients with resected stage I non-small cell lung cancer: a report from the Lung Cancer Study Group. Cancer 1984;54:1802–13.
7. Martini N, Bains MS, Burt ME, et al. Incidence of local recurrence and second primary tumors in resected stage I lung cancer. J Thorac Cardiovasc Surg 1995;109:120–9.
8. Lung Cancer Study Group, Ginsberg RJ, Rubenstein LV. Randomized trial of lobectomy versus limited resection for T1N0 non-small cell lung cancer. Ann Thorac Surg 1995;60:615–22.
9. Kodama K, Doi O, Higashiyama M, et al. Intentional limited resection for selected patients with T1N0M0 non-small cell lung cancer. J Thorac Cardiovasc Surg 1997;114:347–53.
10. Koike T, Yamato Y, Yoshiya K, et al. Intentional limited pulmonary resection for peripheral T1 N0 M0 small-sized lung cancer. J Thorac Cardiovasc Surg 2003;125:924–8.
11. Martin-Ucar AE, Nakas A, Pilling JE, et al. A case-matched study of anatomical segmentectomy versus lobectomy for stage I lung cancer in high-risk patients. Eur J Cardiothorac Surg 2005;27:675–9.
12. Keenan RJ, Landreneau RJ, Maley RH Jr, et al. Segmental resection spares pulmonary function in patients with stage I lung cancer. Ann Thorac Surg 2004;78:228–33.
13. Okada M, Yoshikawa K, Hatta T, et al. Is segmentectomy with lymph node assessment an alternative to lobectomy for non-small cell lung cancer of 2 cm or smaller? Ann Thorac Surg 2001;71:956–61.
14. Yoshikawa K, Tsubota N, Kodama K, et al. Prospective study of extended segmentectomy for small lung tumors: the final report. Ann Thorac Surg 2002;73:1055–8.
15. Patel AN, Santos RS, Hoyos AD, et al. Clinical trails of peripheral stage I (T1N0M0) non-small cell lung cancer. Semin Thorac Cardiovasc Surg 2003;15:421–30.
16. Okada M, Koike T, Higashiyama M, et al. Radical sublobar resection for small-sized non-small cell lung cancer: a multicenter study. J Thorac Cardiovasc Surg 2006;132:769–75.
17. Ginsberg RJ, Hill LD, Eagan RT, et al. Modern thirty-day operative mortality for surgical resections in lung cancer. J Thorac Cardiovasc Surg 1993;86:654–8.
18. Patz EF Jr, Goodman PC, Bepler G. Screening for lung cancer. N Engl J Med 2000;343:1627–33.
19. Tsubota N, Ayabe K, Doi O, et al. Ongoing prospective study of segmentectomy for small lung tumors. Ann Thorac Surg 1998;66:1787–90.
20. Landreneau RJ, Sugarbaker DJ, Mack MJ, et al. Wedge resection versus lobectomy for stage I (T1N0M0) non-small-cell lung cancer. J Thorac Cardiovasc Surg 1997;113:691–8.
21. Okada M, Mimura T, Ikegaki J, et al. A novel video-assisted anatomic segmentectomy technique: selective segmental inflation via bronchofiberoptic jet followed by cautery cutting. J Thorac Cardiovasc Surg 2007;133:753–8.
22. Okada M, Nishio W, Sakamoto T, et al. Effect of tumor size on prognosis in patients with non-small cell lung cancer: the role of segmentectomy as a type of lesser resection. J Thorac Cardiovasc Surg 2005;129:87–93.
23. Cerfolio RJ, Allen MS, Nascimento AG, et al. Lung resection in patients with compromised pulmonary function. Ann Thorac Surg 1996;62:348–51.
24. Miller DL, Rowland CM, Deschamps C, et al. Surgical treatment of non-small cell lung cancer 1 cm or less in diameter. Ann Thorac Surg 2002;73:1545–50.
25. Nakamura K, Saji H, Nakajima R, et al. A phase III randomized trial of lobectomy versus limited resection for small-sized peripheral non-small cell lung cancer (JCOG0802/WJOG4607L). Jpn J Clin Oncol 2010;40:271–4.
26. Wisnivesky JP, Henschke CI, Swanson S, et al. Limited resection for the treatment of patients with stage IA lung cancer. Ann Surg 2010;251:550–4.
27. Shapiro M, Weiser TS, Wisnivesky JP, et al. Thoracoscopic segmentectomy compares favorably with thoracoscopic lobectomy for patients with small stage I lung cancer. J Thorac Cardiovasc Surg 2009;137:1388–93.
28. Okada M, Tsutani Y, Ikeda T, et al. Radical hybrid video-assisted thoracic segmentectomy: long-term results of minimally invasive anatomical sublobar resection for treating lung cancer. Interact Cardiovasc Thorac Surg 2012;14:5–11.
29. Harada H, Okada M, Sakamoto T, et al. Functional advantage after radical segmentectomy versus lobectomy for lung cancer. Ann Thorac Surg 2005;80:2041–5.
30. Santos R, Colonias A, Parda D, et al. Comparison between sublobar resection and 125iodine

brachytherapy after sublobar resection in high-risk patients with stage I non-small-cell lung cancer. Surgery 2003;134:691–7.
31. Lee W, Daly BD, DiPetrillo TA, et al. Limited resection for non-small cell lung cancer: observed local control with implantation of I-125 brachytherapy seeds. Ann Thorac Surg 2003;75:237–42.
32. Fernando HC, Santos RS, Benfield JR, et al. Lobar and sublobar resection with and without brachytherapy for small stage IA non-small cell lung cancer. J Thorac Cardiovasc Surg 2005; 129:261–7.
33. Fernando HC, Landreneau RJ, Mandrekar SJ, et al. The impact of adjuvant brachytherapy with sublobar resection on pulmonary function and dyspnea in high-risk patients with operable disease: preliminary results from the American College of Surgeons Oncology Group Z4032 trial. J Thorac Cardiovasc Surg 2011;142(3):554–62.
34. Fernando HC, Landreneau RJ, Mandrekar SJ, et al. Thirty- and ninety-day outcomes after sublobar resection with and without brachytherapy for non-small cell lung cancer: results from a multicenter phase III study. J Thorac Cardiovasc Surg 2011; 142:1143–51.
35. Okada M, Tauchi S, Iwanaga K, et al. Associations among bronchioloalveolar carcinoma components, positron emission tomographic and computed tomographic findings, and malignant behavior in small lung adenocarcinomas. J Thorac Cardiovasc Surg 2007;133(6):1448–54.
36. Nakayama H, Okumura S, Daisaki H, et al. Value of integrated positron emission tomography revised using a phantom study to evaluate malignancy grade of lung adenocarcinoma: a multicenter study. Cancer 2010;116(13):3170–7.
37. Okada M, Nakayama H, Okumura S, et al. Multicenter analysis of high-resolution computed tomography and positron emission tomography/computed tomography findings to choose therapeutic strategies for clinical stage IA lung adenocarcinoma. J Thorac Cardiovasc Surg 2011;141(6):1384–91.
38. Tsutani Y, Miyata Y, Nakayama H, et al. Prognostic significance of using solid versus whole tumor size on high-resolution computed tomography for predicting pathologic malignant grade of tumors in clinical stage IA lung adenocarcinoma: a multicenter study. J Thorac Cardiovasc Surg 2012;143:607–12.
39. Tsutani Y, Miyata Y, Nakayama H, et al. Prediction of pathologic node-negative clinical stage IA lung adenocarcinoma for optimal candidates undergoing sublobar resection. J Thorac Cardiovasc Surg 2012; 144:1365–71.
40. Tsutani Y, Miyata Y, Nakayama H, et al. Solid tumors versus mixed tumors with a ground-glass opacity component in patients with clinical stage IA lung adenocarcinoma: Prognostic comparison using high resolution computed tomography findings. J Thorac Cardiovasc Surg 2012. [Epub ahead of print].
41. Okada M. Subtyping Lung Adenocarcinoma According to the Novel 2011 IASLC/ATS/ERS Classification: Correlation with Patient Prognosis. Thorac Surg Clin 2013;23(2):179–86.
42. Tsutani Y, Miyata Y, Nakayama H, et al. Oncologic outcomes of segmentectomy compared with lobectomy for clinical stage IA lung adenocarcinoma: Propensity score-matched analysis in a multicenter study. J Thorac Cardiovasc Surg, in press.
43. Nomori H, Okada M. General Knack of Segmjentectomy. In: Nomori H, Okada M, editors. Illustrated Anatomical Segmentectomy for Lung Cancer. First edition. London: Springer; 2012. p. 9–21.

Management of Tumors Involving the Chest Wall Including Pancoast Tumors and Tumors Invading the Spine

Jean Deslauriers, MD, FRCS(C)[a,*], François Tronc, MD[b], Dalilah Fortin, MD, FRCS(C)[c]

KEYWORDS

• Lung cancer • Chest wall invasion • En-bloc resection • Pancoast tumor

KEY POINTS

- Patients likely to require chest wall or spinal resection for the removal of a primary lung cancer need careful preoperative evaluation, including mediastinoscopy.
- Induction chemoradiation has become "standard of care" for such patients.
- Completeness of resection is a key determinant of long-term survival.
- Patients with N_2 disease should not be offered surgery.

INTRODUCTION

In most series, bronchogenic carcinomas involving the chest wall by direct extension encompass approximately 5% to 8% of resectable lung cancer. They include tumors invading the ribs or spine, as well as Pancoast tumors. As a whole, these bronchogenic carcinomas are given the T_3 or T_4 denominator depending on the structures involved.[1]

In the past, such lesions were considered to be incurable, but over the past 30 to 40 years, several investigators have reported series of patients who have undergone successful surgical resection through various approaches. This information originates, however, from reviews that are retrospective and often include a small number of patients. Many questions thus remain partially unanswered, including the role of multimodality regimens and the identification of prognostic factors, such as tumor and nodal status, as well as completeness of resection. These issues may indeed never be completely resolved, because the limited number of patients available for study precludes randomized prospective trials. In the days of the Lung Cancer Study Group, we looked at the possibility of doing randomized trials in patients with Pancoast tumors, but it was estimated that even if we were to randomize all US patients with this type of disease, there would still be too few to carry out a successful trial. Similarly, a prospective clinical trial undertaken in 1980 to study the potential benefit of postoperative radiation therapy in patients with lung cancer and chest wall invasion was never completed because of poor accrual.

This article reviews the literature as well as some data from our own institution in an attempt to shed

Disclosure: The authors declare no conflict of interest.

[a] Division of Thoracic Surgery, Institut universitaire de cardiologie et de pneumologie de Québec (IUCPQ), Laval University, 2725 chemin Sainte-Foy, L-3540, Quebec City, Quebec G1V 4G5, Canada; [b] Department of Thoracic Surgery, Hôpital Louis-Pradel, 28 Avenue Doyen Lépine, Bron, Cedex 69677, France; [c] Department of Thoracic Surgery, Schulich School of Medicine & Dentistry, London Health Science Centre, Critical Care Trauma Centre, Victoria Hospital, Western University, D2-528, London, Ontario N9A 5W9, Canada
* Corresponding author.
E-mail address: jean.deslauriers@chg.ulaval.ca

Thorac Surg Clin 23 (2013) 313–325
http://dx.doi.org/10.1016/j.thorsurg.2013.05.001
1547-4127/13/$ – see front matter

light on some of those questions. We discuss what should be done in terms of preoperative evaluation, what is the role of multimodality therapy, what factors are affecting prognosis after resection, and, finally, what should be the expected survival after surgery.

LUNG CANCER INVADING THE CHEST WALL

Terminology and Historical Highlights

Bronchogenic carcinomas involving the chest wall are peripheral tumors invading the parietal pleura alone or in a more advanced state penetrating the endothoracic fascia and extending to the ribs and sometimes chest wall muscles (**Fig. 1**). Most such tumors will require combined lung and chest wall excision to be completely resected, which is the main determinant of long-term survival.

Frank P. Coleman of Richmond, Virginia, is given credit as being the first to recommend lung resection with "block excision" of the chest wall for lung cancer invading the ribs. In his 1947 historical article,[2] he reported on 4 patients who had had pneumonectomy with chest wall resection. There was 1 postoperative death but the remaining 3 patients were living well and free of disease 5 months to 6 years after the operation. In 1957, Gronquist and colleagues[3] reported on 16 cases encountered at the Mayo Clinic between 1947 and 1954 and concluded that "either pneumonectomy or lobectomy done in association with resection of the chest wall can be a curative procedure, especially if the involvement of the thoracic wall is limited to the parietal pleura." In 1966, Hermes C. Grillo and colleagues,[4] from the Massachusetts General Hospital, suggested that all patients with involvement of the parietal pleura should undergo

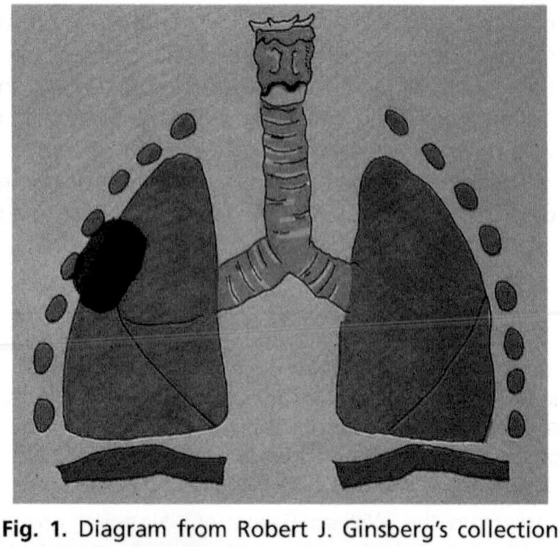

Fig. 1. Diagram from Robert J. Ginsberg's collection depicting a peripheral lung cancer invading the chest wall. (*Courtesy of* R.J. Ginsberg.)

en bloc resection of the lung and chest wall rather than extrapleural resection. In their series, there was no long-term survival in patients who had an extrapleural resection only.

Importance of Preoperative Evaluation

In patients presenting with peripheral lung tumors abutting the chest wall, the 2 main objectives of preoperative evaluation are to determine, before the actual surgery, if a given patient is likely to require chest wall resection and what is the clinical nodal status. The first consideration is important, because patients likely to need chest wall resection could benefit from induction chemoradiation, as patients with Pancoast tumors do, whereas the second consideration is even more important because the presence of lymph node metastases has a disastrous impact on survival in this subset of patients.[5,6]

The most common presenting symptom is chest pain, which in itself is not a prognostic factor but is a strong indicator that chest wall resection will be needed. A bone scan is not very useful in determining chest wall invasion but, in our experience, virtually 100% of patients who have both chest pain and a positive bone scan will need chest wall resection to achieve an R_0 status. By contrast, asymptomatic patients with negative bone scans are likely to require only an extrapleural resection or the tumor may not even be invading the parietal pleura.

Trying to determine the depth of invasion through imaging studies is critical, and radiographic signs, such as an obvious mass invading the chest wall or rib destruction, are clear indicators that the chest wall will have to be resected. Computed tomography (CT) is not a reliable predictor of chest wall invasion, but in an interesting study, Ratto and colleagues[7] showed that obliteration of the extrapleural fat plane was a most sensitive and specific finding. Magnetic resonance imaging (MRI) has the theoretic advantage of being able to determine if the muscle layers are involved, whereas "respiratory dynamic MRI" has the potential to demonstrate independent movements of chest wall and lungs during respiration, thus ruling out parietal pleura invasion. In one study, respiratory dynamic MRI had a sensitivity of 100% and a specificity of 83% to document chest wall invasion.[8]

Once the preoperative evaluation has shown no distant spread, and the local extent of the tumor has been determined, all patients should, in our opinion, undergo a mediastinoscopy, which is still considered the "gold standard" to clinically stage the mediastinum. Depending on tumor location, lymph nodes from different stations should be sampled, and if any are found to be malignant, we think that surgical therapy with or without induction treatments should not be recommended. As Dr Robert J. Ginsberg often said, "you should select before you resect."

Results of Surgery and Role of Adjuvant Therapies

Although some investigators are advocating thoracoscopic surgery to resect tumors invading the chest wall,[9] most surgeons prefer an open approach. The chest is entered away from the tumor and the area of concern is first carefully palpated to determine whether or not there is true invasion of the chest wall.[10] If there are only inflammatory adhesions between tumor and chest wall, an extrapleural resection is probably adequate surgery, but if there is any question of invasion beyond the parietal pleura, the patient should have an en bloc resection of the lung and involved chest wall (**Fig. 2**). Some investigators advocate resecting portions of one intact rib above and below the tumor with a 3-cm to 4-cm lateral margin,[11] but it is generally accepted that a 1-cm margin in all directions is adequate margin.

Depending on the size and site of the defect that has been created, reconstruction is done with or without the use of prosthetic material. Small or even medium-sized defects located posteriorly behind the scapula, for instance, can be reconstructed without prosthetic material, whereas larger defects, especially those located anteriorly or laterally, need to be reconstructed with prosthetic material, most commonly a flexible prosthesis, such as a Gore-Tex patch (W.L. Gore and Associates, Newark, DE) or a Marlex mesh (Bard, Cranston, Rhode Island). When the defect is located at the tip of the scapula, Marc Riquet and colleagues[12] recommend resecting the tip of the scapula to prevent scapula entrapment on the rib below the reconstruction. Operative mortality associated with these procedures is in the range of 5% to 6% and the results of some series published since the beginning of the twenty-first century are listed in **Table 1**. Unfortunately, results are difficult to interpret because most series are heterogeneous and include patients who have had incomplete resections, as well as some who have had adjuvant radiotherapy. Despite these limitations, the overall 5-year survival is in the vicinity of 30%.

In our own series of 125 patients who underwent complete en bloc resection of lung and chest wall between 1980 and 2000, the operative mortality was 5.6% (7/125) and the overall 5-year survival was 31.0%, with a median survival of 448 days (**Fig. 3**). Interestingly, there was no survival difference between patients who had chest pain preoperatively and those who did not ($P = .594$) (**Fig. 4**). We also analyzed the sites of first recurrences (n = 82) (**Table 2**), which were distant in half the patients, suggesting that some consideration should be given to induction chemoradiation with regimens similar to those used in the treatment of superior sulcus tumors.

There have virtually been no reports on the specific role of radiotherapy in patients with lung cancer invading the chest wall, but in a small retrospective series of 35 patients with complete resection done in Toronto between 1969 and 1981, Alec Patterson and colleagues[16] showed that irradiated patients (Preoperative: 5, Postoperative: 8) had a 5-year survival of 56% as compared with 30% in nonradiated patients.

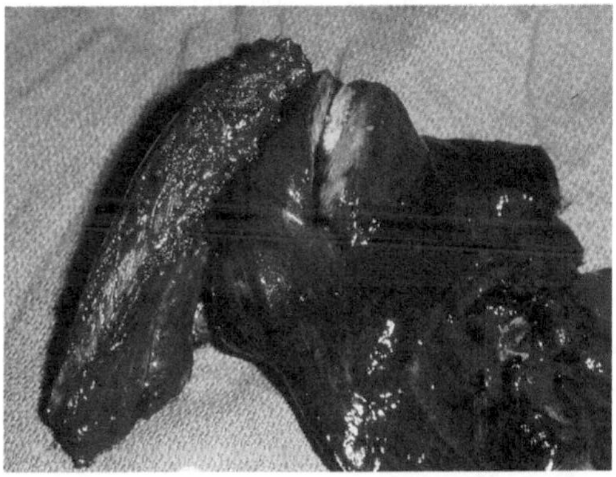

Fig. 2. Right upper lobe with en bloc excision of the chest wall.

Table 1
Results of surgery after en bloc resection of lung cancer invading the chest wall in series reported after the year 2000

Author, Ref, Year	No. Patients	Operative Mortality, %	5-Year Survival, %
Chapelier et al,[13] 2000	100	4.0	18
Magdeleinat et al,[14] 2001	209	7.0	21
Burkhart et al,[15] 2002	94	6.3	39
Doddoli et al,[5] 2005	309	7.8	31
Current (Tronc F, Deslauriers J, 2006)	125	5.6	31

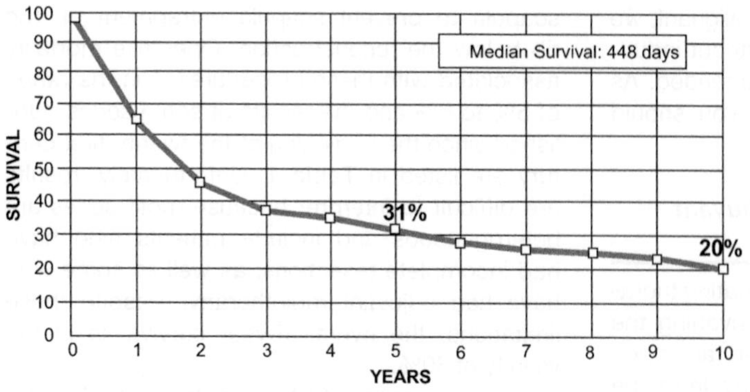

Fig. 3. Overall survival of 125 patients who had complete resection of lung cancer invading the chest wall between 1980 and 2000.

Prognostic Factors

A number of prognostic factors have been identified in association with resected bronchogenic carcinomas invading the chest wall and they are listed in **Table 3**. Among them, incomplete resection is the most consistent factor associated with poor prognosis. Indeed, the most striking finding presented by Downey and colleagues,[6] from the Memorial Sloan Kettering Cancer Center in New York, was that an incomplete resection, even if leaving only microscopic disease, offers no curative benefit. In that series, the survival of incompletely resected patients was indistinguishable from that of patients undergoing no resection at all, with only 4% of incompletely resected patients and 0% of unresected patients being alive 3 years after surgery.

The extent of resection that should be done when the tumor invades only the parietal pleura is a surgical issue that is still controversial, with some surgeons believing that an extrapleural dissection without chest wall resection has a negative impact on survival.[17,18] In Jeff Piehler and colleagues'[17] series from the Mayo Clinic, for instance, there was a 75.0% 5-year survival rate with en bloc resection in contrast to 27.9% after extrapleural resection. Most surgeons believe, however, that if the parietal pleural comes off easily from the endothoracic fascia, there is no need to resect the chest wall.

Several studies have documented that lymph node metastases (N_1 and N_2) are associated with poor survival figures. In 2001, Facciolo and colleagues[11] from Rome reported that the 5-year survival in the subsets T_3N_0 and T_3N_2 were respectively 67.3% and 17.9% (P = .007). Similarly, Downey and colleagues[6] reported that the 5-year survival in R_0 patients with T_3N_0 disease was 49%, in those with T_3N_1 disease it was 27%, and in patients with T_3N_2 disease it was 15% (P<.0003). In our own series, the 5-year survival was 35% for patients with T_3N_0 status compared with 11% for patients with T_3N_2 disease (P = .0025) (**Fig. 5**).

The depth of parietal invasion also appears to be a prognostic factor, and Facciolo and colleagues[11] reported a 5-year survival of 79.1% if only the parietal pleura was involved compared with 54.0% if there was involvement of soft tissues with or without bone invasion (P = .014).

SUPERIOR SULCUS (PANCOAST) TUMORS

Terminology and Historical Highlights

A superior sulcus tumor is a bronchogenic carcinoma developing at the thoracic inlet and typically involving, by direct extension, the lower trunks of

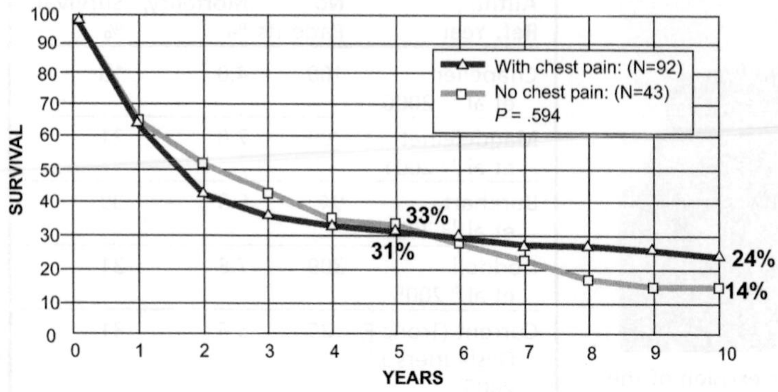

Fig. 4. Survival related to presence or absence of chest pain preoperatively in 125 patients who had complete resection of lung cancer invading the chest wall between 1980 and 2000.

Table 2
Sites of first recurrences (82/125) and time to first recurrence

Site of First Recurrence	No. Patients (%)	Time to Recurrence
Logoregional	35 (43)	251 d
Only site	31	
Local + Distant	4	
Distant	41 (50)	249 d
Second primary	6 (7)	

Data from Tronc F, Deslauriers J. Current series.

the brachial plexus, the intercostal nerves, the stellate ganglion, and the adjacent ribs and vertebrae (**Fig. 6**).[19] The Pancoast syndrome, as it is known today, is characterized by shoulder pain, with or without radiation to the arm, axilla, or scapula; Horner syndrome; and atrophy of the hand muscles. Pain is the most consistent symptom and a critical determinant of the Pancoast syndrome. Indeed, patients who have a carcinoma located at the lung apex but who do not have pain should not be considered to have a Pancoast tumor. This is an important consideration when patients are to be included in clinical trials evaluating the role of multimodality regimens in the treatment of this condition.

Many surgeons believe that superior sulcus tumors are named as such because they are in relation to an apical groove that is formed by the subclavian artery as it crosses over the lung. Anatomically, however, the pulmonary sulcus is a deep groove that runs along the costovertebral gutter from the arch of the first rib to the insertion of the diaphragm at the bottom of the thoracic cage. Tumors of the superior pulmonary sulcus develop in the upper portion of this groove and, by definition, are in a posterior location. They are surrounded by the first rib, lower trunk of the brachial plexus, subclavian blood vessels, and stellate ganglion.

A review of the history pertinent to Pancoast tumors and Pancoast syndrome is most interesting because it illustrates very well the difficulties that can be encountered in accurately determining who should be given credit as being the first to describe a specific entity (**Table 4**). According to our review of the literature, superior sulcus tumors were first reported by Edwin S. Hare from the United Kingdom, who, in a 1838 publication in the *London Medical Gazette*,[20] discussed the case of a patient who had presented with a history of pain, tingling, and numbness in the distribution of the left ulnar nerve and who had been found, at postmortem examination, to have a hard tumor located at the lung apex and extending superiorly toward the origin of the brachial plexus.[21] In 1918, Professor Americo Ricaldoni, an internist at the Facultad de Medicina de Montevideo in Uruguay, reported 2 cases documented by autopsy and described the specific anatomic features of this entity (**Fig. 7**).[22]

In 1924, Henry Pancoast,[23] a radiologist from Philadelphia, called the tumor located at the lung apex and associated with pain in the upper extremity, an apical chest tumor. In his second article,[24] given as the chairman's address at the 83rd Annual Meeting of the American Medical Association (New Orleans, LA, May 1932), he reported on 7 cases of a peculiar neoplastic entity found in the upper portion of the pulmonary sulcus and suggested to name it "superior sulcus carcinoma." Pancoast thought that the neoplasm probably arose from embryonal epithelial rests of the last branchial cleft and he added that death occurred as a result of what seemed to be a comparatively trivial growth without metastasis.

In 1932, Tobias,[25] from Buenos Aires, described very accurately the anatomic and clinical features of this entity and called it "painful apicocostovertebral syndrome" caused by an apical tumor. Like Ricaldoni,[22] Tobias recognized that it originated from the lung and that it was the localization of the tumor that made it specific, rather than its origin. Because of this significant contribution, the syndrome associated with superior sulcus tumors is sometimes called the Pancoast-Tobias Syndrome.

Because of their extensive local invasiveness, Pancoast tumors were long considered incurable until Chardack and MacCallum,[26] reported, in 1956, the case of a patient who survived 6 years

Table 3
Most important prognostic factors in resected bronchogenic carcinomas with chest wall invasion

Factor	Better Prognosis	Worse Prognosis
Completeness of resection	R_0 resection	R_1 or R_2 resection
Extent of resection	Entire chest wall	Extrapleural resection
Pathologic nodal status	N_0	N_2
Depth of parietal invasion	Parietal pleura only	Deep structures

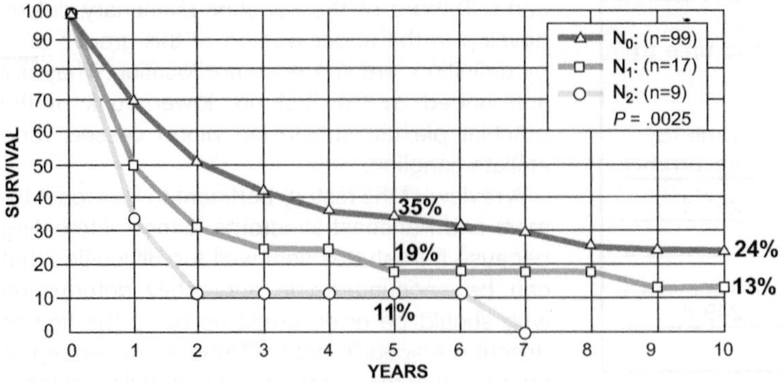

Fig. 5. Survival related to nodal status in 125 patients who had complete resection of lung cancer invading the chest wall between 1980 and 2000.

after surgical resection followed by postoperative radiation. Subsequently, Shaw and colleagues[27] from Dallas found that preoperative radiation facilitated surgical resection and that this combined treatment was potentially curative. Their contribution was important because preoperative radiation followed by surgical resection became the "standard of care" for lung cancer of the superior sulcus until the early 2000s.

Preoperative Evaluation and Clinical Staging

The diagnosis of Pancoast tumor begins when the patient presents with the appropriate symptom complex and the suggestion of an apical mass or apical thickening on standard chest radiographs. Classically, there is a significant delay from the onset of chest pain to diagnosis and often patients will have consulted orthopedists, chiropractitioners, or physiotherapists before the correct diagnosis is made.

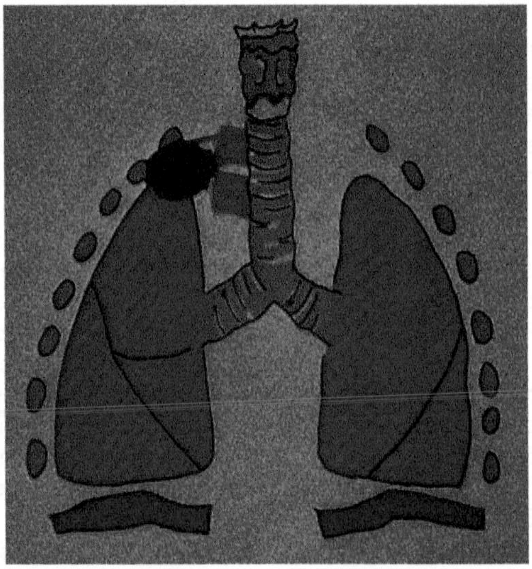

Fig. 6. Diagram from Robert J. Ginsberg's collection depicting a tumor of the superior pulmonary sulcus. (*Courtesy of* R.J. Ginsberg.)

Obtaining a tissue diagnosis is crucial, not only to establish the diagnosis of malignancy and determine the histology of the tumor, but also to rule out rare infections that can also cause a Pancoast syndrome. Because of the peripheral nature of Pancoast tumors, bronchoscopy has a low diagnostic yield, but fine-needle aspiration done under CT guidance through a cervical[28] or posterior triangle approach has a diagnostic yield of 95% to 100%.

A CT scan, or preferably an MRI scan, should then be obtained to determine the degree of tumor invasion into the surrounding structures. Currently, MRI or magnetic resonance angiography (MRA) with gadolinium are the preferred imaging modalities because they allow better visualization of the tumor's relationship to the brachial plexus, subclavian vessels, vertebral bodies, intervertebral foraminas, and surrounding soft tissues. In an early study done by Heelan and colleagues[29] from the Department of Medical Imaging at Sloan Kettering Cancer Center in New York, MRI was found to be more accurate than CT in the evaluation of superior sulcus tumors (94% vs 63%). In general, however, CT and MRI are complementary modalities and both should be done.

Because lymph node status is the most significant factor in determining treatment paradigm and prognosis, mediastinoscopy is a key element of the staging process and should be done in all presumed operable cases. Because superior sulcus tumors have a tendency to spread to supraclavicular nodes across the apical parietal pleura, we also recommend routine ipsilateral ultrasonography and fine-needle aspiration of any suspicious nodes. If positive nodes are identified at mediastinoscopy or cervical ultrasonography, patients are usually not offered surgery.

In most institutions, the surgical resection of Pancoast tumors is done by a team, consisting of a thoracic surgeon and a spine surgeon or neurosurgeon and all patients should be seen by members of this surgical multidisciplinary team

Table 4
Historical highlights in the description of superior sulcus tumors

Author, Ref, Year	Country	Description
Hare,[20] 1838	UK	Documented case of a patient with a tumor at the lung apex.
Ricaldoni,[22] 1918	Uruguay	Described the anatomic features of the tumor.
Pancoast,[23,24] 1924, 1932	USA	Described the clinical features of superior sulcus carcinomas. Thought that the tumor was extrapulmonary in origin.
Tobias,[25] 1932	Argentina	Recognized that the tumor originated from lung tissue and called it "Painful apicocostovertebral syndrome."

before treatment is planned so as to make certain that the tumor is technically resectable. Our own criteria for resectability and nonresectability of superior sulcus tumors are listed in **Table 5**. Vascular and vertebral body involvement have traditionally been contraindications to surgical resection, but, with advances in surgical techniques including those of spinal instrumentation,[30] these tumors can now be resected, although the usefulness of surgery in this subset of patients with T_4 disease is not well documented.

Treatment by Multimodality Regimens

The traditional combined modality of preoperative irradiation (3000–3500 cGy given over 2 weeks) followed by surgery 1 month later, as originally described in 1961 by Shaw and colleagues,[27] was used by most surgeons until the early 2000s. Irradiation was thought to improve resectability by shrinking the tumor, reducing the likelihood of seeding viable cells during resection, blocking the lymphatics around the tumor and, in general, maximizing local control. Surgical results were, however, difficult to interpret because most published series were single-institution retrospective reviews with small numbers of patients and heterogeneous

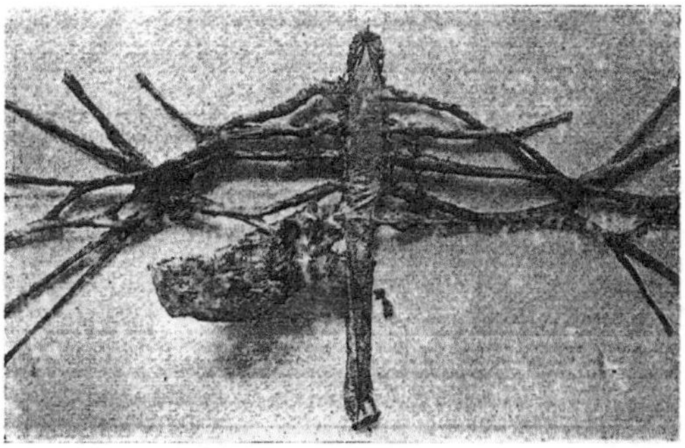

Fig. 7. Description of superior pulmonary sulcus tumors by Professor Americo Ricaldoni from Montevideo in 1918. Anatomy of the tumor invading the lower trunk of the brachial plexus. (*From* Ricaldoni A. Anales de la Facultad de Medicina, Tome III, Lamina IX. 1918.)

populations with regard to tumor stage and treatment protocols. Despite these limitations, better survival rates (approximately 30% at 5 years) and improved local control by preoperative radiation followed by surgery versus radiotherapy or surgery alone has been consistently reported, especially in patients with greater than 50% response to radiotherapy and in those without nodal involvement (pN_0).[31–33]

Although adequate local control can be achieved with preoperative radiation followed by surgery, distant relapses are frequent and a common cause of death. Recently, Valerie Rusch and colleagues[34] reported the results of the Phase II Southwest Oncology Group Trial 9416 of induction chemoradiation followed by surgical resection for non–small cell lung cancer of the superior sulcus in 110 patients. Each patient required mediastinoscopy-negative disease and preoperatively received 2 cycles of cisplatin and etoposide concurrent with 45 Gy of radiation. Patients who responded to treatment (**Fig. 8**) or maintained stable disease underwent thoracotomy 3 to 5 weeks later and, after surgery, were given 2 additional cycles of chemotherapy. Of the 95 patients eligible for surgery, 88 underwent thoracotomy and 83 had a complete resection. Two patients died postoperatively (operative mortality of 2.4%) and pathologic complete response or minimal residual microscopic disease was observed in 61 resected specimens. Five-year survival was 44% for all patients and 54% after complete resection. That study clearly demonstrated that overall survival was markedly improved relative to historical controls of radiation plus resection. Other studies have shown similar results with induction chemoradiotherapy, which has now become now "standard of care" in patients with Pancoast tumors.[34–39]

Surgical Approaches

Surgical resection remains the treatment of choice for superior sulcus tumors. The objective is to resect the upper lobe with the invaded ribs (usually

Table 5
Technical resectability of Pancoast tumors

Involved Structure	Can Be Resected	Should Not Be Resected
Chest wall	Ribs including first rib Limited invasion of vertebral bodies	Marked invasion of vertebral bodies
Neurologic	Sympathetic chain C_8–T_1 nerve root	C_7 nerve root
Vascular	Subclavian vessels	

the first 3 ribs), the transverse processes of invaded vertebrae, and all involved structures, such as the lower trunk of the brachial plexus (C_8–T_1), the stellate ganglion, and the upper dorsal sympathetic chain. As previously mentioned, a combined thoracic and orthopedic or neurosurgical team is essential to optimize resectability. Although some surgeons believe that a wedge resection of the apex is acceptable, most believe that lobectomy results in better survival, similar to what is observed after surgery of other types of non–small cell lung cancer.[40]

As a rule, superior sulcus tumors not invading the thoracic inlet are completely resectable through the classic posterior Shaw-Paulson approach,[27,41] which involves a high posterolateral thoracotomy carried to the level of C_7 at the base of the neck. This approach allows excellent exposure to the posterior chest wall, including the transverse processes and thoracic nerve roots (C_8–T_1) but restricted access to the more anterior structures, such as the subclavian vessels. It also allows standard exposure to the pulmonary hilum and anatomic resection of the involved lobe. Chest wall reconstruction is seldom needed because the scapula covers most of the defect.

Beginning in the late 1970s, several anterior approaches (**Table 6**) have been developed to improve exposure to anterior apical structures, such as the subclavian blood vessels. The first such descriptions originated from Japan[42,43] and included the classic anterior-posterior hook approach described in 1993 by Niwa and colleagues[43] from Nagoya. Niwa and colleagues'[43] operation involved a classic posterolateral thoracotomy, which curved upward anteriorly toward the sternoclavicular joint.

In 1993, Dartevelle and colleagues from Paris[44] described an anterior transcervical thoracic approach to facilitate exposure of the lung apex, as well as that of cervically based structures, such as the brachial plexus and subclavian vessels. Their operation involved an incision along the anterior border of the sternocleidomastoid muscle that continued over the clavicle (hockey-stick incision) (**Fig. 9**). The sternocleidomastoid muscle was divided and the medial half of the clavicle resected, thus exposing the thoracic inlet. In the original series of 29 patients reported by Dartevelle and colleagues,[44] 20 patients needed an additional thoracotomy to remove the involved lobe. With this approach, both the clavicle and first rib are resected, which, on occasion, could cause postoperative alterations in the shoulder mobility and cervical posture. To minimize the incidence of these problems, which, at times, can be clinically significant, Grunenwald and Spaggiari[45] developed a transmanubrial technique done through a manubrial L-shaped transection and first costal cartilage resection. This approach involves the retraction of an osteomuscular flap including but sparing the clavicle, thus preserving the stability of the shoulder girdle. In 1998, Robert Korst and Michael Burt[46] recommended the use of the hemiclamshell approach to resect those tumors.

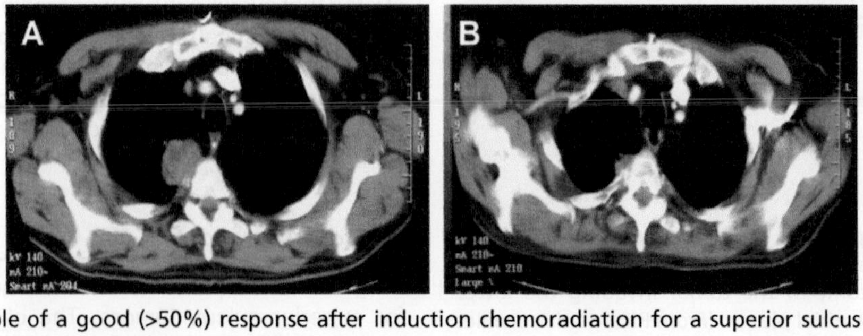

Fig. 8. Example of a good (>50%) response after induction chemoradiation for a superior sulcus tumor of the right upper lobe. (*A*) Pretreatment CT. (*B*) CT done after concurrent chemoradiation and before surgery.

Table 6
Anterior approaches to superior sulcus tumors

Author (Ref, Year)	Procedure
Masaoka et al,[42] 1979	Proximal median sternotomy extended to the anterior fourth intercostal space and to the base of the neck.
Niwa et al,[43] 1993	Anterior-posterior hook approach.
Dartevelle et al,[44] 1993	Anterior transcervical-thoracic approach.
Grunenwald & Spaggiari,[45] 1997	Transmanubrial approach.
Korst & Burt,[46] 1998	Hemiclamshell approach.

According to the investigators who reported results on 42 patients, the hemiclamshell technique has several advantages over other approaches, including excellent exposure to the hilum, facilitating lobectomy. Other advantages are that there is no limit to the size of chest wall that can be resected and, because the clavicle is not divided and the sternoclavicular joint is left intact, patients have less postoperative discomfort and better shoulder stability.

Prognostic Factors and Possible Postoperative Neurologic Complications

Most people agree that in tumors of the superior sulcus, important prognostic factors are the T status (T_3 vs T_4), the completeness of resection (R_0 vs R_{1-2}) and the nodal status (N_0 vs N_{1-2}). In a seminal article on factors determining outcome after surgical resection of T_3 and T_4 lung cancers of the superior sulcus, Valerie Rusch and colleagues[47] from the Memorial Sloan-Kettering Cancer Center showed, in a multivariate analysis, that all of these factors were statistically significant (**Table 7**). The T status seems important and patients with T_4 status due to invasion of the vertebral bodies, subclavian blood vessels, and brachial plexus, have a significantly worse prognosis. Similarly, patients with Horner syndrome do worse than those who do not have Horner syndrome,[40] because the presence of Horner syndrome often implies extensive posterior invasion and unresectability. Surprisingly, the T status (T_3 vs T_4) did not seem to influence survival in Southwest Oncology Group Trial 9416 that validated the role of induction chemoradiation.[34]

Possible postoperative neurologic complications after surgery of Pancoast tumors are listed in **Table 8** and they include Horner syndrome; sensory and motor deficits, which usually resolve with physiotherapy and rehabilitation; and complications related to accidental penetration of the dural sheath.

MANAGEMENT OF LUNG CANCER WITH VERTEBRAL BODY INVOLVEMENT

Recent technical advances, including spinal instrumentation, have allowed more aggressive management of vertebral body invasion by Pancoast or non-Pancoast non–small cell lung cancer (**Table 9**). Traditionally, these tumors were regarded as having a poor prognosis[48] and were felt to be unresectable.

In 1989, Tom Demeester and colleagues[49] reported a series of 12 patients with lung cancer and vertebral body involvement who were treated by

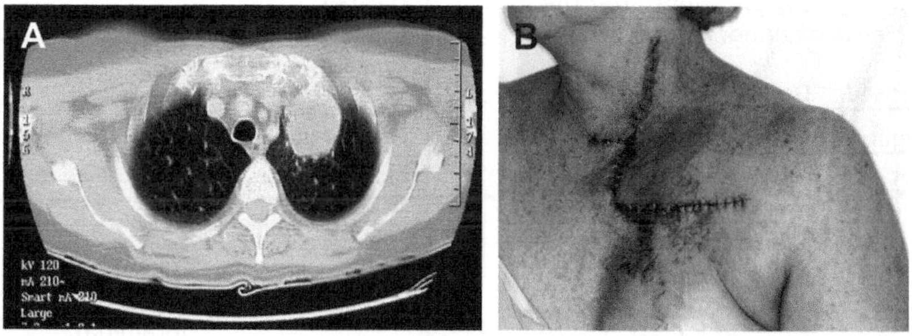

Fig. 9. Dartevelle's transcervical thoracic approach. (*A*) CT scan showing an ideal case for this approach with an anteriorly located apical tumor. (*B*) The incision parallels the lower sternocleidomastoid muscle, courses over the manubrium, and then turns laterally over the clavicle. Note that this patient had a mediastinoscopy at the same time as the resection.

Table 7
Results of the multivariate analysis of prognostic factors influencing overall survival after surgical resection of T_3 and T_4 lung cancers of the superior sulcus

Prognostic Factor	*P* Value	Hazard Ratio Estimated	Hazard Ratio 95% CI
Extent of resection (sublobar vs lobar)	.08	1.4	1.0–2.1
T status (T_3 vs T_4)	.05	1.6	1.0–2.5
Completeness of resection (R_0 vs R_1–R_2)	<01	2.2	1.4–3.3
Nodal status (N_0 vs N_{1-2})	<01	2.1	1.4–3.2

Abbreviation: CI, confidence interval.
Data from Rusch VW, Parekh KJ, Leon L, et al. Factors determining outcome after surgical resection of T3 and T4 lung cancers. J Thorac Cardiovasc Surg 2000;119:1147–53.

preoperative radiation followed by tumor resection and en bloc tangential resection of the vertebral bodies. Five-year survival was 42%. In another series of superior sulcus tumors with vertebral invasion, Gandhi and colleagues[30] from the M.D. Anderson Cancer Center in Houston reported on 17 patients in whom partial vertebrectomy (n = 7), total vertebrectomy (n = 7), or neural foramina or transverse process resection (n = 3) had been done in conjunction with lung cancer resection for superior sulcus tumors. The overall actuarial survival at 2 years was 54%, and additionally, the 2-year survival of patients with R_0 resections was 80% versus 0% for those with positive margins ($P<.0006$). In 2002, Dominique Grunenwald and colleagues[50] from Paris described an even more aggressive approach with en bloc hemi or total vertebrectomy for tumors involving vertebral bodies. The operation, usually done after induction treatment, involved a 2-incision or 3-incision procedure, cervico-thoracic resection of the vertebra (hemivertebrectomy: 15; total vertebrectomy: 4), and bilateral laminectomy in the case of total vertebrectomy. Despite a disappointing predicted 5-year survival of only 14%, the investigators suggested that en bloc resection could be a valid option in selected patients with vertebral involvement by thoracic tumors.

En bloc multilevel hemivertebrectomy has also been advocated by Dartevelle's group[51] for thoracic inlet tumors involving the intervertebral foramina but not the vertebral body. Initial dissection is performed through a transcervical approach followed by posterior midline laminectomy. Among 17 patients treated in this fashion, there was no operative mortality and 5-year survival was 20%. In our own series of 19 patients (14 with preoperative radiation) who underwent partial or total vertebrectomy for lung cancer invading the spine between 1995 and 2001, there was no operative mortality and the 5-year survival was 40% (**Figs. 10** and **11**), indicating that surgery after radiation therapy could be performed with an acceptable morbidity and good survival.

Table 8
Possible neurologic complications after the resection of Pancoast tumors

Structure Excised	Deficit
Stellate ganglion	Horner syndrome
T_1 nerve root	Minimal sensory deficit
C_8–T_1 nerve roots	Sensory deficit of ulnar distribution Motor deficit of intrinsic hand muscles
Entry in dorsal sheath	Spinal fluid leak Meningitis Intradural hematoma with possible paraplegia

Table 9
Surgical series that have reported survival figures after en bloc resection of non–small cell lung cancer invading vertebral bodies

Author, Ref, Year	No. Patients	Survival, %
Demeester et al,[49] 1989	12 (3 Pancoast tumors)	42% (5 y)
Gandhi et al,[30] 1999	17 (all Pancoast tumors)	54% (2 y)
Grunenwald et al,[50] 2002	19	14% (5 y)
Fadel et al,[51] 2002	17 (involvement of intervertebral foramina)	20% (5 y)
Deslauriers & Fortin (2002, current)	19 (all complete resections)	40% (5 y)

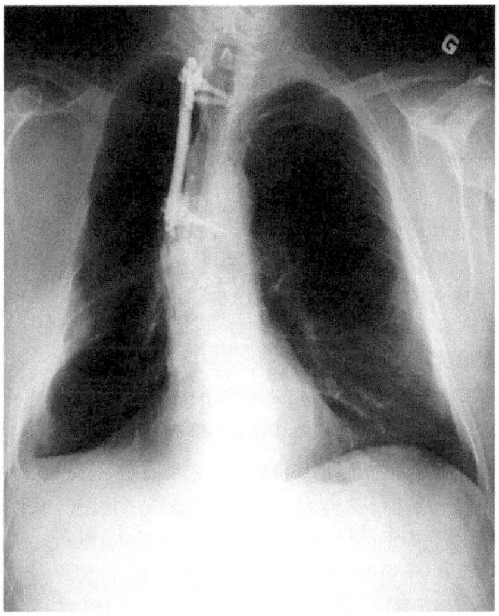

Fig. 10. Radiograph of a patient who had a right upper lobectomy with vertebral body resection 5 years previously. Note the rod that was used to stabilize the spine.

In 2009, the Toronto Group presented a series of 23 consecutive patients[52] who had undergone radical vertebral resection for non–small cell lung cancer invading the spine and who had received nonconcurrent induction chemoradiation (cisplatin and etoposide followed by 45 Gy of radiation). In that retrospective review, the 3-year survival was 58% (median follow-up, 34 months). Patients who had achieved complete pathologic response or near complete response demonstrated significantly better survival than those who did not (3-year survival, 92% vs 20%; $P = .006$).

It thus appears that an aggressive surgical approach to lung cancer invading the spine can be recommended, but surgery should be preceded by induction chemoradiation, as in tumors of the superior pulmonary sulcus. We also stress again the importance of a surgical multidisciplinary approach for the resection of these lesions.

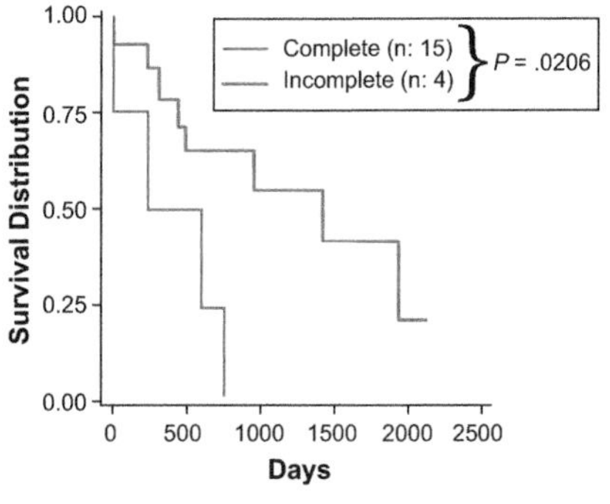

Fig. 11. Survival curve in 19 patients according to completeness of operation.

SUMMARY

From this review, it appears clear that patients with lung cancer invading the chest wall (ribs or vertebral bodies) or those with Pancoast tumors should not be offered surgery if they are likely to have an incomplete resection, even microscopic, or if they have clinical N_2 disease. By contrast, patients in whom complete resection can be done and those with N_0 disease should undergo surgical resection and anticipate good long-term survival. Over the past 15 years, significant progress has been made with regard to surgical approaches and techniques, as well as recognition of the role of induction chemoradiation.

REFERENCES

1. Edge SB, Byrd DR, Compton CC, et al. Lung. In: Edge SB, Byrd DR, Compton CC, et al, editors. AJCC cancer staging handbook. From the AJCC cancer staging manual. 7th edition. Chicago: Springer; 2010. p. 299–323.
2. Coleman FP. Primary carcinoma of the lung with invasion of the ribs. Pneumonectomy and simultaneous block resection of the chest wall. Ann Surg 1947;126:156–68.
3. Gronquist YK, Clagett T, McDonald JR. Involvement of the thoracic wall in bronchogenic carcinoma. Study of 16 cases in which pneumonectomy or lobectomy and simultaneous resection of the thoracic wall were done. J Thorac Surg 1957;33:487–95.
4. Grillo HC, Greenberg JJ, Wilkins EW Jr. Resection of bronchogenic carcinoma involving thoracic wall. J Thorac Cardiovasc Surg 1966;51:417–21.
5. Doddoli C, D'Journo B, Le Pimpec-Barthes F, et al. Lung cancer invading the chest wall: a plea for en-bloc resection but the need for new treatment strategies. Ann Thorac Surg 2005;80:2032–40.
6. Downey RJ, Martini N, Rusch VW, et al. Extent of chest wall invasion and survival in patients with lung cancer. Ann Thorac Surg 1999;68:188–93.
7. Ratto GB, Piacenza G, Frola C, et al. Chest wall involvement by lung cancer: computed tomographic detection and results of operation. Ann Thorac Surg 1991;51:182–8.
8. Akata S, Kajiwara N, Park J, et al. Evaluation of chest wall invasion by lung cancer using respiratory dynamic MRI. J Med Imaging Radiat Oncol 2008;52:36–9.
9. Cerfolio RJ, Bryant AS, Minnich DJ. Minimally invasive chest wall resection: sparing the overlying, uninvolved extrathoracic musculature of the chest. Ann Thorac Surg 2012;94:1744–7.
10. Allen MS. Chest wall resection and reconstruction for lung cancer. Thorac Surg Clin 2004;14:211–6.

11. Facciolo F, Cardillo G, Lopergolo M, et al. Chest wall invasion in non-small cell lung carcinoma: a rationale for en-bloc resection. J Thorac Cardiovasc Surg 2001;121:649–56.
12. Riquet M, Arame A, Le Pimpec-Barthes F. Non-small cell lung cancer invading the chest wall. Thorac Surg Clin 2010;20:519–27.
13. Chapelier A, Fadel E, Macchiarini P, et al. Factors affecting long-term survival after en-bloc resection of lung cancer invading the chest wall. Eur J Cardiothorac Surg 2000;18:513–8.
14. Magdeleinat P, Alifano M, Benbrahem C, et al. Surgical treatment of lung cancer invading the chest wall: results and prognostic factors. Ann Thorac Surg 2001;71:1094–9.
15. Burkhart HM, Allen MS, Nichols FC, et al. Results of en-bloc resection for bronchogenic carcinoma with chest wall invasion. J Thorac Cardiovasc Surg 2002;123:670–5.
16. Patterson GA, Ilves R, Ginsberg RJ, et al. The value of adjuvant radiotherapy in pulmonary and chest wall resection for bronchogenic carcinoma. Ann Thorac Surg 1982;34:692–7.
17. Piehler JM, Pairolero PC, Weiland LH, et al. Bronchogenic carcinoma with chest wall invasion: factors affecting survival following en-bloc resection. Ann Thorac Surg 1982;35:684–91.
18. McCaughan BC, Martini N, Bains MS, et al. Chest wall invasion in carcinoma of the lung. Therapeutic and prognostic implications. J Thorac Cardiovasc Surg 1985;89:836–41.
19. Johnson DE, Goldberg M. Management of carcinoma of the superior pulmonary sulcus. Oncology 1997;11:781–6.
20. Hare ES. Tumor involving certain nerves. London Med Gazette 1838;1:16–8.
21. Konaki R, Putnam JB, Walsh G, et al. The management of superior sulcus tumors. Semin Surg Oncol 2000;18:152–64.
22. Ricaldoni A. Parálisis atrófica radicular inferior. Del plexo braquial por esclerosis epiteliomatosa procedente del domo pleural en el curso de un cáncer latente del pulmón. Anales de la Facultad de Medicina 1918, Tomo III, Lamina IX 1918. 770–97. Spanish.
23. Pancoast HK. Importance of careful, roentgen-ray investigation of apical chest tumors. JAMA 1924; 83:1407–11.
24. Pancoast HK. Superior pulmonary sulcus tumour. Tumour characterized by pain, Horner's syndrome, destruction of bone and atrophy of hand muscles. JAMA 1932;99:1391–6.
25. Tobias JW. Sindrome apico-costo-vertebral doloroso por tumour Apexiano: su valor diagnostic en el cancer primitivo pulmorar. Rev Med Latino Am 1932;17:1522–6 Spanish.
26. Chardack WM, MacCullum JD. Pancoast tumor: five-year survival without recurrence or metastases following radical resection and postoperative irradiation. J Thorac Surg 1956;31:535–42.
27. Shaw RR, Paulson DL, Kee JL Jr. Treatment of the superior sulcus tumor by irradiation followed by resection. Ann Surg 1961;154:29–40.
28. Paulson DL, Weed TE, Rian RL. Cervical approach for percutaneous needle biopsy of Pancoast tumors. Ann Thorac Surg 1985;39:586–7.
29. Heelan RT, Demas BE, Caravelli JF, et al. Superior sulcus tumors: CT and MR imaging. Radiology 1989;170:637–41.
30. Gandhi S, Walsh GL, Komaki R, et al. A multidisciplinary surgical approach to superior sulcus tumors with vertebral invasion. Ann Thorac Surg 1999;68:1778–85.
31. Martinod E, D'Audiffret A, Thomas P, et al. Management of superior sulcus tumors: experience with 139 cases treated by surgical resection. Ann Thorac Surg 2002;73:1534–40.
32. Wright CD, Moncure AC, Shepard JO, et al. Superior sulcus lung tumors. Results of combined treatment (irradiation and radical resection). J Thorac Cardiovasc Surg 1987;94:69–74.
33. Miller JI, Mansour KA, Hatcher CR. Carcinoma of the superior pulmonary sulcus. Ann Thorac Surg 1979;28:44–7.
34. Rusch VW, Giroux DJ, Kraut MJ, et al. Induction chemoradiation and surgical resection for superior sulcus non-small cell lung carcinomas: long-term results of Southwest Oncology Group Trial 9416 (Inter Group Trial 0160). J Clin Oncol 2007;25: 313–8.
35. Attar S, Krasna MJ, Sonett JR, et al. Superior sulcus (Pancoast) tumor experience with 105 patients. Ann Thorac Surg 1998;66:193–8.
36. Suntharalingam M, Sonett JR, Haas ML, et al. The use of concurrent chemotherapy with high-dose radiation before surgical resection in patients presenting with apical sulcus tumors. Cancer J 2000; 6:365–71.
37. Wright CD, Menard MT, Wain JC, et al. Induction chemotherapy compared with induction radiation for lung cancer involving the superior sulcus. Ann Thorac Surg 2002;73:1541–4.
38. Kwong KF, Edelman MJ, Suntharalingam M, et al. High-dose radiotherapy in trimodality treatment of Pancoast tumors results in high pathologic complete response rates and excellent long-term survival. J Thorac Cardiovasc Surg 2005;129: 1250–7.
39. Kappers I, van Sandick JW, Burgers JA, et al. Results of combined modality treatment in patients with non-small cell lung cancer of the superior sulcus and the rationale for surgical resection. Eur J Cardiothorac Surg 2009;36:741–6.
40. Ginsberg RJ, Martini N, Zaman M, et al. Influence of surgical resection and brachytherapy in the

management of superior sulcus tumour. Ann Thorac Surg 1994;57:1440–5.
41. Pitz CC, de la Rivière AB, van Swieten HA, et al. Surgical treatment of Pancoast tumors. Eur J Cardiothorac Surg 2004;26:202–8.
42. Masaoka A, Ito Y, Yasumitsu T. Anterior approach for tumor of the superior sulcus. J Thorac Cardiovasc Surg 1979;78:413–5.
43. Niwa H, Masaoka A, Yamakawa Y, et al. Surgical therapy for apical invasive lung cancer: different approaches according to tumor location. Lung Cancer 1993;10:63–71.
44. Dartevelle PG, Chapelier AR, Macchiarini P, et al. Anterior transcervical-thoracic approach for radical resection of lung tumors invading the thoracic inlet. J Thorac Cardiovasc Surg 1993;105:1025–34.
45. Grunenwald D, Spaggiari L. Transmanubrial osteomuscular sparing approach for apical chest tumors. Ann Thorac Surg 1997;63:563–6.
46. Korst RJ, Burt ME. Cervicothoracic tumors: results of resection by the hemi-clamshell approach. J Thorac Cardiovasc Surg 1998;115:286–95.
47. Rusch VW, Parekh KJ, Leon L, et al. Factors determining outcome after surgical resection of T_3 and T_4 lung cancers. J Thorac Cardiovasc Surg 2000; 119:1147–53.
48. Shahian DM. Contemporary management of superior pulmonary sulcus (Pancoast) lung tumors. Curr Opin Pulm Med 2003;9:327–31.
49. Demeester TR, Albertucci M, Dawson PJ, et al. Management of tumor adherent to the vertebral column. J Thorac Cardiovasc Surg 1989;97:373–8.
50. Grunenwald DH, Mazel C, Girard P, et al. Radical en-bloc resection for lung cancer invading the spine. J Thorac Cardiovasc Surg 2002;103: 271–9.
51. Fadel E, Missenard G, Chapelier A, et al. En-bloc resection of non-small cell lung cancer invading the thoracic inlet and intervertebral foramina. J Thorac Cardiovasc Surg 2002;123:676–85.
52. Anraku M, Waddell TK, de Perrot M, et al. Induction chemoradiotherapy facilitates radical resection of T_4 non-small cell lung cancer invading the spine. J Thorac Cardiovasc Surg 2009;137:441–7.

The Role of Surgery in Patients with Clinical N2 Disease

Reza Mehran, MD

KEYWORDS

• Non–small lung carcinoma • Metastatic mediastinal lymph node • Surgery • Chemotherapy • Radiation therapy

KEY POINTS

- Proper surgical staging is key in the management of patients with suspected mediastinal spread.
- Curative management of lung carcinoma with mediastinal disease is possible.
- The treatment involves a bimodality or trimodality therapy using a combination of systemic therapy, surgery, and radiation therapy, the optimal sequence of which is still unclear.
- Pneumonectomy after chemotherapy and radiation therapy should be used with caution but may have a role in selected patients, with special modifications in the surgical technique.

INTRODUCTION

Patients with N2 non–small cell lung carcinoma (NSCLC) by definition have ipsilateral mediastinal adenopathy and are grouped within stage IIIa disease. Most of these patients are still diagnosed solely using imaging techniques, such as positron emission tomography (PET) and computed tomography (CT) scanning, which causes a significant error in staging if not combined with some form of surgical staging of the mediastinum. N2 adenopathy forms a spectrum of diseases ranging from occult microscopic disease to bulky multistation adenopathy. Proper understanding of the prognosis and treatment implications for each form of mediastinal lymph node metastases has led to the selective use of surgery to treat these patients. This article reviews the role of surgery in the management of patients with N2 mediastinal involvement.

HISTORICAL NOTES

In 1982, Pearson in a retrospective review of his experience at the Toronto General Hospital reported that the survival of patients in whom preoperative mediastinoscopy was positive for N2 nodes was only 9%. The author indicated that in patients with mediastinoscopy-positive nodes, surgery can offer a modest survival benefit only if a complete resection was possible. Pearson established mediastinoscopy as an essential tool in the staging of patients with lung cancer in the days when CT scanning was still not universally available.[1]

In 1988, Mountain[2] developed the staging system of lung cancer that is now the basis of the staging of lung cancer adopted by the American Joint Commission on Cancer 7th edition. The staging identified patients with mediastinal disease as having a poor prognosis when treated with surgery or radiotherapy alone.

In 1990 the addition of chemotherapy to radiotherapy or surgery significantly improved survival of patients with N2 disease, using a cisplatinum-based chemotherapy.

In a highly quoted publication, the Intergroup (IG) trial 0319 in 2009 showed that chemotherapy and radiation therapy given with or without surgery are good options in the treatment of patients with N2 disease as long as a pneumonectomy was avoided.[41]

Department of Thoracic and Cardiovascular Surgery, MD Anderson Cancer Center, 1400 Pressler, FCT 19.5066, Unit 1489, Houston, TX 77030–4009, USA
E-mail address: rjmehran@mdanderson.org

Thorac Surg Clin 23 (2013) 327–335
http://dx.doi.org/10.1016/j.thorsurg.2013.04.007

PRIMARY LUNG CANCER AND MEDIASTINAL LYMPHATIC SPREAD

Spread of primary lung cancer to the mediastinal lymph nodes remains the most important factor influencing prognosis and treatment in patients with potentially resectable lung cancer. Under the present revised lung cancer staging system, the N2 descriptor applies to mediastinal metastatic disease on the ipsilateral side of the primary tumor and are categorized as stage IIIa disease. This article discusses the management of T1, T2, and T3 tumors with N2 involvement. Superior sulcus tumor is not discussed in this article.

N2 can be categorized as clinical or pathologic. Clinical staging is based on imaging studies only, whereas pathologic staging is obtained by direct pathologic assessment of the nodes when sampled in a methodic fashion either by mediastinoscopy, endobronchial ultrasound (EBUS), or at the time of chest exploration.

Using imaging only, there are limitations to the use of size criteria to determine the presence or absence of nodal metastases, because metastases occur in normal-sized nodes and nodal enlargement can be secondary to benign conditions, such as granulomatous disease. To simplify measurements, a lymph node in the paratracheal, hilar, subcarinal, paraesophageal, paraaortic, or subaortic region is generally considered enlarged if the short-axis diameter is greater than or equal to 10 mm.[3]

Pathologic examination still remains the most accurate method of determining metastatic disease. The sensitivity of histopathology improves using immunohistochemistry with antibodies to cytokeratins, or the use of other molecular detectors with reverse transcriptase polymerase chain reaction methodology, but their application clinically is still limited.[4] Paradoxically, some authors believe that micrometastatic disease is associated with an increased risk of recurrence and death and may be even a worse disease than that with gross disease on imaging.[5]

Intraoperative sentinel node mapping with technetium 99m is an accurate way to identify the first site of lymphatic tumor drainage in NSCLC. This method may also improve the precision of pathologic staging. However, at the moment its usefulness in lung cancer is not clear because all patients must have either a mediastinal node dissection or sampling of all nodal stations and when compared with axillary node dissection the procedure carries very little risk of complication.[6]

Another concept that has been reported is the concept of skip nodal metastasis, whereby patients present with N2 disease without having N1 nodal involvement. N2 patients with mediastinal lymph node skip metastasis have a more favorable prognosis compared with N2 patients with continuous infiltration of the regional lymph nodes. Patients with a continuous lymph node involvement show an increased number of infiltrated mediastinal lymph nodes per patient compared with patients with a noncontinuous spread. Skip metastasis is an independent prognostic factor of survival. The presence of skip metastasis seems to subclassify a unique subgroup of N2 disease in NSCLC. However, presently skip nodal disease remains more of a curiosity with no therapeutic implications (**Box 1**).[7]

EPIDEMIOLOGY

More than 1.5 million new cases of lung cancer are diagnosed annually worldwide. The incidence in the United States was 226,160 cases in 2012.[8] About 10% of all patients with NSCLC present with stage IIIA N2 disease. These patients have a worse prognosis because of a higher rate of locoregional and distal recurrences, with an overall 5-year survival rate of about 23%.[9]

Several randomized trials have demonstrated local recurrence rates of 11% to 34% among patients with stage I to III disease after surgery alone for N2 disease and rate of distal metastatic disease as high as 60%, suggesting that additional consolidative therapies are needed in combination with surgery to control local and distal disease. From series that have been reported on prognostic subgroups of N2, it seems that multistation nodal disease has a worse prognosis than single station but the mediastinal location of a single-station disease has no bearing on the prognosis.[8]

DIAGNOSIS OF N2 DISEASE

In patients with localized and clinically resectable NSCLC, the presence and extent of intrathoracic lymph node involvement dictate the treatment strategy and is therefore a crucial part of the patient work up. Since the 1980s, cervical

Box 1
N2, Clinical presentations

- Single station detected only by microscopy or molecular techniques during surgery
- Single station nonbulky on imaging (shortest diameter 1–2 cm on imaging)
- Single station bulky (shortest diameter >2 on imaging)
- Multiple station nonbulky
- Multiple station bulky

mediastinoscopy has been extensively used in the staging of mediastinal lymph nodes. Specificity and false-positive rates of mediastinoscopy can be assumed to be 100% and 0%, respectively. However, in a review of more than 6500 patients undergoing mediastinoscopy between 1985 and 2003, the average sensitivity of mediastinoscopy to detect mediastinal lymph node involvement was approximately 80% and the average false-negative rate was approximately 10%.[10] False-negative results mainly occur in lymph node stations that are not reachable by mediastinoscopy. The yield of the technique is also surgeon dependent. In a study of the pattern of practice in the United States, Little and colleagues[11] found that mediastinoscopy is infrequently performed and lymph nodes are biopsied in less than 50% of patients. Recently, transbronchial and transesophageal ultrasound-guided needle biopsy techniques have provided a valuable adjunct for the evaluation of mediastinoscopic "blind spots," such as stations 5 and 8. The yield of EBUS seems to be equal if not superior to the one of mediastinoscopy.[12]

Several imaging techniques have been used as less invasive staging tools than mediastinoscopy. CT scan of the chest is useful in providing anatomic detail, but the accuracy of chest CT scanning in differentiating benign from malignant lymph nodes in the mediastinum is poor. PET scanning has a much better sensitivity and specificity than chest CT scan for staging lung cancer in the mediastinum, and distant metastatic disease can be detected by PET scanning as well. Integrated PET/CT shows substantially higher accuracy in overall tumor staging over CT and PET interpreted separately. However, the sensitivity of integrated PET/CT to detect malignant nodal involvement is size dependant. It is only 32.4% in nodes less than 10 mm, and 85.3% in nodes greater than or equal to 10 mm.[13]

Therefore, noninvasive staging lacks sensitivity and thus the American College of Chest Physicians recommends that with either test, abnormal findings be confirmed by tissue biopsy to ensure accurate staging. Unfortunately, this is still not a common practice and many patients with "positive" PET/CT scans are erroneously labeled as having advanced disease and treated as such.

Invasive Restaging

The concept of invasive restaging after induction therapy is emerging as a tool in detecting patients who would benefit most from surgery. Surgery seems to be most beneficial for patients who have had a downstaging of their mediastinal disease.[14,15] CT, PET, or remediastinoscopy carry a false-negative rate of 20% to 30%.[16] Repeat mediastinoscopy could be technically difficult and the yield of EBUS after induction therapy could be too low.[10] Hence, presently for those who believe in the concept of surgery only after downstaging, the best approach to evaluate the nodes seems to be an EBUS on initial evaluation followed by mediastinoscopy after induction therapy.

THERAPEUTIC OPTIONS

The optimal treatment of patients with N2 disease is not known despite an extensive amount of literature on the topic. However, some useful trends are apparent and are reviewed in this section. Treatments must be tailored to each patient depending on their performance status and the degree of lymph node involvement. The different treatment strategies tried over the years and still used, and their drawback and advantages, are reviewed in the next sections.

Surgery Alone

Several randomized trials have demonstrated local recurrence rates of 11% to 34% among patients with stages I to III disease after surgery alone.[17–19] The recurrence rates are even higher for patients who have N2 disease at the time of surgery, and can be as high as 60% at 5 years.[20] Therefore, surgery should never be used alone in the treatment of patients with N2 disease.

The anatomic indications for surgery when used in a multimodality approach are very much operator dependent and there is no consensus on the extent of N2 disease that would benefit most from resection. In general, patients who suffer from multistation bulky N2 disease are believed to be inoperable. Those with a single station bulky disease are usually offered surgery but only if there is evidence of clinical response after induction therapy, and then again this is a subject of contention. Presently in North America there is no clear consensus on the surgical management of patients with stage IIIa lung cancer.[21]

Adjuvant Therapy After Surgery

The poor outcomes seen after surgery alone have led clinicians to add systemic and radiation therapy after surgery. There are theoretical advantages to give adjuvant treatments after surgery. First, there is accurate information on staging of the mediastinum and this has important implications in the dose of radiation and fields to be treated. There is pooled evidence in a meta-analysis where patients with N2 diseases treated with chemotherapy and radiation therapy after surgery seemed to have 17% to 20% reduction in the risk of death.[22,23]

The Adjuvant Navelbine International Trialist Association trial,[24] a randomized study comparing the efficacy of adjuvant cisplatin and vinorelbine given sequentially with or without postoperative radiation therapy (PORT) for stage IB-IIIA NSCLC, found that survival was significantly improved in patients with N2 disease who received multimodality treatment. This improvement was unique to the N2 group, because the combined-modality treatment was found to have a detrimental effect on patients with N1 disease.

Adjuvant therapy with systemic and radiation therapy after surgery seems to be the treatment modality recommended for patients with incidental N2 disease discovered at the time of surgery.

Induction Chemotherapy

Because of the lower compliance of patients who have chemotherapy after surgery, investigators started to experiment with induction chemotherapy in patients with known N2 disease. The advantages of induction chemotherapy are in vivo assessment of response to the drugs used, it is better tolerated, patients are more complaint, there is improved parenchymal sparing, and it may theoretically improve survival by better control of the systemic micrometastases.

Based on randomized trials and meta-analyses demonstrating a survival benefit of induction chemotherapy plus surgery versus surgery alone,[25–28] induction chemotherapy for stage IIIA-N2 NSCLC has become a reasonable option for the management of potentially resectable stage IIIA-N2 NSCLC. It is known that nodal response after induction chemotherapy is an important prognostic factor. In one trial, induction chemotherapy produced a 5-year survival rate of 51.6% for patients with disease downstaged to N0, compared with 17.6% for patients with persistent pN1-3 disease.[25]

Similarly, a Swiss study concluded that patients with nodal downstaging to N0-1 after induction therapy had improved disease-free survival and overall survival compared with patients with persistent mediastinal lymph node involvement. The median time to local relapse comparing persistent N2 with N0-1 was 14.4 versus 43.8 months. In patients with pathologic response to chemotherapy, there was a significant reduction in the rate of distant metastasis.[29]

The use of chemotherapy before surgery raised the concern of a possible rise in surgical complications. However, a series of 335 patients undergoing lobectomy or larger resection after chemotherapy showed that the use of preoperative chemotherapy did not significantly affect morbidity or mortality.[30]

The effect of induction chemotherapy seems to be twofold: downstaging of the mediastinal nodes and decrease in the rate of distant metastasis. Although these rates are still unsatisfactory, chemotherapy should always be given upfront in every patient with proven N2 disease who are a candidate for pulmonary resection.

Definitive Chemotherapy and Radiation Therapy Versus Induction Chemotherapy and Radiation Therapy Followed by Surgery

The rate of downstaging of mediastinal nodes after induction chemotherapy alone is low (<20%) and the question remains how to treat most patients who do not get to have a downstaging. There obviously is still a need for better chemotherapy and targeted agents. The addition of radiation therapy to chemotherapy aims at decreasing further the rate of locoregional recurrence.

Radiation therapy given alone in traditional dose and fractionation schedules (1.8–2 Gy per fraction per day to 60–70 Gy in 6–7 weeks) yields poor survival rates and patterns of failure that are locoregional and distant.[31,32] Therefore, radiation therapy should always be used in combination with systemic therapy.

Adding platinum-containing chemotherapy either at systemic doses preceding or at a low radiosensitizing dose concomitant with chest radiotherapy in good performance patients significantly improves the outcome compared with single-modality chest radiotherapy.[33] Definitive-dose thoracic radiotherapy should be no less than the biologic equivalent of 60 Gy in 1.8- to 2-Gy fractions to the planning target volume.[34] Ideally this requires three-dimensional conformal radiotherapy, a technique characterized by beam outlines that match the shape of the planning target volume. Mapping of the planning target volume is improved when using information from the PET/CT scan and from the mapping obtained from surgical mediastinal staging. Planning target volume tailored fields allows the administration of higher total radiation doses, which have been associated with improved local control and better survival.[35]

Three randomized trials have compared chemotherapy and chemoradiotherapy as induction regimen in stage III NSCLC.[36–38] These trials suggest that induction chemoradiotherapy results in better rates of resectability, pathologic downstaging, and pathologic complete remissions than chemotherapy alone but without significantly affecting overall or progression-free survival.

The European Organization for Research and Treatment of Cancer (EORTC) performed a large multicenter randomized trial to compare surgery with radiation therapy in patients with stage IIIa N2 NSCLC who showed response to induction chemotherapy. There was no significant difference in median survival (17.5 months in the radiotherapy arm vs 16.4 months in the surgery arm); 5-year overall survival (14% vs 16%); or progression-free survival. The authors concluded from this bimodality trial that after a radiologic response to induction chemotherapy surgery is not superior to radiotherapy.[39]

In a randomized trial Thomas and colleagues[37] found in patients with stage III NSCLC amenable to surgery that preoperative chemoradiation in addition to chemotherapy increased pathologic response and mediastinal downstaging, but did not improve survival. After induction with chemoradiation, they recommended that pneumonectomy should be avoided. Similarly, in a retrospective study, Higgins and colleagues[40] showed that preoperative chemotherapy and radiation therapy was associated with higher mediastinal complete pathologic response (pCR) rates but did not improve overall survival. The mediastinal pCR rates were significantly greater in those patients undergoing preoperative chemoradiation therapy than in those undergoing chemotherapy alone (65% vs 35%; $P = .02$). This was especially notable in the subgroup of patients with multistation mediastinal involvement (68% vs 11%; $P = .01$).

In a trimodality trial, North American investigators conducted the Inter Group (IG) trial 0139 in which patients with T1-3 NSCLC with biopsy-proved N2 disease and a performance status of 0 to 1 were randomized between induction chemoradiotherapy to 45 Gy followed by either surgery or consolidation radiotherapy to 61 Gy.[41] Both groups received two additional cycles of cis-etoposide subsequently. They found that progression-free survival was significantly better in the surgery group but overall survival did not differ mainly because of a higher postoperative mortality in patients who had a pneumonectomy. The median overall survival was better than the EORTC bimodality trial. In the nonoperative arm the median survival was 22.2 months and 23.6 months in the operative arm. The rate of distal relapse was similar between the two groups and was 37% in the surgical arm versus 42% in the nonsurgical arm. The rate of regional relapse was also similar between the groups despite the fact that the radiation dosage in the surgery arm was suboptimal (45 vs 61 Gy).

In the IG 0319 trial, three factors were found in multivariate analysis to be associated with improved outcome: (1) lobectomy, (2) pathologic downstaging, and (3) completeness of resection. An exploratory analysis in the surgical arm showed a significantly better survival for patients who underwent lobectomy compared with the matched patients in the radiation therapy group. Their conclusion was that chemotherapy plus radiotherapy with resection using a lobectomy or without resection are options for patients with stage IIIa (N2) NSCLC.

In the ECOG (Eastern cooperative oncology group) and IG trials the operative morbidity and mortality was higher than with radiotherapy, suggesting that preference is to be given to the safest approach. This leaves a very unclear role for surgery in the initial management of patients with stage IIIa, N2, NSCLC leaving chemotherapy and radiation therapy as the upfront regimen of choice.

The higher risks of mortality associated with preoperative radiation therapy in patients who need a pneumonectomy have not been seen in two studies where the dosages of radiation were greater than 59 Gy. The postoperative mortality rate was between 0% and 13%.[42,43] Special maneuvers, such as the use of intercostal muscle reinforcement of the stump, may have had a beneficial effect. Pneumonectomy can therefore be safely performed in patients after radiation therapy. In one study, the rate of pCR of the N2 nodes was 84%, although not all of the patients had a surgical confirmation of the N2 disease before initiation of treatments. Despite this impressive sterilization of the mediastinum, 35% of patients had a recurrence and 40% of these recurred locally.[43]

Using the data from some of the studies mentioned previously, Shah and coworkers[44] reported a systematic review and meta-analysis looking at the role of radiation therapy as induction therapy with chemotherapy and found no evidence to support radiation therapy as an induction regimen.

Despite the weak and sometimes contradictory results mentioned in this section, definitive systemic and radiation therapy preferably given concurrently form now the recommended treatment for patients with stage IIIa and N2 disease and there is a National Comprehensive Cancer Network consensus based on high-level evidence suggesting that the intervention is appropriate as sole therapy for the treatment of these patients.[45]

The field of thoracic radiotherapy is rapidly evolving with the development of dose-localization techniques (proton beam therapy, intensity modulated radiation therapy, Stereotactic Body Radiation

Therapy (SBRT), four-dimensional radiation with or without the use of fiducial) which aim at delivering radiation to the tumor with extreme precision and at higher dosages reducing therefore the frequency of radiation-associated injuries.[46] It is hence expected that by using these new technologies that local control of the tumor will further improve in the near future.

The important question still remains as to what to do with the many patients who do not respond to definitive chemotherapy and radiation therapy. One option is the administration of different and more effective systemic or targeted therapies, but the results of these maneuvers are still unknown. Surgery remains an option but many surgeons hesitate to offer surgery after radical doses of radiation have been given. Definitive chemotherapy and radiation therapy therefore although recommended as a treatment option is not an optimal choice for patients with N2 disease.

Induction Systemic Therapy Followed by Surgery, Followed by Post Operative Radiation Therapy (PORT) and Chemotherapy

In general the surgical community believes that selected patients with N2 disease should be given the benefits associated with an R0 resection and surgery as we read earlier is always preferred in patients who did not have radical doses of radiation therapy. This means operating on several patients who could not be downstaged after chemotherapy alone. Persistent pathologic mediastinal nodal involvement after induction chemotherapy followed by surgical resection alone is a negative prognostic factor for stage IIIa-N2 patients with NSCLC because this population has high rates of locoregional and distant failures.

Nine randomized trials examined the impact of PORT on disease-free and overall survival in patients with resected stage I, II, and III NSCLC. These data from more than 2000 patients were individually analyzed by the PORT Meta-analysis Trialists Group.[47] Although the methods of delivery of radiation therapy were very different than now, PORT was shown to have a detrimental effect on overall survival in stage I-II disease. However, for N2 patients there was a small reduction in the rate of local recurrence. The combination of PORT and chemotherapy given concurrently has also been suggested to be beneficial in Radiation Therapy Oncology Group-9705 trial.[48]

Using the Surveillance, Epidemiology, and End Results database, Lally and colleagues[49] investigated the association between survival and PORT in patients with resected NSCLC. In this population-based cohort, PORT use was associated with an increase in survival in patients with N2 nodal disease but not in patients with N0 or N1 nodal disease. These data were verified by Douillard and colleagues[24] who studied the impact of PORT on survival of patients recruited in the Adjuvant Navelbine International Trialist Association (ANITA) study. ANITA is a randomized trial of adjuvant cisplatin and vinorelbine chemotherapy versus observation in completely resected NSCLC stages Ia to IIIb. Use of PORT was recommended for patients with nodal disease but was not randomized or mandatory. This retrospective evaluation suggested similarly a positive effect of PORT in N2 disease especially when patients received adjuvant chemotherapy (median survival, 47.4 vs 23.8 months).

Finally, in a retrospective study evaluating the impact of PORT and chemotherapy in patients who received induction chemotherapy followed by surgical resection, Amini and colleagues[50] found that aggressive consolidative therapies may improve outcomes for patients with persistent N2 disease after induction chemotherapy and surgery. In their study group the rate of locoregional failure rate was only 12%. However, the rate of distal recurrence was still high at 54%. The overall survival of patients who had PORT and chemotherapy was twice as high at 5-year as those who received only PORT (40% vs 20%).

Based on a lower level of evidence (nonrandomized studies) arising from the studies presented in this section, there is a National Comprehensive Cancer Network consensus that the use of Induction chemotherapy followed by surgery and then PORT and systemic therapy is an acceptable method of treating patients with stage IIIa, N2, NSCLC.

At MD Anderson Cancer center we use a trimodality approach for the treatment of N2 disease. All patients who can tolerate surgery and have operable disease follow a treatment scheme as suggested in **Fig. 1**. We favor induction chemotherapy followed by surgical resection. We restage patients with imaging (PET/CT) but we do not use a surgical staging after the induction therapy unless we observe progression of disease. After patients have recovered from surgery they continue with radical doses of radiation therapy to the mediastinum. We give 50 Gy in 25 fractions for completely resected N2 disease. If there was extracapsular extension we go to 60 Gy in 30 fractions. Finally, if the margins were postive, the radiation is increased to 66 Gy in 33 fractions. Gross target volume includes complete extent of ipsilateral mediastinum as defined radiographically. Supraclavicular lymph nodes and lymph nodes in the contralateral hilum are not routinely included in

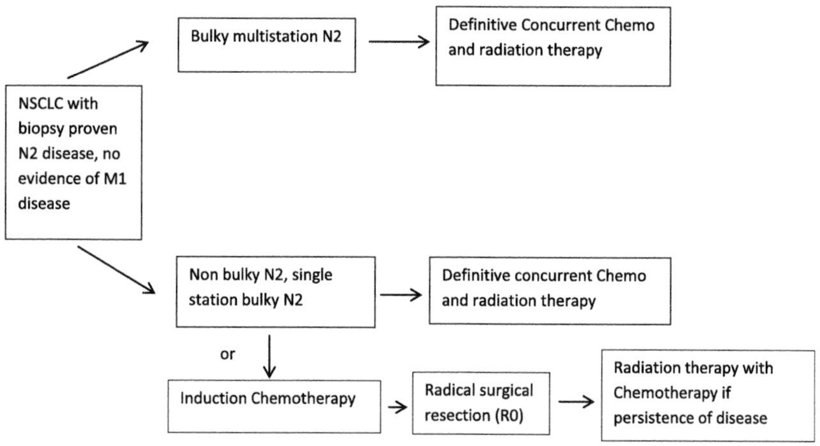

Fig. 1. Suggested treatment schemes for patients with stage IIIa, NSCLC with N2 disease based on best evidence in 2013.

the radiation field and we use intensity-modulated radiation or proton therapy.

In patients with good performance status particularly in those with an incomplete resection the radiation therapy is given concurrently with adjuvant systemic therapy. In those with a more limited performance status the chemotherapy is given either sequentially or omitted. The rational for this aggressive approach is first to try to obtain a downstaging of the nodes before surgery and also hope for an increased resectability of the tumor. We realize that the rate of downstaging is probably higher if radiation is given preoperatively, however, the addition of consolidative therapies after surgery offer a treatment option for patients who have had an incomplete clinical response or an incomplete resection, by being able to deliver radical doses of radiation without interruption. This treatment plan is well tolerated but has yet to be validated by a properly designed clinical protocol.

SUMMARY

The treatment of patients with N2 disease is multidisciplinary. The role of surgery is not clearly established. Patients with bulky multistation N2 disease are considered nonoperable. Those with single station bulky or nonbulky disease have the option of being treated with definitive chemoradiation therapy upfront or with a trimodality treatment involving induction systemic therapy followed by surgery and consolidative radiation and systemic therapy postoperatively. The drawback of a bimodality treatment is how to treat the significant number of patients who do not respond to therapy, hence the preference of the author to use a trimodality approach, although the validity of this treatment plan remains to be visited.

REFERENCES

1. Pearson FG, DeLarue NC, Ilves R, et al. Significance of positive superior mediastinal nodes identified at mediastinoscopy in patients with resectable cancer of the lung. J Thorac Cardiovasc Surg 1982;83: 1–11.
2. Mountain CF. Prognostic implications of the international staging system for lung cancer. Semin Oncol 1988;3:236–45.
3. Toloza E, Harpole L, McCrory D. Noninvasive staging of non-small cell lung cancer: a review of the current evidence. Chest 2003;123:137S–46S.
4. Erhunmwunsee L, D'Amico T. Detection of occult N2 disease with molecular techniques. Thorac Surg Clin 2008;18:339–47.
5. Ricquet M, Bagan P, Le Pimpec Brthes F, et al. Completely resected non-small cell lung cancer: reconsidering prognostic value and significance of N2 metastases. Ann Thorac Surg 2007;84: 1818–24.
6. Liptay MJ, Grondin SC, Fry WA, et al. Intraoperative sentinel lymph node mapping in non-small-cell lung cancer improves detection of micrometastases. J Clin Oncol 2002;20(8):1984–8.
7. Prenzel KL, Mönig SP, Sinning JM, et al. Role of skip metastasis to mediastinal lymph nodes in non-small cell lung cancer. J Surg Oncol 2003; 82(4):256–60.
8. Siegel R, Naishadham D, Jemal A. Cancer statistics, 2012. CA Cancer J Clin 2012;62(1):10–29.
9. Robinson LA, Ruckdeschel JC, Wagner H Jr, et al, American College of Chest Physicians. Treatment of non-small cell lung cancer-stage IIIA: ACCP evidence-based clinical practice guidelines (2nd edition). Chest 2007;132(Suppl 3):243S–65S.
10. Detterbeck FC, Jantz MA, Wallace M, et al. Invasive mediastinal staging of lung cancer: ACCP

evidence-based clinical practice guidelines (2nd edition). Chest 2007;132:202S–20S.

11. Little AG, Rusch VW, Bonner JA, et al. Patterns of surgical care of lung cancer patients. Ann Thorac Surg 2005;80(6):2051–6 [discussion: 2056].
12. Almeida FA. Bronchoscopy and endobronchial ultrasound for diagnosis and staging of lung cancer. Cleve Clin J Med 2012;79(Suppl 1):eS11–6.
13. Billé A, Pelosi E, Skanjeti A, et al. Preoperative intrathoracic lymph node staging in patients with non-small-cell lung cancer: accuracy of integrated positron emission tomography and computed tomography. Eur J Cardiothorac Surg 2009; 36(3):440–5. http://dx.doi.org/10.1016/j.ejcts.2009.04.003.
14. Elias AD, Skarin AT, Leong T, et al. Neoadjuvant therapy for surgically staged IIIA N2 non-small cell lung cancer (NSCLC). Lung Cancer 1997;17:147–61.
15. Cerfolio RJ, Bryant AS, Buddhiwardhan O. Restaging patients with N2 (stage IIIa) non-small cell lung cancer after neoadjuvant chemoradiotherapy: a prospective study. J Thorac Cardiovasc Surg 2006;131:1229–35.
16. De Cabanyes Candela S, Detterbeck F. A systematic review of restaging after induction therapy for stage IIIa lung cancer. J Thorac Oncol 2010;5:389–98.
17. Dautzenberg B, Arriagada R, Chammard AB, et al. A controlled study of postoperative radiotherapy for patients with completely resected non-small cell lung carcinoma. Cancer 1999;86:265–73.
18. Stephens RJ, Girling DJ, Bleehen NM, et al. The role of postoperative radiotherapy in non-small-cell lung cancer: a multicentre randomised trial in patients with pathologically staged T1-2, N1-2, M0 disease. Medical Research Council Lung Cancer Working Party. Br J Cancer 1996;74:632–9.
19. Feng QF, Wang M, Wang LJ, et al. A study of postoperative radiotherapy in patients with non-small cell lung cancer: a randomized trial. Int J Radiat Oncol Biol Phys 2000;47:925–9.
20. Betticher DC, Hsu Schmitz SF, Totsch M, et al. Prognostic factors affecting long-term outcomes in patients with resected stage IIIA pN2 non-small-cell lung cancer: 5-year follow-up of a phase II study. Br J Cancer 2006;94:1099–106.
21. Veeramachaneni NK, Feins RH, Stephenson BJ, et al. Management of stage IIIA non-small cell lung cancer by thoracic surgeons in North America. Ann Thorac Surg 2012;94(3):922–6.
22. van Meerbeeck JP, Surmont VF. Stage IIIA-N2 NSCLC: a review of its treatment approaches and future developments. Lung Cancer 2009;65(3): 257–67.
23. Pignon JP, Tribodet H, Scagliotti GV, et al. Lung adjuvant cisplatin evaluation: a pooled analysis by the LACE Collaborative Group. J Clin Oncol 2008;26:3552–9.
24. Douillard JY, Rosell R, De Lena M, et al, Adjuvant Navelbine International Trialist Association. Impact of postoperative radiation therapy on survival in patients with complete resection and stage I, II, or IIIA non-small-cell lung cancer treated with adjuvant chemotherapy: the Adjuvant Navelbine International Trialist Association (ANITA) Randomized Trial. Int J Radiat Oncol Biol Phys 2008;72(3): 695–701.
25. Roth JA, Fossella F, Komaki R, et al. A randomized trial comparing perioperative chemotherapy and surgery with surgery alone in resectable stage IIIA non-small-cell lung cancer. J Natl Cancer Inst 1994;86:673–80.
26. Garrido P, Gonalez-Larriba JL, Insa A, et al. Long-term survival associated with complete resection after induction chemotherapy in stage IIIA (N2) and IIIB (T4N0-1) non-small-cell lung cancer patients: the Spanish Lung Cancer Group trial 9901. J Clin Oncol 2007;25:4736–42.
27. Dai Y, Han B, Shen J, et al. Preoperative induction chemotherapy for resectable stage IIIA nonsmall-cell lung cancer: a meta-analysis of 13 double-blind, randomized clinical trials. Chin J Lung Canc 2008;11:398–405.
28. Rosell R, Gamez-Codina J, Camps C, et al. A randomized trial comparing preoperative chemotherapy plus surgery with surgery alone in patients with non-small-cell lung cancer. N Engl J Med 1994;330:153–8.
29. Betticher DC, Schmitz SF, Totsch M, et al. Mediastinal lymph node clearance after docetaxelcisplatin neoadjuvant chemotherapy is prognostic of survival in patients with stage IIIA pN2 non-small-cell lung cancer: a multicenter phase II trial. J Clin Oncol 2003;21:1752–9.
30. Siegenthaler M, Pisters K, Merriman K, et al. Preoperative chemotherapy for lung cancer does not increase surgical morbidity. Ann Thorac Surg 2001; 71:1105–12.
31. Rolland E, Le Chevalier T, Auperin A, et al. Sequential radio-chemotherapy (RTCT) versus radiotherapy alone (RT) and concomitant RT-CT versus RT alone in locally advanced non-small cell lung cancer (NSCLC): two meta-analyses using individual patient data (IPD) from randomised clinical trials (RCTs). J Thorac Oncol 2007;2(8):S309–10.
32. Aupérin A, Le Péchoux C, Pignon JP, et al. Concomitant radio-chemotherapy based on platin compounds in patients with locally advanced non-small cell lung cancer (NSCLC): a meta-analysis of individual data from 1,764 patients. Ann Oncol 2006;17(3):473–83.
33. Aupérin A, Rolland E, Curran WJ, et al. Concomitant radio-chemotherapy (RTCT) versus sequential RT-CT in locally advanced non-small cell lung cancer (NSCLC): a meta-analysis using individual

patient data (IPD) from randomised clinical trials (RCTs). J Thorac Oncol 2007;2(8):S310 [abstract: A1–05].

34. Pfister DG, Johnson DH, Azzoli CG. American society of clinical oncology treatment of unresectable non-small-cell lung cancer guideline: update 2003. J Clin Oncol 2004;22:1–24.
35. Zhao L, West BT, Hayman JA, et al. High radiation dose may reduce the negative effect of large gross tumor volume in patients with medically inoperable early stage non-small cell lung cancer. Int J Radiat Oncol Biol Phys 2007;68:103–10.
36. Sauvaget J, Rebischung J, Vannetzel J, et al. Phase III study of neo-adjuvant MVP versus MVP plus chemo-radiation in stage III NSCLC. Proc ASCO 2000;19:495a [abstract: 1935].
37. Thomas M, Rübe C, Hoffknecht P, et al, German Lung Cancer Cooperative Group. Effect of preoperative chemoradiation in addition to preoperative chemotherapy: a randomised trial in stage III non-small-cell lung cancer. Lancet Oncol 2008;9:636–48.
38. Fleck J, Carmargo J, Godoy D, et al. Chemoradiation therapy (CRT) versus chemotherapy (CT) alone as a neoadjuvant treatment for stage III non-small cell lung cancer (NSCLC). Preliminary report of a phase III prospective randomized trial. Proc ASCO 1993. Abstract 1108.
39. Van Meerbeeck JP, Kramer GW, Van Schil PE, et al. Randomized controlled trial of resection versus radiotherapy after induction chemotherapy in stage IIIA-N2 non-small-cell lung cancer. J Natl Cancer Inst 2007;99:442–50.
40. Higgins K, Chino JP, Marks LB, et al. Preoperative chemotherapy versus preoperative chemoradiotherapy for stage III (N2) non-small-cell lung cancer. Int J Radiat Oncol Biol Phys 2009;75(5): 1462–7.
41. Albain KS, Swann RS, Rusch VW, et al. Radiotherapy plus chemotherapy with or without surgical resection for stage III non-small-cell lung cancer: a phase III randomised controlled trial. Lancet 2009; 374(9687):379–86.
42. Sonett JR, Suntharalingam M, Edelman MJ, et al. Pulmonary resection after curative intent radiotherapy (>59 Gy) and concurrent chemotherapy in non-small-cell lung cancer. Ann Thorac Surg 2004;78(4):1200–5.
43. Daly BD, Fernando HC, Ketchedjian A, et al. Pneumonectomy after high-dose radiation and concurrent chemotherapy for nonsmall cell lung cancer. Ann Thorac Surg 2006;82(1):227–31.
44. Shah AA, Berry MF, Tzao C, et al. Induction chemoradiation is not superior to induction chemotherapy alone in stage IIIA lung cancer. Ann Thorac Surg 2012;93(6):1807–12.
45. National Comprehensive Cancer Network. Non-small cell lung cancer. Available at: http://www.nccn.org/professionals/physician_gls/pdf/nscl.pdf.
46. Van Meerbeeck JP, Meersschout S, De Pauw R, et al. Intensity modulated radiotherapy as part of combined modality treatment in locally advanced non-small cell lung cancer. Oncologist 2008;13: 700–8.
47. PORT Meta-analysis Trialists Group. Post operative radiotherapy for non-small cell lung cancer [Cochrane review]. Cochrane Database Syst Rev 2005;2.
48. Bradley JD, Paulus R, Graham MV, et al, Radiation Therapy Oncology Group. Phase II trial of postoperative adjuvant paclitaxel/carboplatin and thoracic radiotherapy in resected stage II and IIIA non-small-cell lung cancer: promising long-term results of the Radiation Therapy Oncology Group–RTOG 9705. J Clin Oncol 2005;23(15):3480–7.
49. Lally BE, Zelterman D, Colasanto JM, et al. Postoperative radiotherapy for stage II or III non-small-cell lung cancer using the surveillance, epidemiology, and end results database. J Clin Oncol 2006; 24(19):2998–3006.
50. Amini A, Correa AM, Komaki R, et al. The role of consolidation therapy for stage III non-small cell lung cancer with persistent N2 disease after induction chemotherapy. Ann Thorac Surg 2012;94(3): 914–20.

Reconstruction of the Bronchus and Pulmonary Artery

Mohsen Ibrahim, MD, PhD[a,*], Giulio Maurizi, MD[a],
Federico Venuta, MD[b,c], Erino Angelo Rendina, MD[a,c]

KEYWORDS

• Sleeve lobectomy • Pulmonary artery • Non–small cell lung cancer

KEY POINTS

- A lateral muscle-sparing incision allows a bronchovascular reconstructive procedure to be performed comfortably and safely.
- In patients undergoing bronchial resection, postoperative use of low-dose steroids is favorable because it reduces secretion retention and atelectasis.
- A main concern in bronchial and vascular reconstructive procedures is avoiding tension on the anastomosis.
- When pulmonary artery reconstruction is required, appropriate anticoagulation management is crucial (1500 U heparin sodium during the resection phase without reversal by protamine sulfate).
- Sleeve lobectomy can be performed safely and effectively after induction therapy, without an increased complication rate.

INTRODUCTION

Sleeve lobectomy (SL) (lobectomy associated with resection and reconstruction of the bronchus, the pulmonary artery [PA], or both) has proved to be a suitable choice for the treatment of centrally located non–small cell lung cancer.[1,2]

SL for lung cancer is indicated when a tumor infiltrates the origin of a lobar bronchus and/or the origin of the lobar branches of the PA (**Fig. 1**) but not to the extent that a pneumonectomy (PN) is required. In addition, SL may be indicated for N1 lymph node infiltration of the bronchus and/or the PA, as is often the case in left upper lobe tumors that require combined bronchovascular reconstruction. Reconstructive procedures may also be indicated after induction therapy when unremovable fibrotic tissue is embedded in the PA and/or the bronchus.

These surgical procedures may be necessary to avoid PN in patients with compromised cardiac and/or pulmonary function, but recent studies have shown that the advantages of sparing lung parenchyma are also evident in patients without cardiopulmonary impairment.[3]

Although bronchovascular reconstruction associated with lobectomy represents operations with higher technical difficulty when compared with standard major lung resection, postoperative morbidity and mortality data from recent experiences reported better overall results in patients undergoing SL than in patients undergoing PN (**Table 1**).[4–15]

Postoperative quality of life has been advocated as one of the strongest factors to consider when making the decision to perform an SL rather than a PN. Several studies have demonstrated that

Conflict of Interest and Source of funding: None declared.
[a] Department of Thoracic Surgery, Sant'Andrea Hospital, Sapienza University of Rome, Via di Grottarossa, 1035, Rome 00189, Italy; [b] Department of Thoracic Surgery, Policlinico Umberto I, Sapienza University of Rome, Rome, Italy; [c] Spencer-Cenci Lorillard Foundation, Rome, Italy
* Corresponding author.
E-mail address: mohsen.ibrahim@uniroma1.it

Thorac Surg Clin 23 (2013) 337–347
http://dx.doi.org/10.1016/j.thorsurg.2013.05.007
1547-4127/13/$ – see front matter

thoracic.theclinics.com

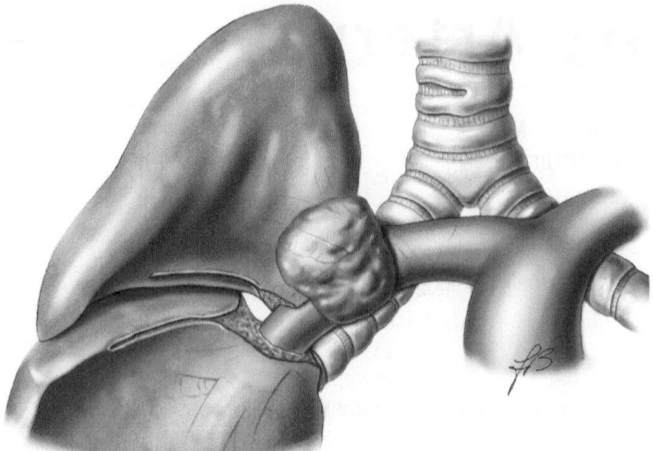

Fig. 1. Tumor infiltrates the origin of the right upper lobar bronchus and the origin of the lobar branches of the PA.

lung parenchyma sparing improves postoperative quality of life due to a greater pulmonary reserve,[12,15] with a statistically significant difference favoring SL based on postoperative loss of FEV1.

Nevertheless, the decision to perform PN or SL is made with the aim of complete resection of the tumor, with free resection margins, while considering both the oncological and physiologic aspects. Many surgeons think that PN, particularly right PN, is a disease itself, with severe postoperative impairment of lung function, cardiac function, and quality of life and, therefore, should be performed only when necessary to obtain full oncological radicality. Since the first sleeve resections were reported in the early 1950s,[16,17] significant technical advances and increasing experience over time have allowed the achievement of excellent clinical and oncologic results, resulting in wide use and consensus in the use of parenchymal-sparing procedures for lung cancer.

BRONCHIAL RESECTIONS

Technical Issues

Bronchial sleeve resections and reconstructions are commonly performed through the same thoracotomy made for standard pulmonary resections (posterolateral or lateral muscle-sparing incisions, which are both suitable for exposure and dissection). The authors' technique starts with the dissection beginning in the anterior hilum and then continuing to complete dissection of the main PA. In cases when bulky disease causes increased difficulty during dissection, the pericardium can be opened on either side to gain

Table 1
Results of reported series comparing SL with PN: morbidity, mortality, and long-term survival

	Pts		Morbidity (%)		Mortality (%)		Surv (5 y) (%)	
Author (y)	**SL**	**PN**	**SL**	**PN**	**SL**	**PN**	**SL**	**PN**
Okada et al,[5] 2000	60	60	13.0	22.0	2.8	2.0	48.0	28.0
Deslauriers et al,[6] 2004	184	1046	—	—	1.6	5.3	52.0	31.0
Bagan et al,[8] 2005	66	151	28.8	29.9	4.5	12.6	72.5	51.2
Ludwig et al,[7] 2005	116	194	38.0	26.0	4.3	4.6	39.0	27.0
Takeda et al,[11] 2006	62	110	45.0	40.9	4.8	3.6	54.1	32.9
Parissis et al,[13] 2009	79	129	16.4	21.6	2.5	8.5	46.8	37.1
Park et al,[14] 2010	105	105	29.5	33.4	1.0	8.6	58.4	32.1
Gomez-Caro et al,[15] 2011	55	21	32.0	33.0	3.6	5.0	61.0	31.0

Abbreviations: Pts, patients; Surv, survival.

improved proximal control. Next, the main PA is surrounded with surgical umbilical tape. The subsequent steps are specific to the type of sleeve resection performed, and each is described independently in the following sections.

Upper SL

Right side

The dissection starts superiorly at the level of the right upper lobe bronchus. The lung is retracted anteriorly, and dissection is continued in the bifurcation between the right upper lobe bronchus and the intermediate bronchus. The lymph node frequently found in this location, is elevated away from the bifurcation to expose the pulmonary arterial branch to the posterior segment of the right lower lobe. Once this branch is identified, the posterior portion of the fissure is completed with a linear stapler. This approach avoids extensive parenchymal dissection in the fissure. The intermediate bronchus is encircled just distal to the right upper lobe takeoff, and surgical umbilical tape is placed to aid airway division at the appropriate site. Once complete resectability is confirmed, ligation and division of the pulmonary arterial branches to the right upper lobe are performed. Similarly, the pulmonary vein branch draining the upper lobe is divided with a vascular stapler, taking care to preserve the middle lobe venous drainage. The minor fissure is completed with a linear stapler. The main stem bronchus is encircled with umbilical tape at its origin.

The bronchial resection phase is then started. The mainstem bronchus is divided just proximal to the right upper lobe takeoff. Once the bronchus has been opened, the decision to proceed with a sleeve resection may be made based on macroscopic or microscopic findings. Subsequently, the intermediate bronchus is divided just distal to the right upper lobe takeoff. These cuts must be perpendicular to the long axis of the airway. A frozen-section examination of the bronchial resection margins is then performed to confirm the radicality of resection. Microscopic tumors found at the bronchial margin require either additional resection of the involved area or PN.

Different techniques have been described for bronchial anastomotic reconstruction. The authors favor the use of interrupted sutures of 4-0 monofilament absorbable material.[18,19] The employment of continuous running suture (complete or partial) has been described by others.[15,20] In the authors' technique (**Fig. 2**), the first suture is placed in an outside-to-inside fashion at the junction of the cartilaginous and membranous bronchi. These initial sutures can be immediately tied to confer improved stability to this point of the anastomosis. Additional sutures are placed at 2-mm intervals to complete the first half of the cartilaginous anastomosis. Once the midpoint of the cartilaginous bronchus is reached, the anastomosis is then completed on the opposite side of the bronchial circumference in a similar fashion. Sutures are then tied, starting from either end of the cartilaginous portion and working toward the middle. Placing and tying the sutures in this order allows compensation for even large-caliber discrepancies. This technique prevents torsion of the bronchial axis and gently stretches and dilates the circumference of the distal bronchus. The anastomosis is then tested with 20 cm water inflation pressure by filling the pleural cavity with saline solution. Needle-hole air leaks are usually ignored; however, air leaks between the cut edges of the bronchus, if small, are reinforced with simple interrupted sutures. A large area of leakage may require replacement of the entire anastomosis. Most investigators recommend protecting the bronchial anastomosis with a viable tissue flap.[21,22] The present authors routinely use an intercostal muscle flap,[21] which has excellent vascularization provided by the intercostal artery; enables preservation of airtightness, even in the event of small anastomotic dehiscence; and minimizes the risk of PA erosion, particularly when an associated vascular reconstruction is performed. Alternatively, the mediastinal fat pad,[22] pericardial tissue, or pleural tissue[20] have been used as viable flaps. For the final success of bronchial reconstruction, it is essential to avoid tension on the anastomosis, which can be achieved by dividing the pulmonary ligament or, more often on the right side, by opening the pericardium around the pulmonary vein.

Left side

Proximal arterial control is obtained taking care to avoid injury to the short apical-posterior segmental branch of the left PA. Dissection is continued along the plane of the artery, and the superior segmental branch to the lower lobe is identified. The posterior fissure is then completed with a linear stapler. The arterial segmental branches to the upper lobe are ligated and divided. The upper pulmonary vein is divided with a vascular stapler. The anterior portion of the fissure is completed with a linear stapler. The mainstem bronchus is encircled proximal to the bifurcation, and umbilical tape is placed. The mainstem bronchus is divided proximal to the bifurcation, and the left lower lobe bronchus is divided at its origin. The origin of the superior segmental bronchus can be quite close to the origin of the lower lobe bronchus, and the lobar

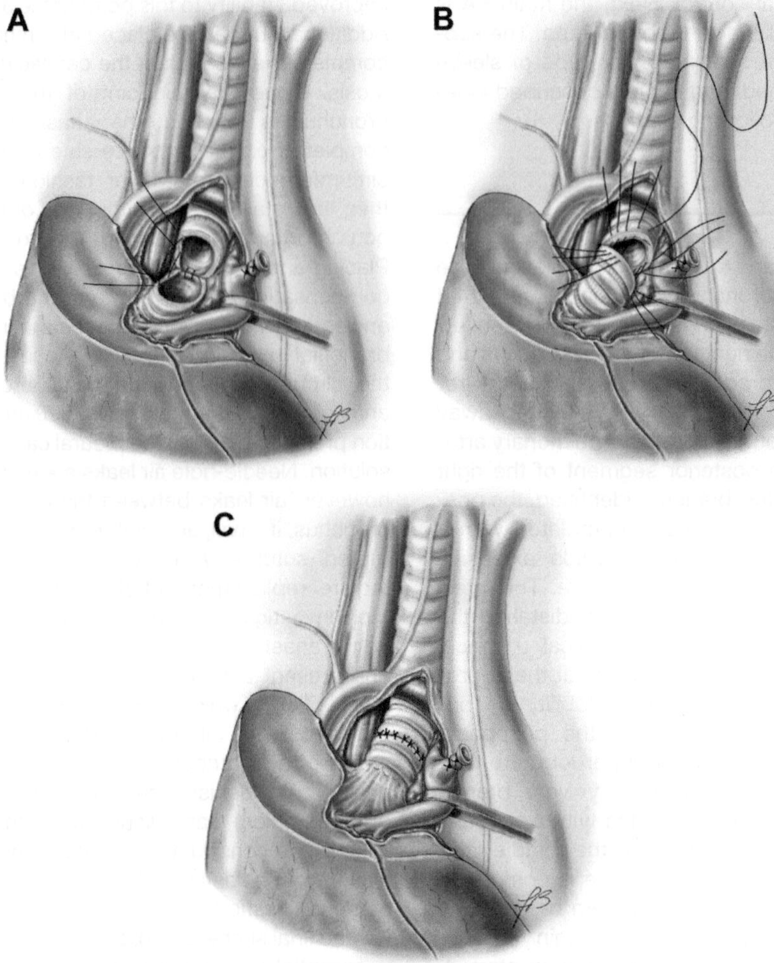

Fig. 2. Right upper bronchial SL. Anastomotic reconstruction (*A, B*). Interrupted sutures have been placed but are still untied. (*C*) Completed bronchial anastomosis.

division must leave the bronchus intact without separating the superior segmental bronchus.

The technique for anastomotic reconstruction has been described previously for right upper SL. Extensive proximal resections can be performed on the left side because of the length of the mainstem bronchus. This anatomic aspect may be responsible for a technically challenging anastomosis because proximal exposure can be partially obscured by the aortic arch. If necessary, the arch can be mobilized and carefully retracted to provide additional exposure. Precise suture placement is particularly important to account for the size discrepancy between the lobar bronchus and the mainstem bronchus.

Middle Lobe Sleeve Resection

Middle lobe sleeve resection is performed infrequently. The bronchus to the middle lobe lies immediately posterior to the middle lobe vein. The bronchus is followed back to its origin. A right-angled clamp is placed around the bronchus intermedius, and this is divided proximally to the middle lobe orifice. The division is slightly angled. The distal division is also angled to preserve the orifice to the superior segment of the lower lobe. The PA lies directly posterior and slightly superior to the bronchus. Therefore, care must be taken to avoid PA injury when dividing the bronchus. The arterial branch to the middle lobe is ligated and divided. After confirmation of negative margins, the airway anastomosis is performed according to the previously described technique.

Lower SL (Y Sleeve)

Right side (sleeve bilobectomy)

Sleeve bilobectomy is performed for an endoluminal lesion in the bronchus intermedius that extends up proximal to the upper lobe orifice. The right mainstem bronchus is divided at this level just proximal to the right upper lobe takeoff, and the right upper lobe bronchus is divided at its origin. The right upper lobe bronchus is then anastomosed to the mainstem bronchus after removal of the middle and lower lobes (the so-called Y sleeve resection). Because of the reorientation of the upper lobe bronchus after removal of the middle and lower lobes, special care must be taken to avoid torsion of the bronchus at the level of the anastomosis.

Left side

For excision of lesions involving the left lower lobe orifice with extension into the mainstem bronchus but sparing the upper lobe orifice, a lower lobectomy with sleeve resection of the left main bronchus can be performed. After completion of the bronchial dissection, umbilical tape is passed around the left mainstem and left upper lobe bronchus. The left upper lobe bronchus is divided at its origin. Next, the mainstem bronchus is divided proximal to the bifurcation and well beyond the extent of the tumor. Once the margins are confirmed microscopically to be negative by frozen-section analysis, anastomotic reconstruction is performed according to the previously described technique. The lingular bronchus may arise proximally to the section line, and care must be taken when dividing the upper lobe bronchus to ensure that it remains intact.

PA RECONSTRUCTION

Technical Issues

Primary or metastatic lung tumors and metastatic N1 lymph nodes with extracapsular extension can infiltrate the PA and involve it to different extents. Limited tangential resection and direct suture are required for partial infiltration of the arterial wall.[23]

More extensive involvement of the PA may require sleeve resection and reconstruction by an end-to-end anastomosis, a patch, or prosthetic/autologous conduit. Moreover, residual tumor or scarring tissue after induction therapy can involve the PA and require a sleeve resection.

However, extended infiltration of the PA, such as a left upper lobe tumor infiltrating the concave surface of the PA from its origin down to the anterobasal artery or, on the right side, posterolateral infiltration from the upper division artery to the artery for the superior segment of the lower lobe, makes PN mandatory to achieve complete tumor resection.

The resection phase and the anastomotic reconstruction have been generally standardized as follows. Achieving full control of the PA is important. The resection step should begin when the PA, bronchus, and pulmonary veins are appropriately prepared. In general, control of the pulmonary veins is much less challenging because they are anatomically distant from tumors that are resectable through a sleeve. However, on the left side, the upper lobe bronchus and the anterior portion of the fissure may have tumor involvement. The superior pulmonary vein can be easily controlled intrapericardially. The dissection in the interlobar fissure is essential for the reconstructive procedure, particularly on the left side. After intravenous injection of 1500 U heparin sodium, the main PA is clamped distantly from the suture line and from the inferior pulmonary vein.

During the reconstructive step of surgery, 3 basic techniques (patch reconstruction, end-to-end anastomosis, and conduit interposition) can be considered based on the PA defect. Running 5-0 monofilament nonabsorbable sutures are used for all of the various PA reconstruction procedures.[24–26] After the suture line is completed, the venous clamp is removed before the suture is tied, and backflow is restored to allow air drainage. The suture is then tied and the arterial clamp is removed. Before closing the chest, it is very important to check the suture line and carefully test lung re-expansion to exclude the possibility of kinking or folding of the PA. At the end of the procedure, particularly if a bronchial sleeve was also performed, it is advisable to interpose viable tissue between the artery and the bronchus. The authors' preference is an intercostal muscle flap.[21] In the postoperative period, anticoagulation therapy (6000 U/d low-molecular-weight heparin) is administered subcutaneously for 7 to 10 days.

Partial Resection and Patch Reconstruction

Patch reconstruction is very versatile and can be used in a variety of circumstances. These circumstances range from limited infiltration involving the origin of segmental arteries to large defects extended longitudinally on one aspect of the PA. The only necessary condition is that the opposite side of the circumference of the PA be free from tumor. If this is not the case, sleeve resection with end-to-end anastomosis or conduit interposition is performed. The arterial reconstruction is performed before the bronchial anastomosis to reduce the arterial clamping time. After the resection, an oval defect oriented along the PA axis ensues, even if the resected portion was round, because of the tension applied on the vessel by the lower lobe. The patch, therefore, is tailored on the resected portion rather than on the PA defect. Various patches can be used; biologic materials, such as azygos vein, autologous pericardial tissue, and bovine pericardial tissue, are preferable because of better biocompatibility. The autologous pericardial tissue is harvested anteriorly to the phrenic nerve, and the pericardial defect is left open. The patch is trimmed appropriately and secured to the artery by 2 stay sutures. The inferior stay suture is not tied; it is used only to keep the patch in place and will be removed when the suture line reaches its level. Some degree of tension is desirable at this stage; it shows that the patch is not exceedingly long, and tension will disappear after unclamping. Suturing must be done very carefully because the edge of the pericardial tissue tends to shrink and curl, and sutures that are too wide apart may result. The pitfalls of harvesting, trimming, and suturing the autologous pericardial tissue are overcome by the use of bovine pericardial tissue, which displays little if any elasticity and has even and stiff edges. The use of autologous or bovine pericardial tissue is recommend because it does not require a separate procedure and the amount of tissue is not limited. The patch is sutured using running 5-0 or 6-0 monofilament nonabsorbable material, proceeding from the top to bottom on the right side, while grasping and stretching the patch, continuing from the bottom to top on the left side (**Fig. 3**).

Sleeve Resection and Reconstruction by End-to-End Anastomosis

PA reconstruction is usually performed after completion of the bronchial anastomosis to minimize the manipulation of the vessel.

When transecting the artery, both proximally and distally, regular and even margins are desirable, even at the cost of some loss of tissue. This practice allows proper placement of the stitches and yields an even inside lumen. In addition, regular suture borders facilitate the correction of the large-caliber discrepancy that usually occurs. In addition, the exposure of the bronchial stumps is optimal when the artery is divided. If the vascular and bronchial procedures are done simultaneously, the bronchial axis is shortened, and the PA stumps are opposable with acceptable tension. On completion of the bronchial anastomosis, the distance between the 2 arterial ends will be markedly decreased, and it can be further reduced by elevating the lower lobe while suturing. Restoration of blood flow and removal of the proximal clamp relieves any residual tension. If the distance between the arterial stumps is deemed excessive, the interposition of a prosthetic conduit is indicated. The anastomosis is performed with running 5-0 or 6-0 monofilament nonabsorbable material. Additionally, the sutures are placed very carefully to avoid stenosis. End-to-end anastomosis can be technically difficult because of the unexpected traction between the stumps and caliber discrepancy (**Fig. 4**).

Sleeve Resection and Reconstruction by a Prosthetic Conduit

Conduit interposition may be useful when a left upper lobe tumor infiltrates the PA extensively but the lobar bronchus is not involved and, therefore, a bronchial sleeve is not indicated. This unusual situation (PA sleeve without bronchial sleeve) may produce a long bronchial segment separating the

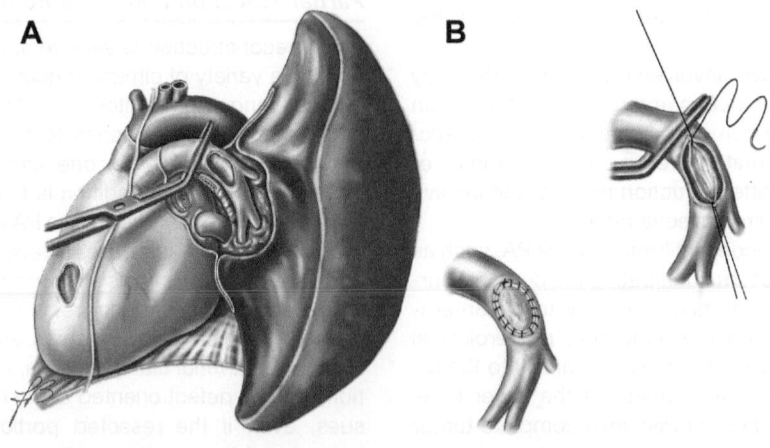

Fig. 3. PA reconstruction. Partial wall resection and patch reconstruction (*A*) after upper lobectomy and partial resection of the PA (an oval defect ensues). Proximal PA stumps is clamped. The pericardial defect is left open. (*B*) The patch is held in place by 2 stay sutures. Completed patch reconstruction of the PA.

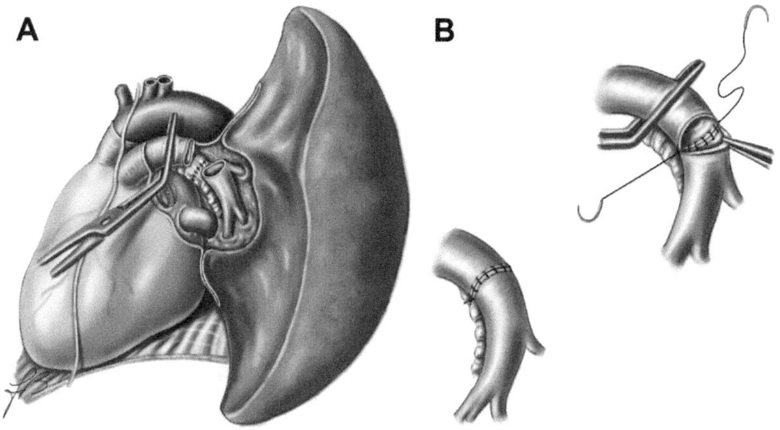

Fig. 4. PA reconstruction. Sleeve resection and reconstruction by end-to-end anastomosis. (*A*) Completed arterial sleeve resection (proximal stump is clamped). The arterial anastomosis is performed after the bronchial suture to minimize manipulation of the vessel. (*B*) Vascular end-to-end anastomosis.

2 widely spaced PA stumps, so that an end-to-end anastomosis is not possible. A prosthetic conduit of synthetic or biologic material, such as autologous pericardial tissue[27] or pulmonary vein portion,[28] can be used. Autologous pericardial tissue or pulmonary vein conduits are fresh and unpreserved, cost-free, and biocompatible. Conversely, bovine pericardial tissue is less cost-effective and less biocompatible but very easy to use. Recently, the authors have preferred the autologous vein conduit when it is feasible to obtain (tumors have not infiltrated the extrapericardial pulmonary vein portion) because it is more useable than pericardial tissue and because other synthetic materials might increase the risk of thrombosis.

When performing upper lobectomy, the pericardium must be opened to gain improved proximal control of the superior pulmonary vein. Subsequently, the superior vein is completely dissected out and sutured proximally with a vascular thoracic-abdominal stapler and ligated distally, thereby dividing it and creating an autologous vein conduit of approximately 2 to 3 cm (preserved in saline solution) (**Fig. 5**). A frozen-section examination of the proximal margin on the vein resection specimen is then performed to confirm the radicality of resection. It is advisable to tailor the length of the conduit from the resected arterial segment because the elasticity of the 2 tissues is comparable. The proximal anastomosis is performed first with running 5-0 monofilament suture (**Fig. 6**). The distal anastomosis is performed last, after the conduit has been trimmed to the appropriate length. It is advisable to parachute the distal end of the conduit, folding it over on itself to obtain some degree of tension, which will disappear after declamping. When the blood flow is restored, the dimension of the conduit will increase. Care must be taken to avoid lengthening the PA, which may cause kinking of the vessel, impaired blood flow, and, ultimately, thrombus formation.

COMMENT

There are some critical and controversial aspects concerning the intraoperative and perioperative management of a bronchial sleeve resection and/or PA reconstruction that are of a different nature and may determine the outcome. To take stock of what we have learned from these lung-sparing operations over time, the authors have analyzed some of the most important aspects independently in the following paragraphs.

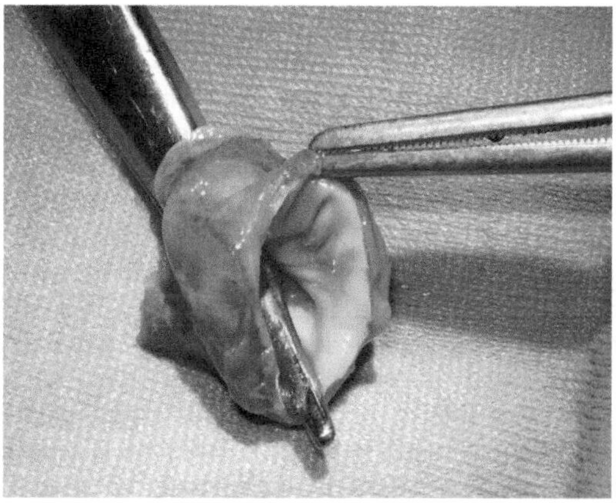

Fig. 5. PA reconstruction. Prosthetic conduit of superior pulmonary vein portion before suturing.

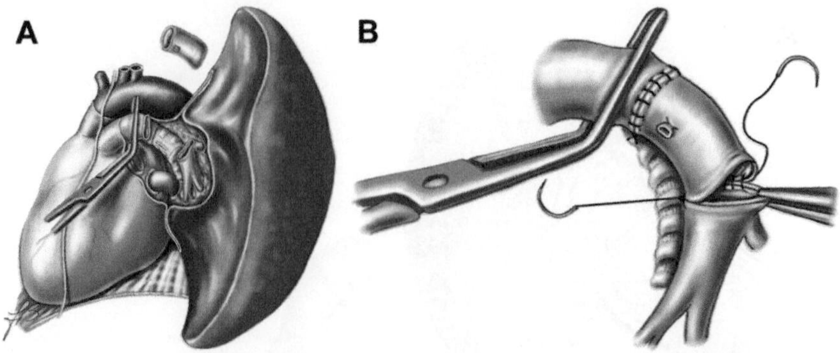

Fig. 6. PA reconstruction. Sleeve resection and reconstruction by autologous superior pulmonary vein conduit. (*A*) After left upper lobectomy, PA sleeve resection is performed (proximal stump is clamped). (*B*) Autologous pulmonary vein conduit of 2 to 3 cm is sutured.

Surgical Incision

Many surgeons are still convinced that wide surgical incisions are preferable for performing complex bronchovascular reconstructions. However, recently some investigators have described video-assisted thoracic surgery (VATS) SL.[29] The authors think that through the improvement of surgical skills and experience, posterolateral thoracotomy might be replaced by a muscle-sparing mini-thoracotomy that allows a reconstructive procedure to be performed comfortably and safely.

Steroids

Another aspect that still remains controversial is the use of postoperative steroids in patients undergoing bronchial resection. The authors think that the postoperative use of low-dose steroids is favorable because it reduces secretion retention and atelectasis, facilitates parenchymal reexpansion, and minimizes the risk of dehiscence and granuloma formation. Aerosolized steroids are also part of postoperative treatment.

Bronchoscopy

When considering the role of bronchoscopy in these complex lung-sparing operations, it is important that an endoscopic examination is performed by one of the operating surgeons in candidates for a sleeve resection. This examination is advantageous at the time of the operation, when the bronchi are incised and divided. It is also useful to have precise knowledge of the preoperative and intraoperative appearance of the airway to detect a stiffness of the bronchial wall that may indicate peribronchial tumor infiltration. This item is crucial in areas where the bronchus is known to be adjacent to the PA, which consequently might be involved.

Routine bronchoscopies are performed at the end of the surgical procedure, before discharge from the hospital, and after 1 and 6 months.

The Use of Viable Tissue Flaps

Bronchoarterial fistula can be effectively prevented by interposing a viable tissue flap between the 2 structures. The use of a mediastinal fat pad, pericardial flap, or pleural flap has been reported.[20,22] However, an intercostal muscle flap is preferable because of its excellent vascularization provided by the intercostal artery.[21]

The preparation of the flap is performed before opening the chest, and the rib retractor is not inserted until the procedure is completed to avoid crushing the intercostal vessels. The periosteum of the fifth rib is incised and then separated from the bone in continuity with the underlying intercostal muscle. Care must be taken to preserve the muscular insertion to the periosteum to avoid injuring the intercostal neurovascular bundle. The intercostal muscle is then incised in the vicinity of the underlying sixth rib, and the anterior insertion of the flap is divided. The pedicle is ligated at its anterior extremity. When the bronchial anastomosis is completed, a large right-angle clamp is slid between the PA and the bronchus, and the suture at the extremity of the flap is slid backward around the bronchial anastomosis and between the bronchus and the PA. The flap is then twisted until its pleural side is in contact with the bronchial anastomosis and the pleura is secured to the bronchus by interrupted absorbable 4-0 sutures.

Avoidance Techniques for Kinking of the PA

A main concern in bronchial and vascular reconstructive procedures is avoiding tension on the anastomosis.

During a patch reconstruction procedure, if some degree of tension exists, it is safer to complete the posterior portion of the suture and subsequently parachute the 2 stumps together while lifting the lower lobe. When a patch reconstruction is associated with a bronchial sleeve, the bronchial axis is shortened, and the length of the artery remains stationary. The PA may tend to kink and fold over on itself. The repositioning of the PA caused by the re-expansion of the lower lobe may increase this risk further. Impairment of blood flow may ensue, and thrombosis may occur. Under these circumstances, it is better to cut away the distorted segment and proceed to an end-to-end anastomosis.

During an end-to-end anastomosis reconstruction, dividing the pulmonary ligament or, more often on the right side, opening the pericardium around the pulmonary vein can be useful to obtain a tension-free suture.

PA Reconstruction with Prosthetic Conduit

The main pitfall in the use of a conduit is sizing its length. Application of the proposed technical issues will prevent this problem. The authors think that the autologous pulmonary vein conduit is preferable for PA reconstruction because it is very easy to use and because other materials might increase the risk of thrombosis. Autologous vein conduit is fresh and unpreserved, cost-free, and biocompatible. Conversely, bovine pericardial tissue is less cost-effective and less biocompatible.

Radiologic Management After PA Reconstruction

Noninvasive radiologic techniques, such as magnetic resonance angiography (MRA) or computed tomography (CT) scan with contrast medium and 3-dimensional (3D) volume rendering, provide outstanding imaging of the PA and may be very useful in demonstrating patency problems even in the immediate postoperative period. In the absence of clinical symptoms, pulmonary angiograms in addition to perfusion lung scans are redundant. In the long term, CT with contrast medium has proved to be a handy, noninvasive diagnostic tool that is useful to evaluate PA patency and distal PA branching as well as the overall oncologic status of patients.

Anticoagulation Management

When PA reconstruction is required, appropriate anticoagulation management is crucial. Initial reports[30] did not clarify this important aspect. Historically, systemic anticoagulation was initiated during the operation (3000–5000 U heparin sodium)[25] and maintained by subcutaneous injection of heparin (15.000 U/d) for 7 to 10 days. The authors now think that intravenous injection of 1500 U heparin sodium during the resection phase without reversal by protamine sulfate at the end of the procedure[26,31] as well as 6000 U/d low-molecular-weight heparin administered subcutaneously for 7 days after surgery is sufficient.

Postoperative Bleeding Avoidance

Because the PA is a low-pressure vessel, leakage from the suture line may pass unnoticed intraoperatively. Also, bleeding may start on the first or second postoperative day after a patch reconstruction. A blood loss of as much as 800 to 1000 mL daily may occur after 1 or 2 days of no drainage, which may last for 1 or 2 days and then stop spontaneously, independently from anticoagulation. Sutures too wide apart may result after unclamping and distention. These sutures would not cause bleeding immediately because the PA is stretched downward by the atelectatic lower lobe, and simple apposition of the tissue edges is enough to counteract the low PA pressure. However, in the postoperative period when the re-expansion of the lower lobe elevates the hilum, rotation and kinking of the PA may distort the suture line and reopen the bleeding site. It is, therefore, very important, especially when using autologous pericardial patches, to check the suture line carefully and test the PA position after re-expansion of the residual lobe.

Induction Therapy

SL can be performed safely and effectively after induction therapy, without an increased complication rate.[32,33] After induction therapy, the bronchus and/or PA can be involved to a various extent either by residual tumor or by desmoplastic reaction, scarring tissue, or fibrosis. Concern over an increased complication rate in these patients has been proved to be excessive and, in the authors' experience, bronchial and PA reconstructive techniques can be performed in this setting safely and effectively. A recent study[33] showed that there was no significant difference in mortality and morbidity rates of patients undergoing SL with and without induction therapy. In addition, the same study demonstrated that after induction therapy, the long-term survival of patients undergoing SL was better than patients undergoing PN.

Comparison Between PA Reconstruction Alone and PA Reconstruction Associated with Bronchial Sleeve

It has been demonstrated[25,26] that the survival of patients undergoing PA reconstruction is

Table 2
Results of studies reporting PA reconstruction

Author (y)	Pts	Morbidity (%)	Mortality (%)	Surv (5 y) (%)
Rendina et al,[25] 1999	52	13.4	0	38.3
Shrager et al,[23] 2000	33[a]	45.0	0	46.7 (4 y)
Lausberg et al,[10] 2005	67	—	1.5	42.9[b]
Nagayasu et al,[35] 2006	29	27.6	17.2	24.2[b]
Cerfolio et al,[31] 2007	42	26.0	2.3	60.0
Alifano et al,[34] 2009	93[c]	29.0	5.4	39.4
Venuta et al,[26] 2009	105	28.5	0.95	44.0

Abbreviations: Pts, patients; Surv, survival.
[a] Only tangential resections.
[b] Overall survival for combined bronchovascular reconstruction.
[c] Tangential resections (n = 88).

comparable, stage-by-stage, to that reported in the major reviews on lung cancer surgery and sleeve resection in the literature. The impact of nodal status on survival is also comparable with that reported for bronchial sleeve and standard resection. In the face of N1 or N2 involvement, once the decision to resect the disease with intent to cure is taken, PA reconstruction can also be proposed as an adequate procedure in this setting. Moreover, there is no significant difference between PA reconstruction alone and PA reconstruction associated with bronchial sleeve in terms of postoperative mortality and morbidity.[34] One apparently new datum that surfaces from the authors' recent study[26] and is different from their previous report[25] is that combined bronchovascular reconstructions may offer better survival. This finding suggests that even these complex lung-sparing operations can be pursued with intent to cure as long as a complete anatomic resection is achieved (**Table 2**).[10,23,25,26,31,34,35]

ACKNOWLEDGMENTS

The authors wish to thank Dr Elisabetta Grigioni for data management and editorial revision.

REFERENCES

1. Ma Z, Dong J, Fan J, et al. Does sleeve lobectomy concomitant with or without pulmonary artery reconstruction (double sleeve) have favorable results for non-small cell lung cancer compared with pneumonectomy? A meta-analysis. Eur J Cardiothorac Surg 2007;32:20–8.
2. Shi W, Zhang W, Sun H, et al. Sleeve lobectomy versus pneumonectomy for non –small cell lung cancer. World J Surg Oncol 2012;10(1):265.
3. D'Andrilli A, Ciccone AM, Ibrahim M, et al. Pneumonectomy versus sleeve resection: M07–02. J Thorac Oncol 2007;2(8):170–1.
4. Gaissert HA, Mathisen DJ, Moncure AC, et al. Survival and function after sleeve lobectomy for lung cancer. J Thorac Cardiovasc Surg 1996; 111:948–53.
5. Okada M, Yamagashi H, Stak S, et al. Survival related to lymph node involvement in lung cancer after sleeve lobectomy compared with pneumonectomy. J Thorac Cardiovasc Surg 2000;119:814–9.
6. Deslauriers J, Grégoire J, Jacques LF, et al. Sleeve lobectomy versus pneumonectomy for lung cancer: a comparative analysis of survival and sites of recurrence. Ann Thorac Surg 2004;77:1152–6.
7. Ludwig C, Stoelben E, Olschewski M, et al. Comparison of morbidity, 30-day mortality, and long term survival after pneumonectomy and sleeve lobectomy for non-small cell lung carcinoma. Ann Thorac Surg 2005;79:968–73.
8. Bagan P, Berna P, Pereira JC, et al. Sleeve lobectomy versus pneumonectomy: tumor characteristics and comparative analysis of feasibility and results. Ann Thorac Surg 2005;80:2046–50.
9. Kim YT, Kang CH, Sung SW, et al. Local control of disease related to lymph node involvement in non-small cell lung cancer after sleeve lobectomy compared with pneumonectomy. Ann Thorac Surg 2005;79:1153–61.
10. Lausberg HF, Graeter TP, Tscholl D, et al. Bronchovascular versus bronchial sleeve resection for central lung tumors. Ann Thorac Surg 2005;79:1147–52.
11. Takeda S, Maeda H, Koma M, et al. Comparison of surgical results after pneumonectomy and sleeve lobectomy for non-small cell lung cancer: trends over time and 20-year institutional experience. Eur J Cardiothorac Surg 2006;29:276–80.
12. Melloul E, Egger B, Krueger T, et al. Mortality, complications and loss of pulmonary function after

pneumonectomy vs. sleeve lobectomy in patients younger and older than 70 years. Interact Cardiovasc Thorac Surg 2008;7:986–9.
13. Parissis H, Leotsinidis M, Hughes A, et al. Comparative analysis and outcomes of sleeve resection versus pneumonectomy. Asian Cardiovasc Thorac Ann 2009;17:175–82.
14. Park JS, Yang HC, Kim HK, et al. Sleeve lobectomy as an alternative procedure to pneumonectomy for non-small cell lung cancer. J Thorac Oncol 2010;5: 517–20.
15. Gomez-Caro A, Garcia S, Reguart N, et al. Determining the appropriate sleeve lobectomy versus pneumonectomy ratio in central non-small cell lung cancer patients: an audit of an aggressive policy of pneumonectomy avoidance. Eur J Cardiothorac Surg 2011;39:352–9.
16. Price-Thomas CP. Conservative resection of the bronchial tree. J R Coll Surg Edinb 1955;1(3):169–86.
17. Allison PR. Course of thoracic surgery in Groningen. Quoted by: Jones PH: Lobectomy and bronchial anastomosis in the surgery of bronchial carcinoma. Ann R Coll Surg Engl 1954;25:20–2.
18. Rendina EA, De Giacomo T, Venuta F, et al. Lung conservation techniques: bronchial sleeve resection and reconstruction of the pulmonary artery. Semin Surg Oncol 2000;18:165–72.
19. Rendina EA, Venta F, Ciriaco P, et al. Bronchovascular sleeve resection. Technique, perioperative management, prevention and treatment of complications. J Thorac Cardiovasc Surg 1993;106(1):73–9.
20. Yildizeli B, Fadel E, Mussot S, et al. Morbidity, mortality, and long-term survival after sleeve lobectomy for non-small cell lung cancer. Eur J Cardiothorac Surg 2007;31(1):95–102.
21. Rendina EA, Venuta F, Ricci P, et al. Protection and revascularization of bronchial anastomoses by the intercostal pedicle flap. J Thorac Cardiovasc Surg 1994;107(5):1251–4.
22. Tsuchiya R. Bronchoplastic techniques. In: Patterson GA, Deslauriers J, Lerut A, et al, editors. Pearson's thoracic and esophageal surgery. 2nd edition. Philadelphia: Churchill Livingstone; 2002. p. 1005.
23. Shrager JB, Lambright ES, McGrath CM, et al. Lobectomy with tangential pulmonary artery resection without regard to pulmonary function. Ann Thorac Surg 2000;70:234–9.
24. Ricci C, Rendina EA, Venuta F, et al. Reconstruction of the pulmonary artery in patients with lung cancer. Ann Thorac Surg 1994;57:627.
25. Rendina EA, Venuta F, De Giacomo T, et al. Sleeve resection and prosthetic reconstruction of the pulmonary artery for lung cancer. Ann Thorac Surg 1999;68:995.
26. Venuta F, Ciccone AM, Anile M, et al. Reconstruction of the pulmonary artery for lung cancer: long-term results. J Thorac Cardiovasc Surg 2009;138(5): 1185–91.
27. Rendina EA, Venuta F, De Giacomo T, et al. Reconstruction of the pulmonary artery by a conduit of autologous pericardium. J Thorac Cardiovasc Surg 1995;110(3):867–8.
28. Cerezo F, Cano JR, Espinosa D, et al. New technique for pulmonary artery reconstruction. Eur J Cardiothorac Surg 2009;36:422–3.
29. Mahtabifard A, Fuller CB, McKenna RJ Jr. Video-assisted thoracic surgery sleeve lobectomy: a case series. Ann Thorac Surg 2008;85(2):729–32.
30. Vogt-Moykopf I, Frits TH, Meyer G, et al. Bronchoplastic and angioplastic operation in bronchial carcinoma: long-term results of a retrospective analysis from 1973 to 1983. Int Surg 1986;71:211.
31. Cerfolio RJ, Bryant AS. Surgical techniques and results for partial or circumferential resection of the pulmonary artery for patients with non-small cell lung cancer. Ann Thorac Surg 2007;83: 1971–7.
32. Rendina EA, Venuta F, De Giacommo T, et al. Safety and efficacy of bronchovascular reconstruction after induction chemotherapy for lung cancer. J Thorac Cardiovasc Surg 1997;114:830.
33. Maurizi G, D'Andrilli A, Anile M, et al. Sleeve lobectomy compared with sleeve lobectomy after induction therapy for non-small lung cancer. J Thorac Oncol 2013;8(5):637–43.
34. Alifano M, Cusumano G, Strano S, et al. Lobectomy with pulmonary artery resection: morbidity, mortality, and long-term survival. J Thorac Cardiovasc Surg 2009;137(6):1400–5.
35. Nagayasu T, Matsumoto K, Tagawa T, et al. Factors affecting survival after bronchoplasty and bronchoangioplasty for lung cancer: single institutional review of 147 patients. Eur J Cardiothorac Surg 2006;29:585–90.

Current Status of Mediastinal Lymph Node Dissection Versus Sampling in Non-small Cell Lung Cancer

Gail E. Darling, MD, FRCS

KEYWORDS

• Staging • Lymph node dissection • Nonsmall cell lung cancer

KEY POINTS

- Systematic lymph node sampling or mediastinal lymph node dissection is adequate for staging of nonsmall cell lung cancer.
- Random sampling is inadequate for staging nonsmall cell lung cancer.
- If systematic lymph node sampling has not been performed before lung resection, either systematic sampling or mediastinal lymph node dissection should be performed at the time of lung resection.
- Pre-resection systematic sampling is indicated for mediastinal nodes that are enlarged on computed tomography, and/or have increased uptake of fluorodeoxyglucose on positron emission tomography–computed tomography.
- Pre-resection systematic sampling of mediastinal nodes is indicated for tumor at increased risk of lymph node metastases including T2 or higher stage tumors, central tumors, or tumors with evidence of N1 involvement.
- Complete resection of nonsmall cell lung cancer requires mediastinal lymph node dissection or systematic sampling.
- Minimum lymph node assessment includes systematic sampling of at least 3 mediastinal nodal stations (N2 nodes), one of which must be the subcarinal nodes (station 7), and removal of 10 to 16 nodes in total including at least stations 10 and 11.

INTRODUCTION

Evaluation of lymph nodes is a key component of management of nonsmall cell lung cancer (NSCLC). However, the approach to lymph node assessment continues to be controversial because some surgeons think that complete lymph node dissection is required, whereas others think that sampling is adequate or even unnecessary in the era of positron emission tomography–computed tomography (PET-CT). This controversy relates to the purpose of lymph node assessment: to contribute to survival or simply to provide staging information. Clearly, assessment of lymph nodes is essential for accurate staging to guide treatment and to predict future prognosis but the questions remain: how many nodes must be removed; which nodal stations must be sampled, and can the surgeon rely on PET-CT? This article addresses the appropriate use of lymph node sampling versus dissection, recommendations for minimum preoperative mediastinal nodal biopsy for staging, and the role of lymph node dissection in improving survival.

Thoracic Surgery, Kress Family Chair in Esophageal Cancer, University of Toronto, Toronto General Hospital, University Health Network, 200 Elizabeth Street, Room 9N-955, Toronto, Ontario M5G 2C4, Canada
E-mail address: gail.darling@uhn.ca

Thorac Surg Clin 23 (2013) 349–356
http://dx.doi.org/10.1016/j.thorsurg.2013.05.002
1547-4127/13/$ – see front matter

TECHNIQUE OF MEDIASTINAL LYMPH NODE DISSECTION

Mediastinal lymph node dissection (MLND) for right-sided tumors includes an en-bloc resection of the lymph node–bearing tissue in the paratracheal space between the superior vena cava anteriorly, the pulmonary artery inferiorly, the esophagus posteriorly, the brachiocephalic trunk superiorly, and the aortic arch medially. In addition, an en-bloc resection of the lower mediastinum is performed including all the lymph node–bearing tissue from the tracheal carina and main stem bronchi superiorly to the diaphragm inferiorly, the pericardium anteriorly, and the esophagus posteriorly. For left-sided tumors, the lower mediastinal dissection is the same but the superior mediastinal dissection extends from the phrenic nerve anteriorly to the vagus nerve posteriorly and to the pulmonary artery inferiorly, including all the tissue between the aortic arch and pulmonary artery. In addition, the ligamentum arteriosum may be divided to access the left paratracheal (4L) nodes (**Fig. 1**).[1]

COMPLETE RESECTION FOR NSCLC

A report from the Complete Resection Subcommittee of the International Association for the Study of Lung Cancer Staging Committee defined complete resection as "microscopically negative resection margins, systematic nodal dissection or lobe specific systematic nodal dissection, no extracapsular nodal extension of tumor and a negative highest mediastinal node." However, the authors further comment that systematic nodal dissection is preferably accomplished by complete removal of mediastinal tissue (ie, MLND); however, excision of at least 3 nodal stations, one of which is the subcarinal station, also fulfills the definition of a systematic nodal dissection.[2] The consensus of the committee was that either approach was acceptable. The term systematic nodal dissection maybe somewhat confusing and it is preferable to use the terms systematic sampling and mediastinal lymph node dissection (**Box 1**).

STAGING OF LYMPH NODES IN NSCLC

Clinical Versus Pathologic Staging

Clinical staging is determined by clinical assessment and diagnostic imaging is determined by CT and PET-CT. Pathologic staging of lymph nodes is determined by the histologic or cytologic examination of lymph nodes obtained by excision at the time of pulmonary resection, or before resection (pre-resection) by mediastinoscopy, mediastinotomy, endobronchial ultrasound (EBUS), endoscopic ultrasound (EUS), or video-assisted thoracic surgery (VATS).

History of Mediastinal Staging

Before the modern era of diagnostic imaging, patients with lung cancer had only a chest radiograph before coming to the operating room for resection. At the time of resection, mediastinal, hilar, and lobar lymph nodes were removed as part of the treatment of the cancer. It became evident that patients who had involvement of mediastinal lymph nodes had worse survival.[3] Many such patients did not benefit from resection of their primary tumor because their cancer recurred within a short period of time. If such patients could be identified before having a thoracotomy, they would be spared the morbidity of an operation from which they would derive no benefit (so-called futile thoracotomy).

The development of the mediastinoscopy by Carlens, which was popularized in North America

Box 1
Definitions

Sampling: Sampling of lymph nodes guided by preoperative or intraoperative findings (also described as random sampling)

Systematic sampling: Sampling of predetermined lymph nodes and lymph node stations

Mediastinal lymph node dissection (MLND): Complete removal of all mediastinal lymph node–bearing tissue based on anatomic landmarks

Extended lymph node dissection: Removal of bilateral paratracheal and cervical lymph nodes by formal dissection

Lobe-specific systematic node dissection: Removal of mediastinal lymph node–bearing tissue based on the location of the tumor

Data from Lardinois D, De Leyn P, Van Schil P, et al. ESTS guidelines for intraoperative lymph node staging in non-small cell lung cancer. Eur J Cardiothorac Surg 2006;30:787–92.

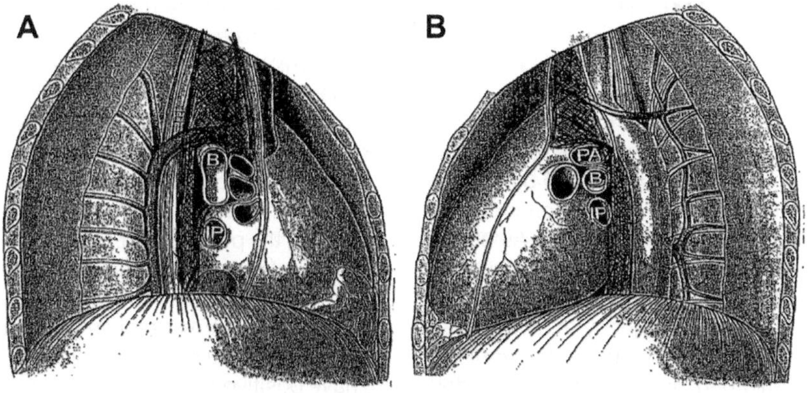

Fig. 1. View of the mediastinum from the right (*A*) and left (*B*) after mediastinal lymph node dissection. Cross-hatched shaded area represents the extent of mediastinal dissection. (*From* Martini N. Mediastinal lymph node dissection for lung cancer. Chest Surg Clin N A 1995; 5:189–203; with permission.)

by Pearson, allowed mediastinal nodes to be histologically evaluated before resection.[4,5] Mediastinoscopy became the gold standard for preresection lymph node staging, allowing the surgeon to sample mediastinal lymph nodes without subjecting the patient to a thoracotomy. If lymph node metastases were identified by histologic evaluation (ie, pathologically staged), the patient could avoid a "futile thoracotomy."

Mediastinoscopy

An adequate mediastinoscopy requires dissection of the left and right paratracheal zones and the subcarinal space. Lymph nodes identified during this dissection are then biopsied by removing either a piece or the entire lymph node. A proper staging mediastinoscopy biopsies ipsilateral and contralateral lymph nodes as well as subcarinal nodes (stations 2R, 4R, 2L, 4L, and 7) (**Fig. 2**). In some patients no nodes will be identified in some of these stations, most commonly station 2L. When this occurs, the operating surgeon should include a statement in the dictated operative note that the station was explored but no node was found. A procedure wherein the surgeon simply palpates the mediastinum or inspects the mediastinum visually with the mediastinoscope is not an adequate mediastinoscopy. A common error in performing mediastinoscopy is performing a biopsy of only an enlarged ipsilateral node. Although this may confirm that the patient has N2 disease, a contralateral node must be biopsied to rule out N3 disease. Furthermore, subcarinal nodes (station 7) and an additional ipsilateral node should be biopsied to determine if the patient has multistation N2 disease. A complete evaluation of the mediastinum is necessary to guide treatment.

Clinical Staging with CT and PET-CT

In the era of staging with CT and PET-CT, are the performance characteristics of CT and PET-CT good enough that surgeons can forgo preresection invasive staging of the mediastinum? Clearly, CT alone is not good enough. The positive predictive value for CT ranges from 0.16 to 0.88 and the negative predictive value ranges from 0.54 to 0.83.[6] On average, the likelihood of an enlarged mediastinal node being histologically positive is only 60%, whereas 20% of normal-sized nodes may harbor metastases.[7] PET performs better with a positive predictive value ranging from 0.40 to 1.00 and a negative predictive value

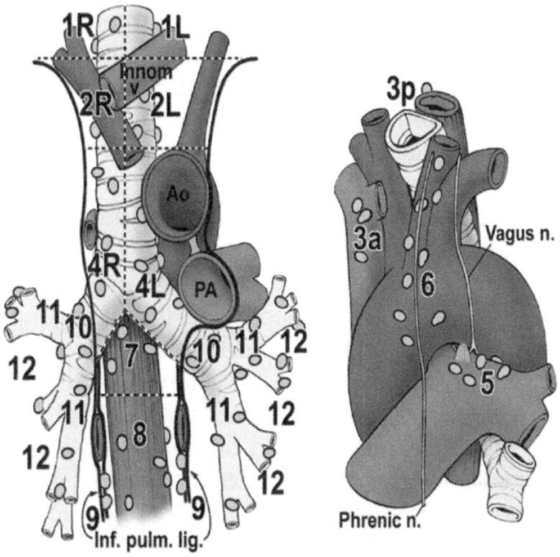

Fig. 2. Lymph node map: stations 1, 2, 3, 4, 5, 6, 7, 8, and 9 are N2 stations. Stations 10, 11, and 12 are N1 stations. Ao, aorta; Inf. pulm. lig., inferior pulmonary ligament; n., nerve; PA, pulmonary artery. (Used with permission of Mayo Foundation for Medical Education and Research, all rights reserved.)

ranging from 0.71 to 1.00.[6] However, the false negative rate for PET is approximately 20% for normal-sized nodes that are PET negative. Conversely, enlarged nodes that are PET positive are falsely positive 15% to 25% of the time.

An evidence-based guideline on the role of invasive mediastinal staging was produced by Cancer Care Ontario.[8] This guideline is in concordance with earlier recommendations from the American College of Chest Physicians.[9] Because the false positive rate for enlarged nodes on CT or "hot" nodes on PET is at least 25%, biopsy of all enlarged or "hot" mediastinal lymph nodes is required. Biopsy of any enlarged nodes is recommended even if increased uptake on PET is not demonstrated. In the patient with normal-sized mediastinal nodes that do not demonstrate increased uptake of fluorodeoxyglucose on PET, invasive staging is still recommended if the patient's tumor is at higher risk for mediastinal lymph node metastases such as those with suspicious N1 nodes, larger tumors (T2 or greater), or central tumors. One may also consider invasive staging in a patient who is high risk for surgery or if the surgeon wants to ensure that sublobar resection or stereotactic body radiotherapy are appropriate options.[10] The one situation where it seems the CT/PET-CT staging may be sufficiently accurate to omit pre-resection staging is small peripheral T1 tumors with a negative PET-CT and no enlarged mediastinal or hilar nodes. In this circumstance the likelihood of positive mediastinal nodes is less than 5%.

Invasive Mediastinal Staging

Invasive mediastinal staging performed before resection has been accomplished historically by mediastinoscopy. More recently EBUS has been used to biopsy mediastinal nodes by transbronchial needle aspiration and seems to be comparable to mediastinoscopy in terms of accuracy.[11] This procedure allows all the same mediastinal nodes to be evaluated cytologically as in mediastinoscopy without the necessity of a general anesthetic and also allows access to the hilar lymph nodes. If EBUS is to be used for staging and to replace mediastinoscopy, a systematic sampling of at least one ipsilateral, one contralateral, and one subcarinal node should be performed just as for mediastinoscopy. Biopsy of mediastinal nodes is also possible using EUS, which allows access to stations 8 and 9.

Pre-resection Staging of Mediastinal Lymph Nodes Versus Intraoperative Staging

The purpose of mediastinoscopy, mediastinotomy, EBUS-transbronchial needle aspiration, and EUS is simply staging of the mediastinal lymph nodes by sampling before resection to rule out N2 or N3 disease, which would preclude resection. Whether mediastinal nodes should be further evaluated by sampling or dissection at the time of thoracotomy or VATS is controversial. Overall, it seems that 10% to 20% of patients will have nodal involvement despite a negative preoperative mediastinoscopy at least in the pre-PET era.[12] In a randomized study of mediastinoscopy compared with CT, 248 patients with negative mediastinoscopy went to thoracotomy but on resampling of mediastinal lymph nodes at the time of thoracotomy, 10% were found to have positive mediastinal nodes.[13] These results suggest that even with negative mediastinoscopy, mediastinal nodes should be systematically sampled or MLND should be performed at the time of pulmonary resection. Even in pT1 NSCLC, N2 disease may occur as found in a study of 968 patients with pT1 NSCLC in which 59 (6.1%) were found to have N2 disease at thoracotomy.[14]

If invasive staging has not been performed before resection, assessment of mediastinal nodes must be performed at the time of resection by either systematic sampling or a complete MLND. Either approach is preferable to (random) sampling, which is inadequate. Proponents of MLND argue that this procedure provides more accurate staging and improves survival because all lymph nodes are removed, thus preventing recurrence from occult metastatic disease in the mediastinal nodes.

Intraoperative MLND Versus Systematic Sampling

MLND removes more lymph nodes than systematic sampling. It seems self-evident that if more lymph nodes are removed, nodal staging should be more accurate. In the American College of Surgeons Oncology Group (ACOSOG) Z0030 trial, the median total number of nodes removed by MLND after rigorous systematic sampling was 18, of which 11 to 12 were N2 nodes.[15] Despite the increased number of nodes examined with MLND, N2 disease was detected in only 3.8% of patients.[16] However, if nonsystematic sampling is performed, the likelihood of missing N2 disease is higher (5%–14%).[17,18]

Survival Benefit of MLND?

Whether MLND improves survival is controversial. Using the SEER database, Varlotto[12] reported a survival advantage for patients with stage I NSCLC undergoing lymphadenectomy compared with those having no lymph node dissection with an increase in 5-year survival from 41.6% to

58.4%. Whether these patients had pre-resection invasive staging is unknown. Of the entire study cohort, 16% had no nodal dissection, 70% of whom had sublobar resections. Assuming that many patients who had a sublobar resection may have had comorbidities precluding anatomic resection, their survival may have been adversely affected by comorbidities, not just the absence of lymph node dissection. Of the group included in the lymphadenectomy group, only 50% of the patients had a dissection of N2 nodes, and 32% had dissection of N1 nodes only.[12] Although the conclusion of this study was that MLND improved survival, clearly the cohorts are not balanced and at best one could conclude that patients having some lymph node dissection had better survival than those who had no lymph node assessment but whether this was due to MLND cannot be determined.

Historical series clearly identified that N2 nodes detected by chest radiograph or mediastinoscopy were associated with a poor prognosis even if resected.[3] Whether N2 disease detected by CT or PET portends the same poor prognosis has not been clearly addressed. Historically, survival for patients with N2 disease who underwent resection ranged from 15% to 40%.[19] In a more recent, single-institution study of patients with unsuspected N2 disease discovered at resection who had a negative CT and PET, 5-year survival was 35% when treated with complete resection and adjuvant therapy.[20] However, multistation N2 disease is associated with a worse prognosis, a factor noted in both historical and recent series.[21] The goal of pre-resection invasive staging is to detect multistation N2 disease (or N3 disease) because of the known poor prognosis and spare the patient the morbidity of a thoractomy. In the era of VATS, mediastinal staging by VATS with intraoperative frozen section before proceeding to resection is not unreasonable because the morbidity of thoracoscopy (VATS) is significantly less that an open thoracotomy.

There have been 4 randomized studies of MLND compared with lymph node sampling addressing the question of whether MLND improves survival. In 3 of these, mediastinal nodes were sampled only if suspicious based on size greater than 1 cm, or hardness, whereas in the ACOSOG Z0030 trial a rigorous systematic sampling was performed before randomization. Wu and coworkers reported on 532 patients with clinical stage I, II, or IIIA NSCLC randomized to MLND or sampling and found improved median survival in the MLND group compared with the sampling group (43 months vs 32 months, $P = .0001$). Invasive staging before resection was not used. As a result, 48% of the patients in the MLND had pathologic stage IIIA disease versus 28% in the sampling arm, which clearly illustrates the benefit of MLND if preresection systematic sampling has not been performed.[18]

In a smaller randomized trial of 169 patients with stage I, II, or IIIA, no difference in survival was found between MLND and MLNS. Only a small number of patients (5.5%) had unsuspected mediastinal lymph node involvement after MLND.[17] Similarly in a randomized study of patients with clinical stage I, small (<2 cm, T1 NSCLC), Sugi and colleagues[22] found no difference in survival between the MLND and sampling but unsuspected N2 disease was identified in 12% and 14% of MLND and sampling groups, respectively.

The largest randomized study was the ACOSOG Z0030 trial in which 1111 patients with early stage NSCLC (T1 or T2) were randomized to MLND or systematic sampling. The entry criteria specified that patients were eligible only if they had a negative systematic sampling by mediastinoscopy or intraoperative systematic sampling at the time of resection. Before randomization, the hilar (station 10) node was also sampled. If all nodes sampled were negative, then the patient was eligible for randomization. Patients randomized to systematic sampling had no further lymph nodes removed from the mediastinum. Systematic sampling consisted of sampling of stations 2R, 4R, 7, and 10R for right-sided tumors and stations 5, 6, 7, and 10L for left-sided tumors. Any enlarged or suspicious nodes were also sampled. Patients randomized to MLND underwent a formal anatomic dissection of the mediastinum removing all lymph node–bearing tissue from the mediastinum. In this way, rigorous staging was performed in all patients and the difference between the 2 arms was only the complete removal of all the lymph node–bearing tissue in the MLND arm. The goal was to determine whether MLND would offer either improved staging or improved survival.

ACOSOG Z0030 analyzed 1023 patients (498 systematic sampling and 525 MLND). In the MLND arm, 3.8% of patients were found to have N2 disease in the MLND specimen; however, there was no difference in overall or disease-free survival between the 2 arms of the trial at 5 years (**Fig. 3**). Furthermore, there was no difference in local, regional, or distant recurrence. The trial demonstrates that in patients with early stage clinical T1 or T2, N0 or nonhilar N1 NSCLC, who have been staged by systematic lymph node sampling, MLND does not improve survival. These results clearly do not apply to patients who have higher T stages nor do they apply to patients who have not had systematic sampling. It is notable however that the systematic sampling used in this

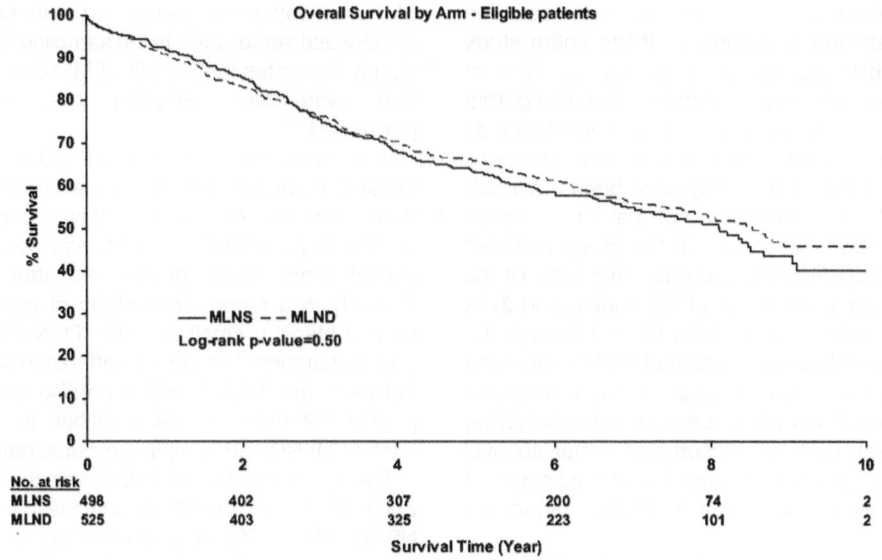

Fig. 3. Overall survival of eligible patients in the ACOSOG Z0030 trial. There is no difference in overall survival between the 2 arms of the trial. MLNS, mucocutaneous lymph node syndrome. (*From* Darling GE, Allen MS, Decker PA, et al. Randomized trial of mediastinal lymph node sampling versus complete lymphadenectomy during pulmonary resection in the patient with N0 or N1 (less than hilar) non-small cell carcinoma. J Thorac Cardiovasc Surg 2011;141:662–70; with permission.)

trial would meet the International Association for the Study of Lung Cancer requirements for a complete resection.[16]

In patients with T3 or T4 tumors, patients who have had neoadjuvant therapy for N2 disease and are undergoing resection, or for those patients who have not had systematic sampling, MLND is appropriate. The benefit of MLND for those who have not had systematic sampling before resection is evident from the Wu trial. In patients with known N1 or N2 disease, there may be a survival benefit. This survival benefit was demonstrated in the subgroup analysis of the Intergroup trial 0115 of adjuvant chemoradiotherapy versus radiotherapy following resection. Patients who had right upper lobe tumors who had MLND had a median survival of 57.5 months compared with 29.2 months for those with right upper lobe tumors who had only sampling. No survival benefit was found for tumors in other lobes.[23] The choice of MLND versus sampling was based on surgeon preference.

Based on these trials, it is apparent that if the patient with a T1 or T2 NSCLC has had systematic sampling and mediastinal and hilar nodes are negative, further lymph node evaluation by MLND does not improve survival. However, if N1 or N2 nodes are positive, or if systematic sampling has not been performed, MLND may provide a survival benefit and should be performed.

Certain aspects of current practice of thoracic surgery are not addressed by these trials. None of these trials used PET-CT for clinical staging. VATS lobectomy was used in only 7% of patients of the ACOSOG Z0030 trial. Many surgeons do not perform pre-resection invasive mediastinal staging if PET-CT with respect to mediastinal nodes is negative irrespective of T stage or primary tumor location. The appropriateness of this depends on the performance characteristics of PET-CT. Based on the Wu data, if pre-resection invasive staging has not been performed, then MLND should be performed at the time of resection. Even though there was no survival benefit for MLND in the ACOSOG Z0030 trial, the authors of the ACOSOG Z0030 trial recommended that MLND should still be performed as part of a complete resection for NSCLC as it provides a thorough assessment of mediastinal nodes. Some have expressed concern that the ACOSOG Z0030 trial results would be interpreted to mean that lymph node dissection is not required; however, all patients had systematic sampling, which would meet the International Association for the Study of Lung Cancer requirements for complete resection.

Minimum Lymph Node Assessment for NSCLC

Although lymph node assessment has been considered an integral part of the management of NSCLC, a pattern of care study in the United States reported that less than 50% of those undergoing pulmonary resection for NSCLC had any lymph node assessment.[24] Several guidelines (ESTS, NICE, SIGN, CCO) have recommended that appropriate lymph node assessment includes systematic sampling of at least 3 mediastinal lymph nodes stations (preferably 5), one of which should be station 7 and at least 10 lymph nodes including both N1 and N2 nodes (ie, systematic sampling).[1,8,25,26] Other authors have reported that 11 to 16 nodes should be evaluated to optimize staging and improve survival.[27–29] Stations 12, 13, and 14 are removed as part of pulmonary lobectomy but N2 lymph nodes as well as N1 nodes stations 10 and 11 must be removed intentionally by the surgeon. Therefore the adequate evaluation of lymph nodes in NSCLC requires diligence on the part of the pathologist in dissection of intralobar nodes and the surgeon in the dissection of interlobar, hilar, and mediastinal nodes.

SUMMARY

Assessment of mediastinal, hilar, and intralobar lymph nodes is an essential part of management of NSCLC. Minimum lymph nodes assessment includes sampling of at least 3 mediastinal node stations, one of which must be station 7 and at least 10 to 16 nodes including N1 and N2 stations. Lymph node assessment is important primarily for staging to guide treatment. However, adequate lymph node evaluation may contribute to survival by identification of N1 disease so that resected patients may benefit from adjuvant chemotherapy. Identification of N2 or N3 disease is important to avoid noncurative surgery as most of these patients will die from systemic disease and therefore require multimodality therapy. Surgery with MLND may improve survival for the exceptional patient with good performance status with single-station N2 disease. For patients who have early stage disease and negative systematic sampling, formal mediastinal lymph node dissection does not improve survival; however, for patients with higher stage disease or those who have not had preresection systematic sampling, mediastinal lymph node dissection may offer some survival benefit.

REFERENCES

1. Lardinois D, De Leyn P, Van Schil P, et al. ESTS guidelines for intraoperative lymph node staging in non-small cell lung cancer. Eur J Cardiothorac Surg 2006;30:787–92.
2. Rami-Porta R, Wittekind C, Goldstraw P. Complete resection in lung cancer surgery: proposed definition. Lung Cancer 2005;49:25–33.
3. Shields TW. The significance of ipsilateral mediastinal lymph node metastasis (N2) in nonsmall cell carcinoma of the lung. J Thorac Cardiovasc Surg 1990;99:48–53.
4. Carlens E. Mediastinoscopy. Dis Chest 1959;36:343.
5. Pearson FG. An evaluation of mediastinoscopy intn the management of presumably operable bronchial carcinoma. J Thorac Cardiovasc Surg 1968; 55:617.
6. Silvestri GA, Gould MK, Margolis ML, et al. Noninvasive staging of non-small cell lung cancer. Chest 2007;132:178S–201S.
7. Gould MK, Kuschner WG, Rydzak CE, et al. Test performance of positron emission tomography and computed tomography for mediastinal staging in patients with non-small cell lung cancer: a meta-analysis. Ann Intern Med 2003;139:879–92.
8. Darling G, Dickie J, Malthaner R, et al. Invasive mediastinal staging of nonsmall cell lung cancer. Available at: http://www.cancercare.on.ca/toolbox/qualityguidelines/clin-program/surgery-ebs/. Accessed January 19, 2013.
9. Detterbeck FC, Jantz MA, Wallace M, et al. Invasive mediastinal staging of lung cancer. Chest 2007;132: 202S–20S.
10. Sarwate D, Sarkar S, Krimsky WS, et al. Optimization of mediastinal staging in potential candidates for stereotactic radiosurgery of the chest. J Thorac Cardiovasc Surg 2012;144:81–6.
11. Yasufuku K, Pierre A, Darling G, et al. A prospective controlled trial of endobronchial ultrasound-guided transbronchial needle aspiration compared with mediastinoscopy for mediastinal lymph node staging of lung cancer. J Thorac Cardiovasc Surg 2011;142(6): 1393–1400.e1.
12. Varlotto JM, Recht A, Nikolov M, et al. Extent of lymphadenectomy and outcome for patients with stage I nonsmall cell lung cancer. Cancer 2009; 115:851–8.
13. The Canadian Lung Oncology Group. Investigation for mediastinal disease in patients with apparently operable lung cancer. Ann Thorac Surg 1995;60: 1382–9.
14. Defranchi SA, Cassivi SD, Nichols FC, et al. N2 disease in T1 nonsmall cell lung cancer. Ann Thorac Surg 2009;88:924–9.
15. Darling GE, Allen MS, Decker PA, et al. Number of lymph nodes harvested from a mediastinal lymphadenectomy. Chest 2010;138:1–6.
16. Darling GE, Allen MS, Decker PA, et al. Randomized trial of mediastinal lymph node sampling versus complete lymphadenectomy during pulmonary resection in the patient with N0 or N1 (less than Hilar) non-small cell carcinoma: results of the ACOSOG Z0030 trial. J Thorac Cardiovasc Surg 2011; 141:662–70.
17. Izbicki JR, Passlick B, Pantel K, et al. Effectiveness of radical systematic mediastinal lymphadenectomy in patients with resectable non-small cell lung

cancer: results of a prospective randomized trial. Ann Surg 1998;227:138–44.
18. Wu Y, Huang ZF, Wang SY, et al. A randomized trial of systematic nodal dissection in resectable non-small cell lung cancer. Lung Cancer 2002;36:1–6.
19. Martini N. Mediastinal lymph node dissection for lung cancer. Chest Surg Clin N Am 1995;5:189–203.
20. Cerfolio RJ, Bryant AS. Survival of patients with unsuspected N2 (stage IIIA) nonsmall-cell lung cancer. Ann Thorac Surg 2008;86:362–6.
21. Kang CH, Ra YJ, Kim YT, et al. The impact of multiple metastatic nodal stations on survival in patients with resectable N1 and N2 nonsmall-cell lung cancer. Ann Thorac Surg 2008;86:1092–7.
22. Sugi K, Nawata K, Fujita N, et al. Systematic lymph node dissection for clinically diagnosed peripheral non-small-cell lung cancer less than 2 cm in diameter. World J Surg 1998;22:290–4.
23. Keller SM, Adak S, Wagner H, et al. Mediastinal lymph node dissection improves survival in patients with stages II and IIIa non-small cell lung cancer. Eastern Cooperative Oncology Group. Ann Thorac Surg 2000;70:358–65.
24. Little AG, Rusch VW, Bonner JA, et al. Patterns of surgical care of lung cancer patients. Ann Thorac Surg 2005;80:2051–6.
25. Scottish Intercollegiate Guidelines Network. Management of patients with lung cancer. A national clinical guideline. Edinburgh (United Kingdom): Scottish Intercollegiate Guidelines Network; 2005.
26. National Collaborating Centre for Acute Care. The diagnosis and treatment of lung cancer. London: National Institute for Health and Clinical Excellence; 2005.
27. Gajra A, Newman N, Gamble GP, et al. Effect of number of lymph nodes sampled on outcome in patients with stage I non-small-cell lung cancer. J Clin Oncol 2003;21:1029–34.
28. Whitson BA, Groth SS, Maddaus MA. Surgical assessment and intraoperative management of mediastinal lymph nodes in non-small cell lung cancer. Ann Thorac Surg 2007;84(3):1059–65.
29. Zhong W, Yang X, Bai J, et al. Complete mediastinal lymphadenectomy: the core component of the multidisciplinary therapy in resectable non-small cell lung cancer. Eur J Cardiothorac Surg 2008;34(1):187–95.

Intraoperative Nodal Staging
Role of Sentinel Node Technology

Shinichiro Miyoshi, MD, PhD

KEYWORDS

• Lung cancer • Lymphadenectomy • Sentinel lymph node • Tracer • Radioisotope

KEY POINTS

- Definition of sentinel lymph node (SLN): an SLN is defined as the first lymph node or group of lymph nodes encountered in lymphatic drainage from a primary tumor.
- Intraoperative SLN biopsy (SLNB) navigation: when metastasis is not found in the SLN, it is most likely not present in more distal lymph nodes. Therefore, an additional lymphadenectomy is considered to be unnecessary.
- Indication: SLNB should be performed for patients with clinical node-negative non–small cell lung cancer (NSCLC) to pathologically determine the presence of SLN metastasis.
- Tracer: although many tracers such as dyes, radioisotopes, magnetite, and iopamidol have been investigated, no appropriate agent that produces high identification and accuracy results has been developed for lung cancer.
- Lobe-specific selective lymph node dissection: a lobe-specific selective lymphadenectomy based on biopsy results of predetermined selective lymph node stations might be considered as an alternative to an SLN lymphadenectomy for early-stage NSCLC.

INTRODUCTION

Lymph node status is a major determinant of stage and survival in patients with non–small cell lung cancer (NSCLC). Although computed tomography (CT) or fluoro-2-deoxy-D-glucose (FDG)-positron emission tomography (PET) scanning have been preoperatively used for diagnosing lymph node status, their sensitivity and specificity are not satisfactory (51% and 85%, 74% and 85%, respectively).[1] A combination of node size and metabolic characteristics shown by FDG-PET/CT has improved the accuracy of staging by showing better anatomic localization of FDG hotspots. However, for most cases, FDG-PET/CT does not eliminate the need for invasive testing.[2] Although mediastinoscopy[3] and recently introduced endobronchial ultrasonography transbronchial needle aspiration techniques[4] are reliable for pathologic diagnosis of lymph node status, neither procedure has the ability to detect all lymph node stations. Lymph node dissection (removal of all ipsilateral lymph node-bearing tissues) is the best method to accurately determine pathologic lymph node status. Thus, a lobectomy with a hilar and mediastinal lymphadenectomy is considered to be the gold standard of surgical care for patients with resectable NSCLC.[5,6]

Recently, sublobar resection, including partial resection and a segmentectomy, has been introduced in association with an increase in number of patients with early-stage lung cancer.[7] The possibility to reduce the extent of the lymphadenectomy procedure has been indicated for patients without metastasis to lymph nodes.[8–13] The question remaining is how to reduce the extent of lymph node dissection without leaving metastatic lymph nodes behind.

Department of General Thoracic Surgery and Breast and Endocrinological Surgery (Surgery II), Okayama University Graduate School of Medicine, Dentistry and Pharmaceutical Sciences, 2-5-1 Shikata-Cho, Kita-ku, Okayama 700-8558, Japan
E-mail address: smiyoshi@md.okayama-u.ac.jp

Thorac Surg Clin 23 (2013) 357–368
http://dx.doi.org/10.1016/j.thorsurg.2013.04.002

For this purpose, a sentinel lymph node (SLN) mapping technique was first introduced for penile carcinoma by Cabanas in 1977,[14] and those concepts have since been more widely applied to melanoma and breast cancer cases.[15,16] The role of sentinel node technology has become established for such superficial malignancies.[17,18]

Little and colleagues[19] first applied an SLN mapping technique for patients undergoing lung resection for NSCLC. Since then, many studies have been performed by lung cancer surgery investigators, which are critically reviewed in this article. As an alternative to SLN biopsy (SLNB), biopsy of lobe-specific selective lymph node stations is also discussed.

HISTORICAL NOTES

Regional node dissection is an accepted part of surgical treatment of many solid tumors. It was first applied to breast cancer in 1894 by Halsted and then later extended to other malignancies, including head and neck cancers, gastrointestinal neoplasms, and melanoma. Lung cancer surgery was started with a successful pneumonectomy by Graham in 1933, and Churchill and colleagues[20] were the first to suggest that a less radical operation such as a lobectomy may be adequate for surgical treatment of lung cancer. Since Cahan's report in 1960,[21] a lobectomy has been used as the standard surgical procedure for lung cancer, in which the extent of mediastinal lymph node dissection (MLND) is determined specific to each lobe with a primary tumor, with the procedure termed a radical lobectomy. However, the magnitude of the operation and the fact that NSCLC recurs in distant sites have reduced the popularity of MLND in Europe and the United States. On the other hand, systematic hilar and mediastinal lymphadenectomy procedures have been widely performed in Japan since Naruke and colleagues[22] created a lymph node map and reported the significance of MLND for lung cancer surgery in 1978.

Cabanas first described the SLNB concept for penile cancer in 1977.[14] However, that method was later found to be unreliable, because the false-negative rate was unacceptably high and the technique difficult to perform.[23] On the other hand, the concept was later adopted for nodal assessment of melanoma and breast cancer,[15,16] and the role of sentinel node technology has now become established for such superficial malignancies.[17,18]

In association with an increase in number of patients with early-stage lung cancer,[7] lung cancer surgical specialists who routinely perform MLND in their patients have generally come to the position that MLND is excessive for patients with N0 disease. On the other hand, surgeons who did not perform MLND for all of their patients have presented it as acceptable for patients with lymph node metastasis, who should benefit from the technique. Thus, the SLN mapping technique was first applied to patients undergoing lung resection for NSCLC by Little and colleagues.[19]

DEFINITION OF SLN AND ITS BENEFITS

The SLN is defined as the first lymph node or group of lymph nodes encountered in lymphatic drainage from a primary tumor.[14] An SLN mapping technique can identify lymphatic drainage path from the site of the primary tumor to the individual lymph nodes within the lymphatic basin and indicate which nodes are most likely to contain metastatic cancer cells. Intraoperative mapping permits selective identification, removal, and intraoperative evaluation by frozen section analysis of SLNs, allowing accurate pathologic staging during the operation. When metastasis is not found in SLNs, it most likely is not present in more distal lymph nodes. Thus, by using a minor procedure, surgeons can identify patients with metastatic nodal disease who would most likely benefit from a standard lymphadenectomy and in those who do not have nodal metastases, thus improving morbidity related to radical lymphadenectomy. An additional benefit of SLN detection is application of more sensitive pathologic detection techniques to specified nodes. In addition, immunohistochemistry (IHC) and reverse transcription-polymerase chain reaction techniques have increased the accuracy of detection of micrometastasis.[24,25]

INDICATIONS

An SLNB should be performed in most patients with clinical node-negative NSCLC, especially clinical T1N0M0 (c-T1N0M0). Thoracic surgeons who have been routinely performing radical lymphadenectomy including hilar and mediastinal lymph nodes for all patients with resectable NSCLC are searching for a reliable method to reduce the extent of lymphadenectomy for such patients with early-stage NSCLC without leaving metastatic lymph nodes behind, in the hope of avoiding lymphadenectomy-related complications in patients who do not need that radical procedure. On the other hand, thoracic surgeons who do not routinely perform lymphadenectomy for all patients would like to select patients with radiologically occult N1 or N2 disease during surgery, because they would benefit from a lymphadenectomy, and subsequently perform adjuvant therapy to avoid postoperative local and distant recurrence. According to the annual registry report of the Japanese Association for Thoracic Surgery,[26] 77% of 32,801 patients who underwent surgery for NSCLC in 2010 had c-T1N0M0 disease, of whom 90% were pathologic T1N0M0, theoretically indicating that they did not require a lymphadenectomy.

TRACERS AND INJECTION METHODS

Several tracers have been extensively investigated for use in intraoperative SLN mapping of NSCLC; the results are summarized in **Table 1**.

Dyes

Morton and colleagues[15] conducted studies of cats to determine ideal dyes and techniques for identifying regional lymphatics, with several substances examined for their potential usefulness as a tracking dye. These substances included methylene blue, isosulfan blue, patent blue-V, cyalume, and fluorescein dyes. Among the substances tested in cats for their accuracy in identifying the regional lymphatic drainage pattern, patent blue-V and isosulfan blue were found to produce the best results and were also shown to possess several characteristics useful for mapping regional lymphatics. When injected intradermally, they rapidly enter the lymphatics and show minimal diffusion into the surrounding soft tissue. The bright blue coloration of these dyes is also readily visible and allows easy identification of the lymphatic channel. Furthermore, these investigators found that dye injected into each area of the skin drained reliably only to the SLN, then later to lymph nodes further up the lymphatic chain. Based on their results, they used patent blue-V and isosulfan blue for intraoperative mapping of regional lymphatics in patients with clinical stage I melanoma. In addition, Giuliano and colleagues[16] used isosulfan vital dye for intraoperative mapping of regional lymphatics in patients with potentially curable breast carcinoma.

Isosulfan blue dye was initially used in patients with NSCLC by Little and colleagues.[19] In that study, a total of 5 mL was injected in divided doses into each quadrant of lung tissue immediately surrounding the tumor after a thoracotomy. At the completion of lung resection, paratracheal, subaortic, subcarinal, and inferior pulmonary ligament lymph node groups were all resected en bloc. During performance of the resection, the first lymph node, if any, to stain blue was considered the SLN and separately subjected to a histologic examination. SLNs were identified in only 17 (47%) of the 36 patients studied. Sugi and colleagues[27] and Rzyman and colleagues[28] also reported that the blue dye staining method for SLN identification was inadequate and should not be recommended for clinical use. In those studies, the blue dye technique was considered to have limited potential because of the original dark color of the anthracotic pulmonary lymph nodes.

Radioisotopes

Technetium 99m sulfur colloid

The accuracy of technetium 99m (Tc 99m) sulfur colloid injection has been reported to exceed 90% in breast carcinoma cases.[29,30] Tc 99m sulfur colloid was first used for SLN mapping in patients with primary lung cancer by Liptay and colleagues.[31] Intraoperative injection of a colloid suspension was performed directly into lung masses at the time of the thoracotomy, with a total of 2 mCi administered in a 4-quadrant injection pattern. Divided doses of 0.5 mCi suspended in 0.5 mL of solution were injected at the outer margins of the tumor, then a standard dissection was performed to complete anatomic resection of the tumor. Readings were taken with a handheld γ probe counter, and the values for counts per second of the primary tumor and intrathoracic nodal stations were documented. Initially, the tumor specimen and nodal stations were surveyed in the thorax. Radiolabeled nodes were also examined off the operative field and separately from the tumor specimen. The migration of the Tc 99m sulfur colloid solution was considered successful if a specific nodal station registered a count per second greater than 3 times the background value. A lymph node station with the highest count per second and ex vivo measurement greater than 3 times the intrathoracic background was classified as an SLN, and reported as such to the surgical pathology department. The particle size of Tc 99m sulfur colloid is 40 nm and its migration time to an SLN was found to be short, at from 10 to 15 minutes.[32]

After the initial scintigraphic readings and standard anatomic lung resection with ipsilateral mediastinal node dissection were completed, a repeat examination with a γ probe was performed to assess residual radioactivity and potentially overlooked lymph nodes. The remaining radioactivity levels were recorded and repeated resection of nodal stations performed if indicated by the handheld γ counter readings and visual inspection. Seventy-eight (86%) of 91 patients studied had an SLN identified and underwent complete resection. Sixty-nine of those 78 patients with SLNs were classified as true-negative, with no

Table 1
Reports of SLN mapping

Type of Tracers	Reference	Name of Tracers	Injection	No. of Patients	SLN Identification Rate (%)
Dye	Little et al,[19] 1999	Isosulfan blue dye	Intraoperative	36	47
	Sugi et al,[27] 2003	Isosulfan blue dye	Intraoperative	18	50
	Sugi et al,[27] 2003	ICG	Intraoperative	16	6
	Rzyman et al,[28] 2006	Patent blue	Intraoperative	42	36
	Rzyman et al,[28] 2006	Methylene blue	Intraoperative	68	22
Radioisotope	Liptay et al,[31] 2000	Tc 99m sulfur colloid	Intraoperative	45	82
	Liptay et al,[32] 2002	Tc 99m sulfur colloid	Intraoperative	91	86
	Schmit, 2002	Tc 99m + isosulfan blue dye	Intraoperative	31	81
	Nomori et al,[34] 2002	Tc 99m tin colloid	Preoperative, CT-guided	46	87
	Melfi, 2003	Tc 99m sulfur colloid	Preoperative, CT-guided	16	96
	Melfi, 2003	Tc 99m sulfur colloid	Intraoperative	10	
	Sugi et al,[27] 2003	Tc 99m tin colloid	Preoperative, CT-guided	14	64
	Lardinois et al,[33] 2003	Tc 99m nanocolloid	Preoperative, BFS	20	95
	Ueda et al,[35] 2004	Tc 99m tin colloid	Preoperative, CT-guided	15	NA
	Rzyman,[28] 2006	Tc 99m: Nanocoll N, Nanocic N, tin colloi N, filtered Nanocic N	Intraoperative	110	84–100
	Liptay,[49] 2009	Tc 99m sulfur colloid	Intraoperative	39	62
	Kim et al,[36] 2012	Tc 99m MSA	Preoperative	48	96
	Kim et al,[36] 2012	Tc 99m MSA	Intraoperative	34	97
Magnetite	Nakagawa,[38] 2003	Furumoxides	Intraoperative	38	82
	Minamiya et al,[39] 2006	Furumoxides	Intraoperative	20	80
NIRF ICG	Yamashita et al,[43] 2011	NIRF ICGI	Intraoperative	31	81
	Gilmore et al,[42] 2012	NIRF ICG	Intraoperative		90
Iopamidol	Takizawa et al,[47] 2012	Iopamidol	Preoperative, BFS	13	92

Abbreviations: BFS, bronchofiberscopy; ICG, indocyanine green; MSA, neomannosyl human serum albumin; NA, not available; NIRF, near-infrared fluorescent; Tc, technetium.

metastasis found in other intrathoracic lymph nodes without concurrent SLN involvement. In 9 patients, the SLN was the only positive node, and in 7 of those, the SLN was found to have only micrometastatic disease in IHC findings.

An intraoperative injection is used for collapsed lungs; however, migration of the radionuclide may be affected during preparation of the structures to be removed. Thus, a preoperative injection is performed on the ventilated lungs, which have a physiologic status. Based on these concepts, Lardinois and colleagues[33] applied preoperative bronchoscopic radioisotope injection for SLN mapping in patients with NSCLC. The patients were initially intubated with a single-lumen endotracheal tube, then bronchoscopy with a fiberoptic endoscope was performed through the endotracheal tube. When the tumor was bronchoscopically visible, a protected needle was inserted through the endoscope, and the needle tip was inserted in a transbronchial manner at the tumor margin. When the tumor was not visible endoscopically, the needle was inserted at the carina of the most distal pulmonary subsegment that could be reached endoscopically in the proximity of the tumor according to its location on preoperative CT scan images. The SLN identification rate of this technique using bronchofiberscopy was 95% (19/20), which was higher than that of an intraoperative technique.

Tc 99m tin colloid

Under Japanese law, a radioisotope can be injected only in an approved radioisotope room. Nomori and colleagues[34] chose Tc 99m tin colloid as a tracer and injected it according to the following procedure. (1) In the CT room, the site for radioisotope injection was marked on the skin, and the angle and depth of the needle required to reach the peritumoral region were determined. (2) The day before surgery, in the radioisotope room, a 23-gauge needle was introduced from the marked point on the skin to the peritumoral region, according to the angle and depth measured. (3) The Tc 99m tin colloid at 6 to 8 mCi suspended in a volume of 1 to 1.5 mL was injected with a single shot. (4) Lymphoscintigraphy was performed 5 minutes after the injection and again the next morning just before surgery. The Tc 99m tin colloid has a particle size about 1000 nm in diameter, which is larger than that of the Tc 99m sulfur colloid, and requires more than 6 hours to reach the SLN. This long migration time permits injection on the day before surgery. SLNs were identified in 40 (87%) of 46 patients studied and no false-negative SLNs were detected in 14 patients with N1 or N2 disease (0%). Furthermore, in vivo and ex vivo counting showed 88% concurrence for identification of SLNs in the mediastinum. On the other hand, this concurrence ratio was extremely low for identification of SLNs in the hilum or interlobar SLNs,[35] because of the shine-through effect from the tumor and background radioactivity aerosolization.

Tc 99m neomannosyl human serum albumin

To produce an agent that more accurately represents the physiologic flow of lymphatic drainage and accumulation in the SLN, receptor-binding agents with smaller molecular size targeting mannose-binding proteins in the lymph nodes have been identified and designed. Kim and colleagues[36] developed a novel mannose receptor-binding agent for SLN identification termed Tc 99m neomannosyl human serum albumin (Tc 99m MSA), with a molecular diameter of 6 $\times$ 8 nm, and performed the first clinical trial for both reliability and feasibility of SLN identification using this new radioactive agent in 42 patients with stage I NSCLC. From the time course monitored by lymphoscintigraphy in that study, the radioisotope was taken up by lymph nodes from 30 minutes after injection and the levels of detection did not change over the course of 1 day. Therefore, these investigators proposed that Tc 99m MSA be injected either just before or during the operation. In their next study,[37] a total dose of 1 mCi of Tc 99m MSA in a 0.2-ml solution was administered to the peritumoral region under CT guidance in the CT room at 1 to 2 hours before surgery or soon after a thoracotomy. In the intraoperative injection group, the investigators waited 5 minutes after injection of the radiotracer before proceeding, in order to avoid surgical destruction of the lymphatic system of the pleura, as well as the bronchi and vessels. The SLN identification rates in both groups were high: 95.8% in the preoperative group and 97.1% in the postoperative group. However, radiolabeled nodes were examined only at the back table after dissection.

Other Tracers

Other investigators have developed new techniques to overcome many of the formidable limitations of dye and radioactive tracers for SLN mapping.

Magnetite

Nakagawa and colleagues[38] developed a novel method that uses magnetite, which is ferumoxide, a colloidal superparamagnetic iron oxide of nonstoichiometric magnetite, as a tracer. Five milliliters of ferumoxide was injected around the tumor intraoperatively, then lung resection and lymph node dissection were performed 15 minutes later. Magnetic force within the lymph nodes was measured using a highly sensitive handheld magnetometer ex vivo. Although the results were promising, the magnetic force was measured only at the back table, not in the thorax. Therefore, these investigators developed a new more sensitive and sterilizable magnetometer for in vivo SLN mapping,[39] although the in vivo SLN detection rate was only 80%. **Fig. 1** shows those intraoperative measurement procedures.[40]

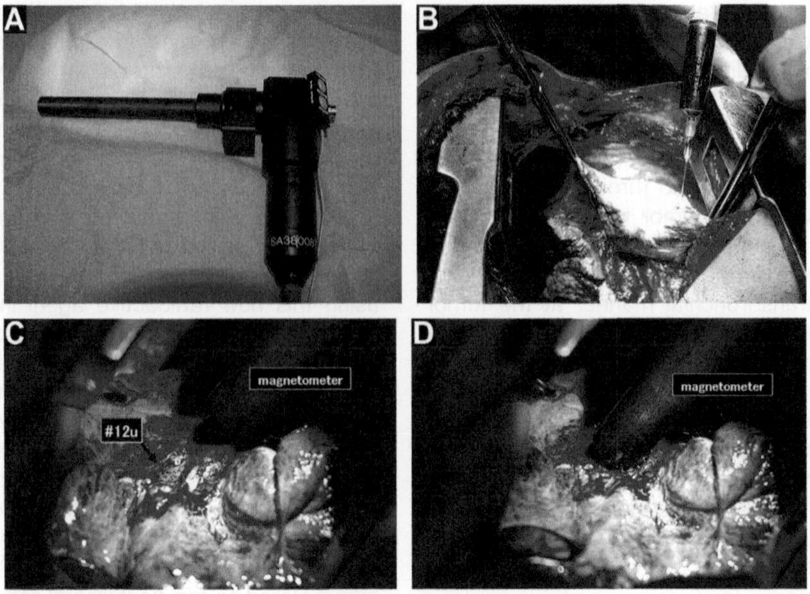

Fig. 1. Detection of magnetite in SLNs using a newly developed sterilizable magnetometer. (*A*) Sterilizable portable magnetometer. (*B*) Injection of ferumoxide (5 mL) around the tumor. (*C*) Intraoperative measurement of magnetic force within a lymph node (12u) to identify the SLN. (*D*) The magnetometer is moved close to the lymph node (12u). (*Courtesy of* Jun-ichi Ogawa, MD, PhD, Division of Thoracic Surgery, Department of Surgery, Akita University School of Medicine, Hondo Akita City, Japan.)

Near-infrared fluorescent indocyanine green

When indocyanine green (ICG), one of the most common and safe dyes for use in humans, was used as a tracer to detect SLN in patients who have lung cancer, the detection rate was only 6.3%[27] and the injected ICG was not visible in anthracotic lymph nodes with a naked eye. ICG is known to absorb infrared rays in vivo by binding with serum protein. When a near-infrared (NIR) fluorescence imaging system was developed to detect NIR fluorescence emitted from ICG, which migrates to draining lymph node basins, the role of ICG for SLNB in NSCLC was reexamined.[41,42]

Invisible NIR light penetrates tissue and illuminates fluorescent objects up to a depth of 1 cm in solid tissue. By maintaining separation of visible and NIR fluorescent light, it is possible to simultaneously acquire color and NIR fluorescence images, which can then be overlaid. Thus, a single intraoperative procedure is available to visualize SLNs, with the surgical field remaining unaltered. Phase 1 trial findings established the feasibility of SLN mapping in patients with lung cancer and showed that NIR mapping can be achieved in real time using a minimally invasive intraoperative approach. Additional studies are now under way to assess optimal ICG dosing, as well as the effects of SLNB results on adjuvant therapy plans and overall outcomes in patients with early NSCLC staged using this technology. Yamashita and colleagues[43,44] applied this technique for SLN mapping in cases of video-assisted thoracoscopic surgery segmentectomy and lobectomy and reported an SLN identification rate of 80.7%. **Fig. 2** shows an image obtained with a video-assisted thoracoscopic ICG fluorescence imaging system of the SLN at the interlobar node station (11i) in a case of primary lung adenocarcinoma of the right lower lobe.

Iopamidol

In 2004, Suga and colleagues[45] reported a method of SLN identification using CT-guided percutaneous injection of iopamidol into peritumoral lung tissue. These investigators successfully identified SLNs in all 9 patients with preoperative NSCLC without any complications. However, in 2006, the same group[46] reported that cerebral air embolism can occur using this method.

Takizawa and colleagues[47] developed a novel method of CT lymphography with transbronchial injection of iopamidol, a water-soluble extracellular CT contrast agent. With their method, an ultrathin bronchoscope is inserted into the target bronchus under the guidance of virtual bronchoscopic navigation images, then CT images of the chest are obtained at 0.5 and 5 minutes after injection of 2 or 3 mL of iopamidol through a microcatheter. SLNs were identified when the maximum CT attenuation value of the lymph nodes on postcontrast CT images was increased by 30 Hounsfield units or more compared with the precontrast

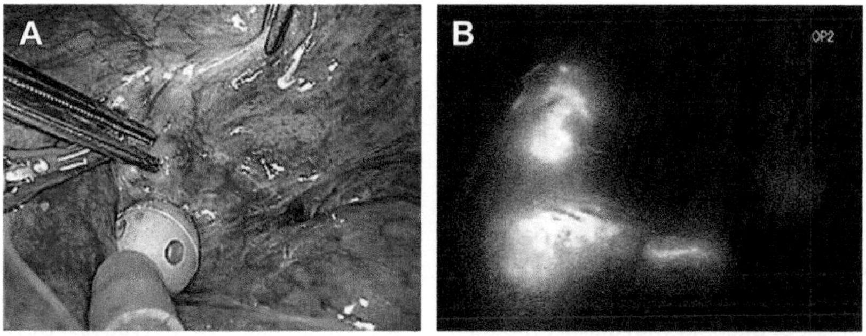

Fig. 2. Video-assisted thoracoscopic ICG fluorescence imaging system showing SLNs at an interlobar node station (11i) in primary lung adenocarcinoma of the right lower lobe. (*A*) A thoracoscope equipped with a normal light does not reveal the green dye staining, because of anthracosis. (*B*) Fluorescence imaging system visualizing SLNs. (*From* Yamashita S, Tokuishi K, Anami K, et al. Video-assisted thoracoscopic indocyanine green fluorescence imaging system shows sentinel lymph nodes in non–small-cell lung cancer. J Thorac Cardiovasc Surg 2011;141:142; with permission.)

images, with those found in 12 (92.3%) of 13 patients with clinical stage I NSCLC. Although the number of patients studied was small, the SLN identification rate was high. A representative CT lymphography image is shown in **Fig. 3**.

COMMENTS AND CONTROVERSIES

SLN Mapping

In 2005, an American Society of Clinical Oncology Expert Panel conducted a systematic review[17] of literature presented to February 2004 regarding

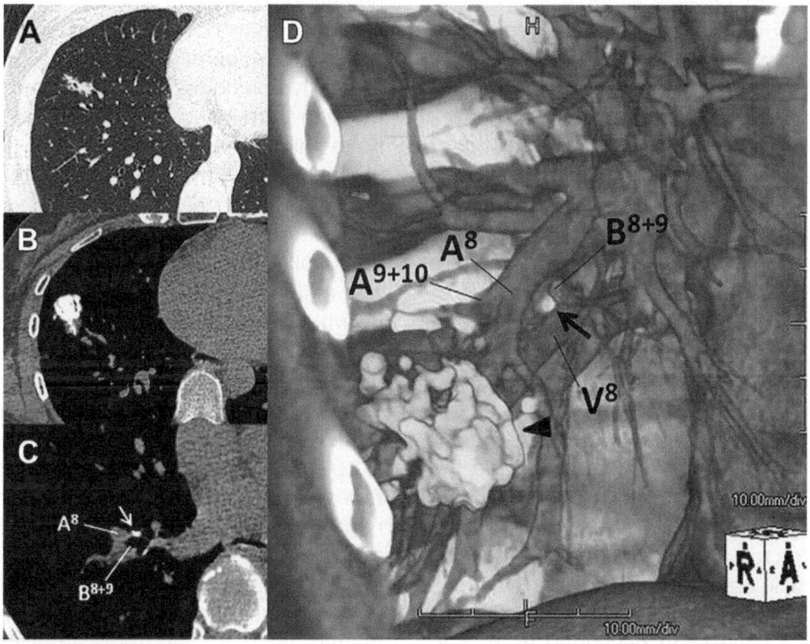

Fig. 3. CT lymphography (CTLG). (*A*) A tumor (diameter 1.6 cm) is shown in right station 9a in a prelymphography CT image. (*B*) Iopamidol is delivered into peritumoral lung tissue of right station 9. (*C*) An oval lymph node (*arrow*) is clearly enhanced in a post-CTLG image. (*D*) Three-dimensional CT image rendered by 1-mm-thick multidetector CT image slices obtained at 0.5 minutes after CTLG, clarifying the position of an SLN and the hilum structure. Sentinel node (*arrows*); iopamidol injected into peritumoral lung tissue (*arrowhead*). (*From* Takizawa H, Kondo K, Toda H, et al. Computed tomography lymphography by transbronchial injection of iopamidol to identify sentinel nodes in preoperative patients with non-small cell lung cancer: a pilot study. J Thorac Cardiovasc Surg 2012;144:97; with permission.)

the use of SLNB for early-stage breast cancer, which included 1 prospective randomized controlled trial, 4 limited meta-analyses, and 69 single-institution and multicenter trials. According to that review, SLNs were identified using radiocolloid, blue dye, or both, for an identification rate of 95% and false-negative rate of 7.3%. The conclusions were as follows. SLNB is an appropriate initial alternative to routine staging axillary lymph node dissection (ALND) for patients with early-stage breast cancer with clinically negative axillary nodes. Completion ALND remains standard treatment of patients with axillary metastases identified by SLNB. Appropriately identified patients with negative SLNB results obtained under the direction of an experienced surgeon do not require completion ALND. Isolated cancer cells detected by a pathologic examination of the SLN with use of specialized techniques are of unknown clinical significance. Although such specialized techniques are often used, they are not a required part of an SLN evaluation for breast cancer. Previous findings suggest that an SLNB is associated with lower morbidity.

Furthermore, the National Surgical Adjuvant Breast and Bowel Project conducted a randomized phase 3 trial,[48] in which the investigators enrolled 5611 patients with breast cancer with clinically negative nodes and compared the results of SLNB followed by ALND with SLNB followed by ALND only if the SLN was positive. These investigators concluded that overall survival, disease-free survival, and regional control were statistically equivalent between the groups. When the SLN is negative, SLN surgery alone with no further ALND is an appropriate, safe, and effective therapy for breast cancer with clinically negative lymph nodes.

An important question relates to the status of SLN navigation surgery in lung cancer compared with that of SLN navigation surgery in breast cancer. The search continues for the best tracer to identify SLNs with a high identification rate.

Regarding the SLN identification rate, more than 90% is required for clinical use. According to the summary in **Table 1**, radioactive tracers with a smaller particle size are promising,[28,36] because the identification rate has been reported to exceed 90%. The particle sizes of Tc 99m MSA, Nanocoll (human albumin), Nanocis (sulfur colloid), and filtered Nanocis have been described as 6×8, less than 80, 32 to 178 nm, and 50 nm, respectively. When these small radioactive tracers are injected intraoperatively, in vivo and ex vivo radioactivity measurements show only a slight influence from the shine-through effect on sensitivity and negative predictive value (NPV), which are concordant in 92% of the cases.[28] Furthermore, timing of the injection, before or after a thoracotomy, is not important. Therefore, intraoperative injection is recommended because of lower cost and increased efficiency.[36]

Because the number of patients in the pilot studies reviewed here is small, as shown in **Table 1**, it is difficult to evaluate the validity of SLN mapping techniques in clinical practice. Only Rzyman and colleagues[28] studied more than 100 patients and reported that a radioguided method using tracers with small particle size had a high identification rate, high sensitivity rate, and high NPV (100%, 87%, and 93%, respectively) when IHC findings were considered. When standard hematoxylin-eosin staining was applied, the sensitivity and NPV of SLN mapping was lower (74% and 89%, respectively). Although IHC is not a required part of SLN evaluation for breast cancer, it may be mandatory for NSCLC.

The greatest concern with an SLNB is the potential of a false-negative result, which could increase the potential for local recurrence in the thorax. According to a report by Rzyman and colleagues,[28] the false-negative rate was 8% in cases that used Nanocoll (n = 31), 17% in those that used Nanocis (n = 49), and 0% in those that used filtered Nanocis (n = 15). Although a false-negative rate of 7.3% is acceptable for breast cancer, that may not be low enough for NSCLC, because a reoperation for removal of residual metastatic lymph nodes is not easy and the response rates to currently available anticancer drugs are not as high as with breast cancer.

Because SLN mapping with radioactive technetium in NSCLC has been shown to be feasible in several single-institution reports, the Cancer and Leukemia Group B designed a phase 2 trial to test a standardized version of Liptay's method,[49] in which 8 surgeons participated and 46 of a planned 150 patients were enrolled. Of those patients, 43 had cancer and underwent an attempted complete resection, with 39 undergoing SLN mapping. One or more SLNs were identified in 24 (61.5%) of those 39 patients, with accurate indication (no other nodes positive for cancer if SLN negative) in 20 (83.3%). Overall, the SLN mapping procedure was found to be accurate in 20 (51.2%) of 39 patients. This trial was terminated early based on disappointing accuracy, slower than expected accrual, and reduced National Cancer Institute funding. Its failure was considered to be a result of the requirement of a strong collaboration among nuclear medicine, radiology, surgery, and pathology disciplines, as well as the learning curve required for the procedure. The investigators concluded that their multi-institutional attempt at validating this technique was unsuccessful. Thus, an ideal tracer for SLN mapping in NSCLC remains to be shown.

Lobe-Specific Selective Lymph Node Stations and Selective Lymphadenectomy

Systematic hilar and mediastinal lymphadenectomy procedures have been widely performed for all stages of resectable NSCLC patients in Japan since Naruke and colleagues[22] reported the significance of MLND. However, in association with an increase in the number of patients with early-stage lung cancer, the possibility of reducing the extent of a mediastinal lymphadenectomy procedure has been noted for these patients.[9–13]

We previously conducted an investigation to determine which mediastinal lymph node stations should be examined during surgical intervention to diagnose N2 or less disease in patients with NSCLC.[9] For the primary tumors, 3 mediastinal lymph node stations were selected for each lobe, as shown in **Table 2**, and defined as lobe-specific selective mediastinal lymph node stations. Although the concept of selective mediastinal lymph node stations is similar to that of SLN, we consider it to be more practical and convenient than an SLN examination using a tracer-guided SLNB technique, because selective mediastinal lymph node stations can be examined pathologically during surgical intervention without the need for special equipment.

As a next step, a prospective study of selective mediastinal dissection from intraoperative biopsy of the selective mediastinal lymph node stations was conducted.[12] We pathologically investigated 1 representative lymph node at each of the 3 stations using frozen sectioning immediately after completing dissections of the interlobar, hilar, and selective mediastinal lymph node stations in 69 patients with NSCLC. For patients whose selective lymph nodes were found to be negative, additional MLND was not performed. During 41 $\pm$ 25 months of follow-up, mediastinal lymph node recurrence was observed in only 1 patient, who had tumor invasion to the neighboring lobe beyond the interlobar fissure. The cancer-specific 5-year survival rate was 96.6% in patients with pathologic stage IA and 67.4% in those with pathologic stage IB disease. These results suggested that selective MLND is applicable to patients with NSCLC whose selective lymph node stations are not metastatic. We recently revised the original method for selective mediastinal lymph node stations to obtain greater accuracy and usefulness, and the extent of this selective lymphadenectomy procedure is shown in **Table 2**.

Okada and colleagues[13] also evaluated the possibility of lesser MLND for early-stage lung cancer. These investigators defined their selective mediastinal dissection procedure as follows. Dissection of the upper mediastinum for upper-lobe tumors is performed, although that is not needed for lower-lobe tumors with intact hilar and lower mediastinal nodes. Also, dissection of the lower mediastinum for an upper-lobe tumor is not routinely required when the nodes in the hilum and upper mediastinum are negative. The investigators compared disease-free and overall survival rates between patients who underwent curative-intent surgery with selective MLND and those who underwent a complete mediastinal lymphadenectomy (historic control). All patients in both groups had clinicosurgical stage I disease. Three stations (numbers 10, 11, and 12) of the N1 lymph nodes and 1 lobe-specific station of the N2 nodes were examined by frozen section to select the type of dissection. There was no significant difference in survival rate, and the investigators concluded that selective MLND for clinicosurgical stage I NSCLC was effective for complete dissection. Ishiguro and colleagues[50] conducted a large-scale retrospective

Table 2
Lobe-specific selective lymph node stations for intraoperative biopsy and extent of selective lymphadenectomy

	Selective Lymph Node Stations			
Tumor Location	Previous	Revised	Selective Lymphadenectomy	
Right upper lobe	2, 3, 4	10, 2, 3, 4	(12u, 11s)	10, 2, 3, 4
Right lower lobe	3, 7, 8	11i, 11s, 7, 8	(12l, 9)	11i, 11s, 7, 8
Left upper lobe	4, 5, 7			
Left superior segment		4, 5, 6	(12u, 11, 10)	4, 5, 6
Left lingular segment		11, 5, 7	(12u, 10)	11, 5, 7
Left lower lobe	4, 7, 8	11, 7, 8	(12l, 9)	11, 7, 8

cohort study and applied a propensity score, and those findings supported the conclusions of Okada and colleagues.[13] More recently, Matsumura and colleagues[51] attempted to clarify the reasonable extent of lymph node dissection during an intentional segmentectomy for small peripheral NSCLC.

Although large multicenter trials are warranted, lobe-specific selective mediastinal dissection might be considered as an alternative for curative surgery for early-stage NSCLC until SLN mapping techniques have become better established for breast cancer and melanoma cases.

SUMMARY

In cases of superficial malignancies such as melanoma or breast cancer, intraoperative lymph node mapping with an SLNB is an effective and minimally invasive alternative to inguinal or ALND for early-stage tumors. For primary lung cancer, although much effort has been made to investigate a variety of tracers, such as dyes, radioisotopes, magnetite, and iopamidol, for discerning SLNs, an appropriate agent that produces high identification and accuracy rates has yet to be developed. Further studies are needed to find an ideal tracer for practical use in patients with NSCLC.

REFERENCES

1. Silvestri GA, Gould MK, Margolis ML, et al. Noninvasive staging of non-small cell lung cancer. Chest 2007;132:178S–201S.
2. Lardinois D, Wedeer W, Hany TF, et al. Staging of non-small-cell lung cancer with integrated positron-emission tomography and computed tomography. N Engl J Med 2003;348:2500–7.
3. Detterbeck FG, Jantz MA, Wallance MB, et al. Invasive mediastinal staging of lung cancer. ACCP evidence based clinical practice guideline (2nd edn). Chest 2007;132:202S–20S.
4. Yasufuku K, Nakajima T, Fujiwara T, et al. Role of endobronchial ultrasound-guided transbronchial needle aspiration in the management of lung cancer. Gen Thorac Cardiovasc Surg 2008;56(6): 268–76.
5. Watanabe Y, Hayashi Y, Shimizu J, et al. Mediastinal nodal involvement and the prognosis of non-small cell lung cancer. Chest 1991;100:422–8.
6. Naruke T, Goya T, Tsuchiya R, et al. The importance of surgery to non-small cell carcinoma of the lung with mediastinal lymph node metastasis. Ann Thorac Surg 1988;96:440–7.
7. Okada M. Radical sublobar resection for lung cancer. Gen Thorac Cardiovasc Surg 2008;56:151–7.
8. Asamura H, Nakayama H, Kondo H, et al. Lymph node involvement, recurrence, and prognosis in resected small, peripheral, non-small-cell lung carcinomas: are these carcinomas candidates for video-assisted lobectomy? J Thorac Cardiovasc Surg 1996;111:1125–34.
9. Miyoshi S, Maebeya S, Suzuma T, et al. Which mediastinal lymph nodes should be examined during operation for diagnosing N0 or N1 disease in bronchogenic carcinoma? Haigan 1997;37:475–84.
10. Okada M, Tsubota N, Yoshimura M, et al. Proposal for reasonable mediastinal lymphadenectomy in bronchogenic carcinomas: role of subcarinal nodes in selective dissection. J Thorac Cardiovasc Surg 1998;116:949–53.
11. Naruke T, Tsuchiya R, Kondo H, et al. Lymph node sampling in lung cancer: how should it be done? Eur J Cardiothorac Surg 1999;16(Suppl 1):S17–24.
12. Yoshimasu T, Miyoshi S, Oura S, et al. Limited mediastinal lymph node dissection for non-small cell lung cancer according to intraoperative histologic examinations. J Thorac Cardiovasc Surg 2005;130:433–7.
13. Okada M, Sakamoto T, Tuki T, et al. Selective mediastinal lymphadenectomy for clinico-surgical stage I non-small cell lung cancer. Ann Thorac Surg 2006;81:1028–33.
14. Carbanas RM. An approach for the penile carcinoma. Cancer 1977;39:456–66.
15. Morton DL, Duan Ren W, Wong SG, et al. Technical details of intraoperative lymphatic mapping for early stage melanoma. Arch Surg 1992;127:392–9.
16. Giuliano AE, Kirgan DM, Guentha JM, et al. Lymphatic mapping and sentinel lymphadenectomy for breast cancer. Ann Surg 1994;220:391–401.
17. Lyman GH, Giuliano AE, Somerfield MR, et al. American Society of Clinical Oncology guideline recommendations for sentinel lymph node biopsy in early-stage breast cancer. J Clin Oncol 2005; 23:7703–20.
18. Wang SL, Balch CM, Hurley P, et al. Sentinel lymph node biopsy for melanoma: American Society of Clinical Oncology and Society of Surgical Oncology joint clinical practice guideline. J Clin Oncol 2012;30:2912–8.
19. Little AG, DeHoyos A, Kirgan DM, et al. Intraoperative lymphatic mapping for non-small cell lung cancer: the sentinel node technique. J Thorac Cardiovasc Surg 1999;117:220–34.
20. Deslauries J. Mediastinal lymph nodes: Ignore? Sample? Dissect? The role of mediastinal node dissection in the surgical management of primary lung cancer. Gen Thorac Cardiovasc Surg 2012; 60:724–34.
21. Cahan WG. Radical lobectomy. J Thorac Cardiovasc Surg 1960;39:555–72.

22. Naruke T, Suemasu K, Ishikawa S. Lymph node mapping and curability at various levels of metastasis in resected lung cancer. J Thorac Cardiovasc Surg 1978;76:832–9.
23. Lam W, Alnajjar HM, La-Touche S, et al. Dynamic sentinel lymph node biopsy in patients with invasive squamous cell carcinoma of the penis: a prospective study of the long-term outcome of 500 inguinal basins assessed at a single institution. Eur Urol 2013;63:657–63.
24. Slade MJ, Smith BM, Sinnett HD, et al. Quantitative polymerase chain reaction for the detection of micrometastases in patients with breast cancer. J Clin Oncol 1999;17:870–9.
25. Jannink I, Fan M, Nagy S, et al. Serial sectioning of sentinel nodes in patients with breast cancer: a pilot study. Ann Surg Oncol 1998;5:310–4.
26. Kuwano H, Amano J, Yokomise H. Thoracic and cardiovascular surgery in Japan during 2010; Annual report by the Japanese Association for Thoracic Surgery. Gen Thorac Cardiovasc Surg 2012;60:673–9.
27. Sugi K, Fukuda M, Nakamura H, et al. Comparison of three tracers for detecting sentinel lymph nodes in patients with clinical N0 lung cancer. Lung Cancer 2003;39:37–40.
28. Rzyman W, Hagen OM, Dziadziusko R, et al. Blue-dye intraoperative sentinel lymph node mapping in early non-small cell lung cancer. Eur J Surg Oncol 2006;32:462–5.
29. Krag DN, Weaver D, Ashikaga T, et al. The sentinel node in breast cancer: a multicenter validation study. N Engl J Med 1998;339:941–6.
30. Cox CE, Pendas S, Cox JM, et al. Guidelines for sentinel node biopsy and lymphatic mapping of patients with breast cancer. Ann Surg 1998;227:645–53.
31. Liptay MJ, Masters GA, Winchester DJ, et al. Intraoperative radioisotope sentinel lymph node mapping in non-small cell lung cancer. Ann Thorac Surg 2000;70:384–9.
32. Liptay MJ, Grondin SC, Fry WA, et al. Intraoperative sentinel lymph node mapping in non-small-cell lung cancer improves detection of micrometastases. J Clin Oncol 2002;20:1984–8.
33. Lardinois D, Brack T, Gaspert A, et al. Bronchoscopic radioisotope injection for sentinel lymph-node mapping in potentially respectable non-small-cell lung cancer. Eur J Cardiothorac Surg 2003;23:824–7.
34. Nomori H, Horio H, Naruke T, et al. Use of technetiumu-99m tin colloid for sentinel lymph node identification in non-small cell lung cancer. J Thorac Cardiovasc Surg 2002;124:486–92.
35. Ueda K, Suga K, Kaneda Y, et al. Radioisotope lymph node mapping in nonsmall cell lung cancer: can it be applicable for sentinel node biopsy? Ann Thorac Surg 2004;77:426–30.
36. Kim HK, Kim S, Sung HK, et al. Comparison between preoperative versus intraoperative injection of Technetium-99m neomannosyl human serum albumin for sentinel lymph node identification in early stage lung cancer. Ann Surg Oncol 2012;19:1343–9.
37. Kim S, Kim HK, Kang DY, et al. Intra-operative sentinel- lymph node identification using a novel receptor-binding agent (technetium-99m neomannosyl human serum albumin, 99mTc-MSA) in stage I non-small cell lung cancer. Eur J Cardiothorac Surg 2010;37:1450–6.
38. Nakagawa T, Minamiya Y, Katayose Y, et al. A novel method for sentinel lymph node mapping using magnetite in patients with non-small cell lung cancer. J Thorac Cardiovasc Surg 2003; 126:563–7.
39. Minamiya Y, Ito M, Katayose Y, et al. Intraoperative sentinel lymph node mapping using a new sterilizable magnetometer in patients with non-small cell lung cancer. Ann Thorac Surg 2006;81:327–30.
40. Minamiya Y, Ogawa J. The current status of sentinel lymph node mapping in non-small cell lung cancer. Ann Thorac Cardiovasc Surg 2005; 11:67–72.
41. Khullar O, Frangioni JV, Grinstaff M, et al. Image-guided sentinel lymph node mapping and nanotechnology-based nodal treatment in lung cancer using invisible near-infrared fluorescent light. Semin Thorac Cardiovasc Surg 2009;21: 309–15.
42. Gilmore DM, Khullar OV, Colson YL. Developing intrathoracic sentinel lymph node mapping with near-infrared fluorescent imaging in non-small cell lung cancer. J Thorac Cardiovasc Surg 2012;144: S80–4.
43. Yamashita S, Tokuishi K, Anami K, et al. Video-assisted thoracoscopic indocyanine green fluorescence imaging system shows sentinel lymph nodes in non-small cell lung cancer. J Thorac Cardiovasc Surg 2011;141:141–4.
44. Yamashita S, Tokuishi K, Miyawaki M, et al. Sentinel node navigation surgery by thoracoscopic fluorescence imaging system and molecular examination in non-small cell lung cancer. Ann Surg Oncol 2012;19:728–33.
45. Suga K, Yuan Y, Kaneda Y, et al. Computed tomography lymphography with intrapulmonary injection of iopamidol for sentinel lymph node localization. Invest Radiol 2004;39:313–24.
46. Ueda K, Kaneda Y, Sudo M, et al. Cerebral air embolism during imaging of a sentinel lymphatic drainage in the respiratory tract. Ann Thorac Surg 2006;81:721–3.
47. Takizawa H, Kondo K, Toda H, et al. Computed tomography lymphography by transbronchial injection of iopamidol to identify sentinel nodes in preoperative patients with non-small cell lung

cancer: a pilot study. J Thorac Cardiovasc Surg 2012;144:94–9.
48. Krag DN, Anderson S, Julian TB, et al. Sentinel-lymph-node resection compared with conventional axillary-lymph-node dissection in clinically node-negative patients with breast cancer: overall survival findings from the NSABP B-32 randomised phase 3 trial. Lancet Oncol 2010;11:927–33.
49. Liptay MJ, D'amico TA, Nwogu C, et al. Intraoperative sentinel node mapping with technetium-99 in lung cancer: results of CALGB 140203 multicenter phase II trial. J Thorac Oncol 2009;4:198–202.
50. Ishiguro F, Matsuo K, Fukai T, et al. Effect of selective lymph node dissection based on patterns of lobe-specific lymph node metastases on patient outcome in patients with resectable non-small cell lung cancer: a large-scale retrospective cohort study applying a propensity score. J Thorac cardiovasc Surg 2010;139:1001–6.
51. Matsumura Y, Hishida T, Yoshida J, et al. Reasonable extent of lymph node dissection in intentional segmentectomy for small-sized peripheral non-small-cell lung cancer. J Thorac Oncol 2012;7:1691–7.

Can Stereotactic Ablative Radiotherapy in Early Stage Lung Cancers Produce Comparable Success as Surgery?

Shervin M. Shirvani, MD, MPH[a], Joe Y. Chang, MD, PhD[a], Jack A. Roth, MD[b,*]

KEYWORDS

• SABR • SBRT • NSCLC • Stage I • Comparative effectiveness

KEY POINTS

- Stereotactic ablative radiotherapy (SABR) uses highly focused, ablative doses of radiation to treat early stage lung cancer and is a possible alternative to surgery.
- Results in medically inoperable stage I lung cancer are promising; however, SABR has not been directly compared with surgery and also carries its own risks.
- For patients who are medically inoperable, the preponderance of available data suggests that SABR is superior to conventional radiation.
- With SABR, inoperable patients can expect a high rate of local control and lung cancer–specific survival with minimal toxicity.
- Prospective studies are needed to assess the role of SABR in patients with both operable and inoperable stage I lung cancer.

INTRODUCTION: A HISTORICAL PERSPECTIVE ON STEREOTACTIC ABLATIVE RADIOTHERAPY

Stereotactic ablative radiotherapy (SABR), also called *stereotactic body radiotherapy* (SBRT), delivers high doses of radiation to a tumor in 5 or fewer fractions. The essential feature is that multiple low-dose radiation fields delivered from varying angles are made to converge on an overlap region that harbors the neoplastic growth (**Fig. 1**).[1,2] Furthermore, the dose distribution is fine-tuned so that the dose steeply decreases a few millimeters beyond this intended treatment volume, thus sparing nearby normal structures from harmful toxicity (see **Fig. 1**; **Fig. 2**).

SABR represents a stark departure from traditional radiation therapy. Conventional radiotherapy is delivered via daily treatments given over the course of multiple weeks. The reason for this practice, called *fractionation*, is rooted in the biologic phenomenon of differential DNA repair. Normal tissues can efficiently repair damaged genetic material in between daily treatments, but tumor cells, because of their intrinsic dysfunction, are less capable of DNA repair following radiation. Therefore, this differential capacity for repair provides radiation oncologists a means to separate

[a] Department of Radiation Oncology, The University of Texas MD Anderson Cancer Center, 1515 Holcombe Boulevard, Houston, TX 77030, USA; [b] Department of Thoracic and Cardiovascular Surgery, The University of Texas MD Anderson Cancer Center, 1515 Holcombe Boulevard, Houston, TX 77030, USA
* Corresponding author.
E-mail address: jroth@mdanderson.org

Thorac Surg Clin 23 (2013) 369–381
http://dx.doi.org/10.1016/j.thorsurg.2013.05.009

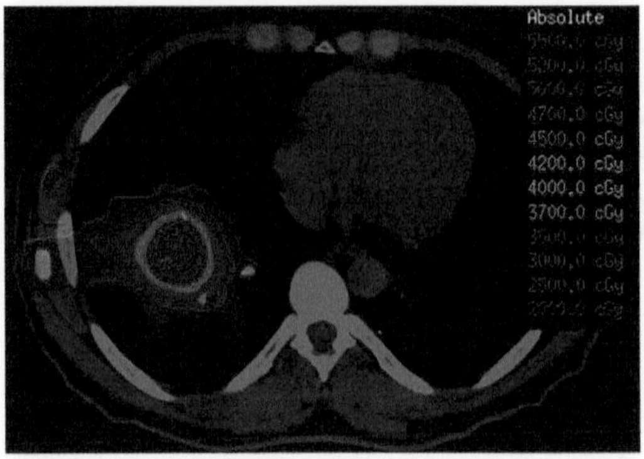

Fig. 1. Multiple radiation beams (9 beams, not shown) converging on target to generate an overlap region at target that receives an ablative dose (purple and red: 50 Gy and more in 4 fractions) while minimizing dose exposure to healthy lung, heart, esophagus, and spinal cord.

the effects of radiation on cancer cells from its effects on normal tissues. Indeed, conventional radiotherapy as practiced for several decades has depended on this phenomenon to improve the toxic-therapeutic ratio.

If the number of fractions is reduced so that patients receive a few large doses instead of many small doses, neither tumor cells nor normal cells are able to repair the amount of DNA damage that accrues. In these cases, the radiation dose is said to be ablative. Historically, the use of ablative radiation regimens, such as those used in SABR, had few applications because of the potentially devastating consequences of ablating normal structures. This concern was particularly appropriate in the era of 2-dimensional radiation planning during which radiation was directed at tumor targets via the use of orthogonal plain films. Although this technique allowed the radiation oncologist to aim radiation portals away from prominent bony structures, such as the vertebral column, it was difficult to routinely visualize, much less avoid, many critical tissues, such as the esophagus, bronchial tree, brachial plexus, or major vessels. Therefore, conventional fractionation remained the chief method for sparing normal tissues from the effects of radiotherapy.

More recently, the advent of modern radiation planning using conformal techniques and computed tomography (CT)-based simulation has given radiation oncologists the ability to sculpt radiation dose distributions in a customized fashion for each patient. Through the use of multiple beam angles and, in some cases, intensity modulation of beamlets within each beam, contemporary radiation plans can be shaped to conform to a tumor target as well as to bend around nearby normal structures. In this era of visualizing and dose painting, anatomic avoidance of normal structures can augment or even take the place of fractionation for normal tissue sparing. It is in this context that ablative stereotactic regimens have found firm clinical footing.

When first introduced, stereotactic radiation was limited to immobile tumors within the central nervous system. Tumors inside the lung or in the abdomen beneath the diaphragm were considered to be poor targets for SABR because of their motion during respiration. The dynamic nature of these targets meant that a catastrophic event could take place if, during breathing, a tumor was carried out of an ablative dose region and replaced by a vital normal tissue. Ultimately, this problem was solved through the development of 4-dimensional (4D) CT imaging at the turn of the millennium. With this technology, both the tumor and adjacent tissues could be visualized across a respiratory cycle. Therefore, dose distributions

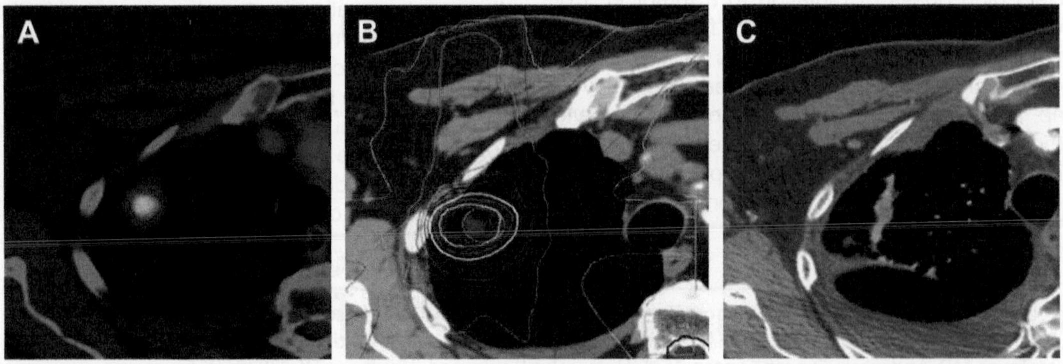

Fig. 2. (*A*) Positron emission tomography/computed tomography (CT) demonstrating right upper lobe nodule confirmed to be non–small cell lung cancer in a patient who was not a candidate for surgery. (*B*) Treatment with SABR to a dose of 50 Gy in 4 fractions (*white isodose line*). (*C*) Surveillance CT scan 6 months following treatment. The tumor has been replaced by a linear consolidation.

could be designed to cover the tumor and avoid normal structures during all phases of breathing rather than at a single time point.

Once these technological advances in imaging and treatment planning became generally available, SABR was widely implemented in both academic and community centers. The main appeal of SABR is that the treatment precludes the need for general anesthesia or an invasive procedure and can be delivered quickly over 1 to 5 daily treatments. In the context of lung cancer, SABR quickly found a niche as a last-resort therapy for patients deemed to be medically inoperable, a population whose options were otherwise limited to palliative chemotherapy, hospice, or marginally effective conventional radiotherapy. The fact that these patients were found to have excellent outcomes with SBRT has become one of the drivers for further exploration of this technology for healthier patient populations.

Currently, SABR has emerged as a standard definitive therapy for patients who are too frail for surgery or who refuse an operation; multiple population-based studies have convincingly demonstrated superiority of this technology over conventional radiation. The important next question is whether there is a role for SABR in patients that are fit to undergo an operation. Herein the authors review the technical parameters necessary for high-quality SABR treatment, review pitfalls and challenges, and assess the current evidence for SABR in the treatment of non–small cell lung cancer (NSCLC). Finally, the authors review comparative effectiveness studies and future trials that address the question of whether SABR should be the first-line treatment of patients who are fit to undergo an operation.

TECHNICAL REQUIREMENTS FOR HIGH-QUALITY SABR IN THE THORAX

Four critical steps are necessary for patients to be offered SABR to treat early stage lung cancer:

1. Positioning and immobilization
2. Respiratory compensation
3. Tumor coverage while respecting normal tissue constraints
4. Confirmation of accuracy at the time of radiation delivery[3]

Positioning Patients

Proper positioning and immobilization of patients are the fundamental requirements for any type of radiotherapy, whether conventional or ablative. Because the biologic characteristics of radiation preclude a second chance at therapy in most cases, it is critical to avoid tumor miss through variations in patient position from one daily treatment to the next. The necessary reproducibility in position is usually accomplished by aligning patients with several reference points.[4] Typically, patients are instructed to raise their arms to grasp a T-shaped bar while the trunk and abdomen are placed on a vacuum-sealed bag extending from the head to the pelvis. The bag is customized to the contour of the patient's body at simulation, and several points of alignment are indexed to the treatment couch and gantry using in-room lasers directed at marks on the patient's body and vacuum bag. For apical tumors, customized masks are also fabricated to immobilize the head, neck, and shoulders. A patient who is unable to undergo positioning and immobilization in rigorous fashion should not be offered SABR.

Compensating for Tumor Motion

During the respiratory cycle, lung tumors have been observed to move along all directional axes (anterior-posterior, superior-inferior, or medial-lateral); additionally, the tumors can be stretched and/or deformed.[5,6] Capturing the entire tumor in the radiation field throughout this motion is critical because otherwise an opportunity for cure is squandered. In the contemporary era, the path of a tumor during a respiratory cycle is delineated with 4D CT planning.

With this technique, tomographic visualization of the tumor's motion is obtained by acquiring oversampled CT images while simultaneously monitoring the patient's respiration. The CT images can then be assigned to different bins representing the different phases of the respiratory cycle. The 4D image is then created by reconstructing 3-dimensional (3D) images from each respiratory-phase bin and then playing all of the phases in proper sequence.[7] These images provide the position of the tumor and surrounding structures at all times during respiration.

Armed with this data, the radiation oncologist can customize the SABR plan by choosing one of several options (free-breathing, respiratory-gating, or breath-holding scans) for treatment planning and radiation delivery.[4,5,8] In one hypothetical example, an elderly man with an inferiorly located peripheral tumor may be selected to undergo SBRT. One possibility for treatment is to obtain a 4D simulation and contour the location of the tumor at every point in the respiratory cycle. The radiation oncologist can then choose to treat a region that encompasses the entirety of the tumor's path (called the *internal treatment volume*). In another example, a patient may have a 1-cm tumor that is located 2 cm inferior to the left main-stem bronchus. The treating physician may wish to deliver the ablative dose of radiation but fears causing unacceptable injury to the airways. To avoid this problem, the physician instructs the patient to hold his breath at full inspiration while wearing specialized goggles that provide visual feedback of his diaphragmatic excursion. The patient undergoes simulation at full inspiration at both treatment planning and during daily treatments. With this maneuver, the ablative region covers the tumor while it is well away from the mediastinum and left main-stem bronchus.

Coverage of the Tumor

With regard to tumor coverage, variations in the planning approach to dose prescription likely account for some of the differences in local control rates observed in clinical trials. As Senan and colleagues[2] pointed out in a recent review, a dose prescribed to the center of the tumor can result in an inadequate dose to the lesion's periphery and, therefore, worse local control.[1] Thus, the full dose should ideally be prescribed to a volume that encompasses the entire tumor. Furthermore, the goal should be to deliver a biologically effective dose (BED) greater than 100 Gy to this region. If the lesion is peripherally located and at least 2 cm from critical normal structures, an adequate BED can be achieved with 54 to 60 Gy delivered in 3 fractions or 48 to 50 Gy in 4 fractions prescribed to the 60% to 90% isodose line. If the lesion is more centrally located, the dose and fractionation of 54 to 60 Gy in 3 fractions may ablate normal tissues and result in unacceptable toxicities. In these cases, the physician should consider an altered regimen for SABR with a lower BED or else abandon SABR altogether in favor of surgery.

Verifying the Accuracy of Dose Delivery

The stakes for inaccurate delivery of SABR at the time of treatment are especially high. Missing or undertreating the tumor target could result in local progression and metastatic seeding from a once-curable local disease. At the same time, treating a normal structure inadvertently can result in significant injury or, in the worst case, a fatal complication. The traditional verification strategy in conventional radiation has been to use portal films before each treatment and compare them with radiographs from the treatment planning simulation to ensure that bony landmarks are properly aligned. However, this method is wholly inadequate for ablative radiation, which requires millimeter precision. Rather than using surrogate bony landmarks, it is necessary to directly visualize the lesion at the time of treatment. To that end, systems currently in use include real-time 3D imaging at the time of treatment delivery using technologies, such as a cone-beam CT mounted in the radiation gantry. Another image-guided verification strategy is the use of implanted fiducial markers, which signal the location of the tumor. As accuracy and precision improve with these technologies, the safety margin (planning treatment volume) of the radiation field may be decreased to assist in sparing of critical normal tissues.

If these procedures are instituted with rigorous quality-assurance measures, well-selected patients with early stage lung cancer can expect excellent treatment, recovery, and eradication of their lesion with SABR. Ultimately, it may be necessary to have regulatory standards and external credentialing to enforce high-quality standards at centers that elect to offer SABR.

TOXICITIES AND CHALLENGES FOR SBRT

Adverse Effects

Despite showing great promise in prospective studies, SABR is not without risks. Ablative doses of radiation can cause considerable damage to normal tissues, resulting in severe complications and diminished quality of life. Therefore, anatomic selection of candidates is imperative in order for the benefits of SABR to be meaningful for the individual patient.[3] Three anatomic groups with distinct risks have been identified.

The group that is easiest to treat consists of patients with lesions located in the periphery of the lung but away from the chest wall. For these tumors, ablative doses of radiation are well tolerated because the lung is a parallel organ, which provides latitude for the loss of functional alveolar units around the neoplasm. With current technology, expertise, and quality assurance, grade 3 to 4 toxicity rates now occur in the range of 0% to 10% for these anatomically favorable patients.[9–14] Radiation pneumonitis is the most frequent toxicity observed, and investigators have recommended limiting the ipsilateral lung mean dose to less than 9 Gy to avoid this adverse effect.[14]

If the lesion is centrally located, SABR entails a substantially higher risk. Ablative doses in this region can result in severe injury to mediastinal structures, such as the airways and great vessels, abrogating any advantages over surgery. In fact, a phase II study of 70 patients with both peripherally and centrally located tumors treated to 60 to 66 Gy in 3 fractions found 2-year freedom from severe toxicity rates of only 54% for patients with centrally located tumors compared with 83% in patients with peripherally located tumors.[15] The most common toxicities included pleural effusion, pneumonia, and a decline in pulmonary function. Even more alarming, 4 of the 6 deaths in the trial were likely related to treatment; all of these deaths were in patients with centrally located tumors. The investigators recommended that this dose-fraction regimen not be used in patients with tumors near the central airways. Other rare toxicities associated with SBRT to central structures include tracheal/bronchial injury, esophageal ulceration, and spinal cord myelopathy.[16–18] Tumors near the brachial plexus also carry the risk for severe injury. In a series of 36 patients with tumors at the lung apices treated with a 3-fraction regimen to a median dose of 57 Gy, the rate of brachial plexopathy was 19.4%.[19] Patients reported neuropathic pain, arm weakness, and, in one case, paralysis of the extremity. Risk was associated with receiving more than 26 to 40 Gy to the brachial plexus. However, recent studies showed that SABR of 50 Gy in 4 fractions with respecting normal tissue tolerance or adaptive SABR regimens based on location provide excellent local control without severe toxicities.[20,21] Currently, the Radiation Therapy Oncology Group (RTOG) is conducting a phase I study to evaluate the maximum tolerable SABR dose in centrally located lesions. With modern techniques that incorporate appropriate patient selection, treatment planning, and adherence to dose constraints, these events should not occur with measurable frequency.

Rib fractures and chest wall pain are other potential complications of SABR in patients with tumors close to the chest wall.[22–24] A large institutional series of 265 patients with tumors within 2.5 cm of the chest wall reported a 17% rate of chronic chest wall pain.[24] Notably, obesity and diabetic state were associated with the development of chronic pain in this study. Because 30 to 35 Gy seems to be the inflection point at which incidences of chest wall pain and rib fracture increase, the volume of the chest wall that receives this dose should be limited.[23,24]

Table 1 lists examples of organ dose limitations used in major trials in North America, Europe, and Asia. These values will likely change as clinical experience with SABR increases. Moreover, the incidence of the aforementioned toxicities

Table 1
Dose constraints used in major trials of SBRT

Organ	RTOG 0618 (3 Fractions)	Dutch ROSEL[a] Trial (3 Fractions)	Dutch ROSEL Trial (5 Fractions)	International STARS[b] Trial (4 Fractions)	JCOG 0403
Spinal cord	≤18 Gy	≤18 Gy	≤25 Gy	20 Gy ≤1 mL 15 Gy ≤10 mL	≤25 Gy
Esophagus	≤27 Gy	≤24 Gy	≤27 Gy	35 Gy ≤1 mL 30 Gy ≤10 mL	40 Gy ≤1 mL 35 Gy ≤10 mL
Lung	V20 ≤10%	V20 ≤5%–10%	V20 ≤5%–10%	V20 ≤20% V10 ≤30% V5 ≤50%	V15 ≤25% 40 Gy ≤100 mL MLD ≤18 mL
Brachial plexus	≤24 Gy	≤24 Gy	≤27 Gy	Point ≤40 Gy 35 Gy ≤1 mL 30 Gy ≤10 mL	Not limited
Heart	≤30 Gy	≤24 Gy	≤27 Gy	40 Gy ≤1 mL 35 Gy ≤10 mL	48 Gy ≤1 mL 40 Gy ≤10 mL
Trachea	≤30 Gy	≤30 Gy	≤32 Gy	35 Gy ≤1 mL 30 Gy ≤10 mL	40 Gy ≤10 mL
Bronchi	≤30 Gy	≤30 Gy	≤32 Gy	40 Gy ≤1 mL 35 Gy ≤10 mL	40 Gy ≤10 mL
Skin	≤24 Gy	Not limited	Not limited	40 Gy ≤1 mL 35 Gy ≤10 mL	Not limited

Doses represent limits at any point in the organ at risk unless otherwise specified.

Abbreviations: JCOG, Japanese Clinical Oncology Group; MLD, Mean Lung Dose.

[a] Randomized clinical trial of surgery versus radiosurgery in patients with stage IA NSCLC who are fit to undergo primary resection.

[b] Randomized study of lobectomy versus CyberKnife (Accuray, Sunnyvale, CA, USA) for operable lung cancer.

depends on both the total dose and the size of each daily fraction. By modulating these factors, one can turn down the intensity of ablation (probably at some cost to local control) to achieve acceptable risks of adverse effects. In one series, 27 patients with centrally and superiorly located tumors were treated with a regimen of 50 Gy in 4 fractions (instead of the more common 60–66 Gy in 3 fractions). The rates of subsequent complications were modest despite the tumors' central location: four patients (15%) developed grade 2 pneumonitis, 3 patients (11%) developed grade 2 to 3 skin toxicity and/or chest wall pain, and 1 patient developed brachial plexus neuropathy.[20] For lesions especially adjacent to at-risk normal structures, a more prolonged course of 70 Gy in 10 fractions can be used.[12] The ideal dose and fractionation for each anatomic scenario is a topic of active clinical investigation.

Posttreatment Surveillance

A different kind of challenge for SABR also deserves mention. In the follow-up period, it is often difficult to distinguish postradiation changes from tumor recurrence. On CT, parenchyma changes, such as fibrosis and persistent radiation pneumonitis, can take on a spectrum of manifestations, from diffuse consolidation and ground-glass opacities to focal consolidation and scarring. This wide spectrum of radiographic changes can render tools like the Response Evaluation Criteria in Solid Tumors (RECIST) criteria inadequate for assessing local response. Focal consolidation poses an especially difficult diagnostic challenge (see **Fig. 2**). PET may also fail to distinguish postradiation effects from viable tumor because treated regions can have persistent ^{18}fluorodeoxyglucose avidity for up to a year following SABR.[25,26] More recent studies have suggested strict positron emission tomography (PET) criteria, such as a threshold for standardized uptake volume (ie, >5) more than 6 months after SABR, to help select the best patients for confirmatory biopsy.[27]

Despite these diagnostic challenges, an absence of progression is generally a sign of successful treatment in the short-term, whereas PET positivity becomes a more reliable test for true recurrence in the long-term. Active study in the radiology community will likely generate additional quantitative and qualitative features that will aid in discriminating between SABR effects and relapse. Identifying these recurrences is important because emerging studies suggest that salvage surgery following SABR may be feasible.[28] Future studies are expected to further guide clinical decision making in these settings.

OUTCOMES FOR INOPERABLE PATIENTS: SABR AND CONVENTIONAL RADIATION

Selecting Inoperable Patients

The broad adoption of SABR for early stage lung cancer has currently been limited to patients who are unfit for surgery. Such patients are frequently seen for 2 reasons. First, the median age of patients with NSCLC is 71 years, making this a disease that affects mainly elderly patients with coincident chronic illnesses. Second, the most common risk factor is chronic tobacco exposure, which can afflict patients with multiple medical conditions, including chronic obstructive pulmonary disease, coronary artery disease, cerebrovascular disease, and several other malignancies. This combination of advanced age and comorbidities has made surgery challenging for typical patients with lung cancer.

Perioperative mortality for lobectomy depends on multiple factors, such as age, sex, comorbidities, performance status, degree of dyspnea, and American Society of Anesthesiologists score.[29] Using the Thoracic Surgery Scoring System, a tool that incorporates all of these predictive factors, a healthy 55-year-old man without significant comorbidities or dyspnea at baseline has a predicted mortality rate of 0.38% following lobectomy for early stage NSCLC mortality.[29–31] For the more common scenario of a 70-year-old man with mild to moderate comorbidities, the predicted operative mortality is 2% to 3%. A mortality of 2.7% was observed in the Cancer and Leukemia Group B 39 802 trial, a prospective, multi-institutional study performed to assess the feasibility of video-assisted thoracic surgery lobectomy.[32] Finally, in the oldest patients with moderate to severe comorbid conditions, the Thoracoscore model predicts a mortality rate that approaches 20%. In these patients, it is reasonable to find an alternative to surgery regardless of the fact that early stage lung cancer represents a potentially curable condition.

In addition to the assessment of comorbidities, pulmonary function testing provides useful information on the patients' ability to tolerate the physiologic consequences of lung resection. For patients with compromised pulmonary function, a Technetium (99mTc) microalbumin aggregated lung perfusion study can be obtained to predict postoperative pulmonary function. A predicted postoperative forced expiratory volume in the first second of expiration (FEV_1) less than 35% (or less than 0.8 L) or a predicted postoperative DLCO (Diffusion capacity of the lung for carbon monoxide) less than 40% indicate a higher risk of death and morbidity. Patients not considered operable because of poor pulmonary function when evaluated by a thoracic surgeon may be considered candidates for SABR.

Comparison of SBRT with Conventional Radiation

Traditionally, patients at a high risk of perioperative mortality have been treated with either palliative care or definitive radiotherapy using conventional radiation. However, conventionally fractionated radiation therapy directed at lung tumors is associated with disappointing local control rates of 30% to 50% and long-term survival rates of only 10% to 30%.[33,34] The likely explanation for these grim results is that the highest BED conventionally fractionated regimens can deliver is 80 Gy, a level not sufficient for the complete eradication of all neoplastic cells (**Box 1**). With SABR, a BED of 100 Gy or higher can be delivered safely to small tumor volumes by taking advantage of the anatomic avoidance strategies discussed earlier.

In fact, in contrast to the poor results of conventional fractionation, multiple prospective studies of SABR have demonstrated high local control of the primary lesion with published rates of 70% to 98% (**Table 2**).[9–14] The most important study among them is the RTOG Trial 0236, which was the culmination of applying the lessons learned from the SABR experiences of early adopters. This study accrued 59 patients with early stage NSCLC between 2004 and 2006 and treated their lung tumors to 54 Gy in 3 fractions using the SABR technique.[9] The results were impressive. Only one local failure within 2 cm of the original lesion and 3 additional failures within the involved lobe were observed, resulting in an actuarial local control rate of 98.0% and regional control rate of 90.7% at 3 years. With the publication of these results, the standard of care for inoperable patients began to shift from conventional radiation or palliation to SABR.

Although the results of RTOG 0236 were far better than historical outcomes associated with conventional radiation, the trial did not directly compare the different radiotherapy approaches. Comparative effectiveness research has helped to fill this gap. In the Netherlands, 2 recent studies have implied that SABR is superior to conventional radiation. The first by Palma and colleagues[35] was limited to 2 specialized centers in the Netherlands, with a study interval through 2007; the second study by Haasbeek and colleagues[36] extended the analysis to 4605 elderly patients in the entire Netherlands Cancer Registry, with a study interval through 2009. In both investigations, the investigators compared the rates of elderly patients receiving treatment and their survival before and after the introduction of SABR. In both studies, the investigators found that the proportion of patients with the disease who ultimately received definitive treatment increased. Moreover, they found that the overall survival had improved in this population, despite the fact that there was no evidence that stage migration had occurred. Further analysis revealed that this improvement in survival was limited to the cohort of patients who underwent SABR and that the survival associated with surgical strategies was essentially unchanged. Based on these findings, the investigators concluded that the introduction of SABR accounted for improvements in both access to treatment and successful cure among elderly patients with early stage NSCLC who were treated with radiation.

An important caveat of the Dutch studies is that individual treatment data were unavailable in these registries to separately analyze those receiving SABR versus those receiving conventional radiation. Therefore, the conclusion that transitioning from conventional radiation to SABR was responsible for the observed trends was somewhat circumstantial. More recently, Shirvani and colleagues[37] used population-based data from the United States Surveillance Epidemiology and End

Box 1
Biologically effective dose

A useful concept for understanding radiotherapy is the BED. Although a thorough discussion of radiobiology is beyond the scope of this article, an essential principle is that radiotherapy effects depend on 2 parameters: the total dose delivered and the size of the dose delivered in each session (called the *fraction size*).

Because of this phenomenon, one cannot compare the relative intensities of different regimens using only the total dose. Instead, it is useful to calculate a single quantity that takes into account both the fraction size (FS) and the total dose (TD). This quantity is the BED and is calculated using the following equation:

$$BED = TD \times (1+FS/(\alpha/\beta))$$

The other quantity in the equation, the α/β ratio, is a radiobiological parameter that reflects the radio sensitivity of the relevant tissue, whether it is the tumor or a normal structure. As discussed in this article, early studies have shown that a BED greater than 100 Gy is necessary to optimize the success rate of non–small cell tumor ablation with SABR.

Table 2
Selected studies of SBRT for early stage NSCLC

Trial	Stage	Dose and Number of Fractions	3-Year Local Control	3-Year Overall Survival
Inoperable				
Timmerman et al,[9] 2010	T1-T2 N0	54 Gy, 3 Fractions	97.6%	72.0% (2 y)
Nagata et al,[10] 2005	T1-T2 N0	48 Gy, 4 Fractions	94.0%	T1: 83.0%; T2: 72.0%
Xia et al,[12] 2006	T1-T2 N0	70 Gy, 10 Fractions	95.0%	78.0%
Chang et al,[14] 2012	T1-T2 N0	50 Gy, 4 Fractions	98.5% (2 y)	78.2% (2 y)
Operable				
Nagata et al,[17] 2010	T1 N0	48 Gy, 4 Fractions	68.5%	76.0%
Lagerwaard et al,[21] 2008	T1-T2 N0	60 Gy/3, 5, or 8 Fractions	93.0%	84.7%

Results (SEER)–Medicare database to specifically compare SABR with conventional radiation. Using data from patients treated between 2001 and 2007, this retrospective study adjusted for a spectrum of covariables, including age and comorbidities, as well as the use of staging techniques, including PET and mediastinal lymph node sampling. In both traditional multivariable and propensity-score matched models, the investigators found that conventional radiation was associated with significantly inferior overall survival and lung cancer–specific survival with a hazard ratio of 2 when measured against SABR.

These population-based studies strongly suggest that SABR is responsible for improved outcomes for inoperable patients over the last 10 years. As it happens, 2 ongoing trials are also comparing conventional radiotherapy and SABR in the prospective, randomized setting: the Scandinavian SPACE (Scandinavian Stereotactic Precision And Conventional Radiotherapy Evaluation) study and the Trans-Tasman CHISEL (Hypofractionated Radiotherapy [Stereotactic] Versus Conventional Radiotherapy for Inoperable Early Stage I Non-small Cell Lung Cancer [NSCLC]) study. Although it is certainly possible that the publication of these trials will contradict the retrospective evidence, the available data unequivocally support the use of SABR over conventional radiation in inoperable patients, provided that anatomic dose constraints can be met.

OUTCOMES FOR OPERABLE PATIENTS: SABR AND SURGERY

The Rationale for SABR in Operable Patients

Although the evidence for SABR over conventional radiation has resulted in a major change in the standard of care for inoperable patients, the more interesting and controversial question is whether patients who are operable should instead undergo SABR. Several considerations make this question worth asking. First, as described in the last section, surgery entails a mortality risk that is greater than that observed with SABR. Secondly, anatomic resection techniques also entail the risk of surgical morbidity. Systematic reviews of VATS lobectomy and thoracotomy lobectomy demonstrate complication rates of 16.4% and 31.2%, respectively.[38] These morbidities include atrial fibrillation, postoperative pneumonia, and persistent air leakage from a chest tube. Despite these risks, most of these complications are manageable and do not result in long-term impairment; the operative mortality for most series is less than 2%.[39]

Nonetheless, many patients who can tolerate resection based on residual pulmonary function measurements may still develop functional impairment after lobectomy and also face a continuing risk of second primary lung cancer. Thus, with lung preservation as an important consideration, SABR has emerged as an alternative even for patients deemed to be operable. In this section, current nonrandomized evidence comparing the 2 strategies is reviewed. Finally, important considerations regarding the design and execution of randomized trials is discussed.

Nonrandomized Evidence Comparing Surgery with SABR

Comparisons of historical data have suggested outcomes for SABR patients that approach the success rate of surgery. For instance, a review of medically operable patients who received SABR in a multi-institutional study in Japan showed 5-year local recurrence and overall survival rates of 8.4% and 70.8%, respectively, if a BED of 100 Gy was achieved.[40] These outcomes are comparable to the 5-year rates observed in the lobectomy arm of the North American Lung Cancer Study Group 821 trial (6% and 70%, respectively).[41] Although some commentators have noticed this interesting convergence, others have been appropriately skeptical of historical comparisons.

Currently, 3 categories of evidence have been used to compare SABR with surgery in a more rigorous way: single-arm prospective trials of operable patients who elected for SABR, single-institution retrospective comparisons of surgery and SABR, and population-based studies with multivariable adjustment. Currently, no randomized trial data that directly compares surgery with SABR are available. In fact, randomized trials to address this question have been beset by accrual difficulties, driven by patient and physician attitudes toward the perceived relative benefits of the 2 therapies. It is hoped that the cumulative evidence reviewed here will help in convincing both physicians and patients to actively participate in such trials.

With regard to the first category of evidence, groups in Japan and the Netherlands have prospectively evaluated patients who were deemed operable but who nonetheless elected to undergo SABR. Nagata and colleagues[17] reported initial outcomes from the Japanese Clinical Oncology Group 0403 trial, a prospective phase II study in which stage IA operable patients received 48 Gy in 4 fractions. The 65 patients in this study were elderly (median age, 79 years) but were generally in good health, with inclusion criteria of good performance status (0–2), Pa_{O_2} 60 mm Hg or more, and FEV1 700 mL or more. Moreover, each patient had to be individually assessed by a thoracic surgeon who confirmed the patient's ability to undergo an operation. With a median follow-up of 45.4 months, the 3-year overall survival rate was 76.0%, and the 3-year local progression-free survival rate was 68.5%. Grade 3 toxicities included chest pain (1.5%), dyspnea (3.1%), hypoxia (1.5%), and pneumonitis (3.1%). No grade 4 toxicities or deaths were observed.

The Dutch prospective study followed "potentially operable" patients who also underwent SABR instead of surgery.[42] These patients were slightly younger, with a median age of 76 years. The 3-year local control and overall survival rates were 93.0% and 84.7%, respectively, and toxicity was mild, with severe (grade $\geq$3) radiation pneumonitis and rib fractures occurring in 2% and 3% of patients, respectively. Given their promising outcomes, the investigators of both studies contend that it is very unlikely that these potentially operable patients would have been better served had they undergone wedge resection or lobectomy. A third single-arm study of operable patients is being conducted in the United States by the RTOG.

In the second category of evidence, investigators from the William Beaumont Hospital group published a single-institution, retrospective comparison of surgery and SABR.[43] Between 2003 and 2008, borderline operable patients at this institution were treated with either SABR or wedge resection. These patients were not candidates for lobectomy because of cardiopulmonary comorbidities. A review of this center's experience demonstrated that SABR and wedge resection had the same rate of distant metastases and cause-specific survival, but a nonsignificant trend was observed for a decreased risk of local and regional recurrence in the SABR group. An important limitation of this study is that statistical adjustment was not implemented to correct for baseline differences between the 2 patient cohorts, making it hard to disregard the role of selection bias when interpreting the results.

Investigators from Washington University in St. Louis presented another institutional retrospective comparison.[44] In this study, baseline differences were adjusted for using propensity-score matching. Using this methodology, the investigators observed equal rates of local recurrence and disease-specific survival when comparing SBRT patients with matched surgical patients. Of note, the surgical cohort included both wedge resection and lobectomy patients.

The final category of evidence is population-based studies from Europe and the United States. The first, by Palma and colleagues,[45] used a cancer registry in North Holland to compare elderly patients older than 75 years treated with either surgery or SABR. Patients were matched by age, stage, gender, and treatment year. Long-term overall survival was not statistically different between the groups. However, 30-day mortality was 8.3% in the surgical group versus 1.7% after SBRT. This population-based registry did not contain data for comorbidities and other pertinent patient characteristics, and so statistical adjustment for these factors could not be performed.

Shirvani and colleagues[37] used the SEER-Medicare database to compare SABR with both wedge resection and lobectomy in a cohort of patients older than 65 years. Importantly, this study corrected for a spectrum of covariables, including patient characteristics (age, gender, stage, comorbidity burden); tumor features (stage, histology); diagnostic interventions (mediastinal staging, PET); and demographic characteristics (income, education level). However, performance status and pulmonary function data were unavailable. Like the Dutch study, short-term mortality was considerably better with SABR (<1%) than with either lobectomy or wedge resection (both 4%). In traditional multivariable analysis, lobectomy was associated with the best long-term survival, whereas SABR and wedge resection were not significantly different from one another. However, because the investigators were concerned that traditional multivariable analysis did not adequately adjust for large baseline differences in age, comorbidities, and rates of mediastinal sampling, they also performed propensity-score matching. In the matched analysis, the lobectomy and SBRT cohorts had much more balanced baseline characteristics and were found to have statistically similar overall survival and lung cancer–specific survival.

Toward a Randomized Trial: Challenges and Progress

Unfortunately, attempts to compare surgery with SABR directly have been met with slow progress. Two issues have prevented rapid accrual into such trials. First, the large discrepancy between the therapies has made it difficult for physicians and patients to be free of bias when considering enrollment. After all, one is a radical surgery, whereas the other is a noninvasive outpatient procedure. A second issue is that these strategies entail differences not only in the actual treatment but also in both the up-front staging and downstream follow-up.

With regard to up-front staging, claims data demonstrate that most of the SABR patients are staged with PET, whereas surgical patients typically undergo additional pathologic staging with mediastinal nodal sampling.[37] The false-negative rate of PET scanning is 10% to 30%, which has major implications for stage migration and regional recurrence rates when comparing the 2 treatments. In the period after therapy, surgical patients are typically dispositioned to pathologic confirmation and/or salvage therapy at the first sign of recurrence. On the other hand, SABR patients with imaging changes after treatment are often followed for 6 to18 months to distinguish scar tissue from actual recurrence.[46,47]

Given these divergent practice patterns, it is not surprising that oncologists have been reluctant to enter patients into trials that entail such profoundly different experiences. Therefore, an important challenge for prospective randomized trials is to establish consistent protocols before and after treatment that allow for a fair comparison of the therapies without seeming to compromise patient care.

To make matters more complicated, emerging trends in early stage lung cancer treatment may further cloud the choice between surgery and SABR. The introduction of prognostic biomarkers and molecularly targeted agents may influence the type of definitive local therapy that is required.[48,49] Ultimately, these discoveries will likely stratify patients into ever smaller bins, with the importance of local and regional control dependent on the characteristics of the specific subset. For example, among those with an early metastatic phenotype that is sensitive to systemic agents, adequate sterilization of the lobe with drug therapy may obviate lobectomy, favoring SABR for control of the primary. For patients with a predominantly local, drug-resistant phenotype, on the other hand, surgery that removes both the lobe and regional nodes may be a superior strategy than SABR.

For now, 3 trials have been attempted for the broader population of patients with early stage NSCLC. The ROSEL (Trial of Either Surgery or Stereotactic Radiotherapy for Early Stage [IA] Lung Cancer) trial in the Netherlands sought to randomize stage IA patients into surgery and SABR arms but was ultimately closed early because of poor accrual. The STARS (Randomized Study to Compare CyberKnife to Surgical Resection In Stage I Non-small Cell Lung Cancer) clinical trial is comparing lobectomy to SABR in operable patients. More recently, the American College of Surgeons Oncology Group has opened trial Z4099 to compare SABR and sublobar resection for high-risk operable patients. In light of rates of accrual and the recent openings of these trials, results from these trials will likely not become available until 2018 or later.

In summary, the available evidence suggests that SABR may turn out to be an appropriate option in patients unable to undergo surgery. A growing body of retrospective and population-based research has failed to unequivocally establish superiority for surgery, and prospective studies of SABR suggest very good outcomes among patients who were eligible for an operation. Furthermore, a recent Markov decision analysis incorporating published single-arm outcomes suggested that SABR may not only offer comparable overall survival but also similar quality-adjusted life expectancy too.[50] However, although these results are promising for SABR, it should not be forgotten that lobectomy represents a mature, standard-of-care therapy with excellent outcomes validated over long follow-up. Thus, the proper interpretation of the evidence that favorably compares SABR with surgery is that it is hypothesis generating. Physicians should look to these findings as confirmation that there is clinical equipoise between SABR and surgical options and that enrollment of patients into random allocation clinical trials that seek to decisively answer this question is justified.

SUMMARY

Patients with early stage lung cancer often present as a therapeutic challenge as a result of advanced age, poor performance status, and comorbidities. For patients who are medically inoperable, the preponderance of available data suggests that SABR is superior to conventional radiation. With SABR, inoperable patients can expect a high rate of local control and lung cancer–specific survival with minimal toxicity as long as anatomic constraints are respected and quality-assurance protocols for reliable immobilization, accurate tumor targeting, and precise verification of dose delivery are followed. For operable patients, preliminary studies suggest that SABR could be as efficacious as surgery. However, changes in practice patterns for these patients should be based on the publication of ongoing randomized trials. In the meantime, lobectomy remains the standard intervention for patients with early NSCLC who are in good health and have adequate pulmonary function.

REFERENCES

1. Chang J. Stereotactic ablative radiotherapy for stage I NSCLC: successes and existing challenges. J Thorac Dis 2011;3(3):144–6.
2. Senan S, Palm D, Lagerwaard F. Stereotactic ablative radiotherapy for stage I NSCLC: recent advances and controversies. J Thorac Dis 2011; 3(3):189–96.
3. Shirvani SM, Chang JY. Scalpel or SABR for treatment of early-stage lung cancer: clinical considerations for the multidisciplinary team. Cancers 2011;3(3):3432–48.
4. Chang JY, Roth JA. Stereotactic body radiation therapy for stage I non-small cell lung cancer. Thorac Surg Clin 2007;17(2):251–9.
5. Chang JY, Dong L, Liu H, et al. Image-guided radiation therapy for non-small cell lung cancer. J Thorac Oncol 2008;3(2):177–86.
6. Liu H, Choi B, Zhang J, et al. Assessing respiration-induced tumor motion and margin of internal target volume for image-guided radiotherapy of lung cancers. Int J Radiat Oncol Biol Phys 2005; 63(Suppl 1):S30.
7. Nehmeh S, Erdi Y, Pan T, et al. Four-dimensional (4D) PET/CT imaging of the thorax. Med Phys 2004;31:3179–86.
8. Rosenzweig K, Hanley J, Mah D, et al. The deep inspiration breath-hold technique in the treatment of inoperable non-small-cell lung cancer. Int J Radiat Oncol Biol Phys 2000;48(1):81–7.
9. Timmerman R, Paulus R, Galvin J, et al. Stereotactic body radiation therapy for inoperable early stage lung cancer. JAMA 2010;303(11):1070–6.
10. Nagata Y, Takayama K, Matsuo Y, et al. Clinical outcomes of a phase I/II study of 48 Gy of stereotactic body radiotherapy in 4 fractions for primary lung cancer using a stereotactic body frame. Int J Radiat Oncol Biol Phys 2005;63(5):1427–31.
11. Uematsu M, Shioda A, Suda A, et al. Computed tomography-guided frameless stereotactic radiotherapy for stage I non-small cell lung cancer: a 5-year experience. Int J Radiat Oncol Biol Phys 2001;51(3):666–70.
12. Xia T, Li H, Sun Q, et al. Promising clinical outcome of stereotactic body radiation therapy for patients with inoperable stage I/II non-small-cell lung cancer. Int J Radiat Oncol Biol Phys 2006;66:117–25.
13. Stauder MC, Macdonald OK, Olivier KR, et al. Early pulmonary toxicity following lung stereotactic body radiation therapy delivered in consecutive daily fractions. Radiother Oncol 2011;99:166–71.
14. Chang JY, Liu H, Balter P, et al. Clinical outcome and predictors of survival and pneumonitis after stereotactic ablative radiotherapy for stage I non-small cell lung cancer. Radiat Oncol 2012;7:152.
15. Timmerman R, McGarry R, Yiannoutsos C, et al. Excessive toxicity when treating central tumors in a phase II study of stereotactic body radiation therapy for medically inoperable early-stage lung cancer. J Clin Oncol 2006;24(30):4833–9.
16. Nagata Y, Wulf J, Lax I, et al. Stereotactic radiotherapy of primary lung cancer and other targets: results of consultant meeting of the International Atomic Energy Agency. Int J Radiat Oncol Biol Phys 2011;79(3):660–9.
17. Nagata Y, Hiraoka M, Shibata T, et al. A phase II trial of stereotactic body radiation therapy for operable TINOMO non-small cell lung cancer: Japan Clinical Oncology Group (JCOG0403). Int J Radiat Oncol Biol Phys 2010;78:S27.
18. Joyner M, Salter BJ, Papanikolaou N, et al. Stereotactic body radiation therapy for centrally located lung lesions. Acta Oncol 2006;45(7):802–7.
19. Forquer JA, Fakiris AJ, Timmerman RD, et al. Brachial plexopathy from stereotactic body radiotherapy in early-stage NSCLC: dose-limiting toxicity in apical tumor sites. Radiother Oncol 2009;93(3):408–13.
20. Chang JY, Balter PA, Dong L, et al. Stereotactic body radiation therapy in centrally and superiorly located stage I or isolated recurrent non-small-cell lung cancer. Int J Radiat Oncol Biol Phys 2008;72(4):967–71.
21. Lagerwaard FJ, Haasbeek CJ, Smit EF, et al. Outcomes of risk-adapted fractionated stereotactic

radiotherapy for stage I non-small-cell lung cancer. Int J Radiat Oncol Biol Phys 2008;70(3):685–92.
22. Voroney JP, Hope A, Dahele MR, et al. Chest wall pain and rib fracture after stereotactic radiotherapy for peripheral non-small cell lung cancer. J Thorac Oncol 2009;4(8):1035–7.
23. Dunlap NE, Cai J, Biedermann GB, et al. Chest wall volume receiving >30 Gy predicts risk of severe pain and/or rib fracture after lung stereotactic body radiotherapy. Int J Radiat Oncol Biol Phys 2010;76(3):796–801.
24. Welsh J, Thomas J, Shah D, et al. Obesity increases the risk of chest wall pain from thoracic stereotactic body radiation therapy. Int J Radiat Oncol Biol Phys 2011;81(1):91–6.
25. Matsuo Y, Nakamoto Y, Nagata Y, et al. Characterization of FDG-PET images after stereotactic body radiation therapy for lung cancer. Radiother Oncol 2010;97(2):200–4.
26. Henderson MA, Hoopes DJ, Fletcher JW, et al. A pilot trial of serial 18F-fluorodeoxyglucose positron emission tomography in patients with medically inoperable stage I non-small-cell lung cancer treated with hypofractionated stereotactic body radiotherapy. Int J Radiat Oncol Biol Phys 2010;76(3):789–95.
27. Zhang X, Balter P, Pan T, et al. PET/CT and outcome in lung cancer treated with stereotactic body radiation therapy. Int J Radiat Oncol Biol Phys 2010;78(3):S16.
28. Neri S, Takahashi Y, Terashi T, et al. Surgical treatment of local recurrence after stereotactic body radiotherapy for primary and metastatic lung cancers. J Thorac Oncol 2010;5(12):2003–7.
29. Falcoz PE, Conti M, Brouchet L, et al. The Thoracic Surgery Scoring System (Thoracoscore): risk model for in-hospital death in 15,183 patients requiring thoracic surgery. J Thorac Cardiovasc Surg 2007;133(2):325–32.
30. Chamogeorgakis TP, Connery CP, Bhora F, et al. Thoracoscore predicts midterm mortality in patients undergoing thoracic surgery. J Thorac Cardiovasc Surg 2007;134(4):883–7.
31. Chamogeorgakis T, Toumpoulis I, Tomos P, et al. External validation of the modified Thoracoscore in a new thoracic surgery program: prediction of in-hospital mortality. Interact Cardiovasc Thorac Surg 2009;9(3):463–6.
32. Swanson SJ, Herndon JE 2nd, D'Amico TA, et al. Video-assisted thoracic surgery lobectomy: report of CALGB 39802–a prospective, multi-institution feasibility study. J Clin Oncol 2007;25(31):4993–7.
33. Dosoretz DE, Galmarini D, Rubenstein JH, et al. Local control in medically inoperable lung cancer: an analysis of its importance in outcome and factors determining the probability of tumor eradication. Int J Radiat Oncol Biol Phys 1993;27(3):507–16.
34. Kaskowitz L, Graham MV, Emami B, et al. Radiation therapy alone for stage I non-small cell lung cancer. Int J Radiat Oncol Biol Phys 1993;27(3):517–23.
35. Palma D, Visser O, Lagerwaard FJ, et al. Impact of introducing stereotactic lung radiotherapy for elderly patients with stage I non-small-cell lung cancer: a population-based time-trend analysis. J Clin Oncol 2010;28(35):5153–9.
36. Haasbeek CJ, Palma D, Visser O, et al. Early-stage lung cancer in elderly patients: a population-based study of changes in treatment patterns and survival in the Netherlands. Ann Oncol 2012;23(10):2743–7.
37. Shirvani SM, Jiang J, Chang JY, et al. Comparative effectiveness of 5 treatment strategies for early-stage non-small cell lung cancer in the elderly. Int J Radiat Oncol Biol Phys 2012;84(5):1060–70.
38. Whitson BA, Groth SS, Duval SJ, et al. Surgery for early-stage non-small cell lung cancer: a systematic review of the video-assisted thoracoscopic surgery versus thoracotomy approaches to lobectomy. Ann Thorac Surg 2008;86(6):2008–16 [discussion: 16–8].
39. Nguyen NP, Garland L, Welsh J, et al. Can stereotactic fractionated radiation therapy become the standard of care for early stage non-small cell lung carcinoma. Cancer Treat Rev 2008;34(8):719–27.
40. Onishi H, Shirato H, Nagata Y, et al. Hypofractionated stereotactic radiotherapy (HypoFXSRT) for stage I non-small cell lung cancer: updated results of 257 patients in a Japanese multi-institutional study. J Thorac Oncol 2007;2(7 Suppl 3):S94–100.
41. Ginsberg R, Rubinstein L. Randomized trial of lobectomy versus limited resection for T1 N0 non-small cell lung cancer. Lung Cancer Study Group. Ann Thorac Surg 1995;60:615–22.
42. Lagerwaard FJ, Verstegen NE, Haasbeek CJ, et al. Outcomes of stereotactic ablative radiotherapy in patients with potentially operable stage I non-small cell lung cancer. Int J Radiat Oncol Biol Phys 2012;83(1):348–53.
43. Grills IS, Mangona VS, Welsh R, et al. Outcomes after stereotactic lung radiotherapy or wedge resection for stage I non-small-cell lung cancer. J Clin Oncol 2011;28(6):928–35.
44. Crabtree TD, Denlinger CE, Meyers BF, et al. Stereotactic body radiation therapy versus surgical resection for stage I non-small cell lung cancer. J Thorac Cardiovasc Surg 2010;140(2):377–86.
45. Palma D, Visser O, Lagerwaard FJ, et al. Treatment of stage I NSCLC in elderly patients: a population-based matched-pair comparison of stereotactic radiotherapy versus surgery. Radiother Oncol 2011;101(2):240–4.

46. Dunlap NE, Yang W, McIntosh A, et al. Computed tomography-based anatomic assessment overestimates local tumor recurrence in patients with mass-like consolidation after stereotactic body radiotherapy for early-stage non-small cell lung cancer. Int J Radiat Oncol Biol Phys 2012;84(5):1071–7.
47. Huang K, Dahele M, Senan S, et al. Radiographic changes after lung stereotactic ablative radiotherapy (SABR)–can we distinguish recurrence from fibrosis? A systematic review of the literature. Radiother Oncol 2012;102(3):335–42.
48. Chen HY, Yu SL, Chen CH, et al. A five-gene signature and clinical outcome in non-small-cell lung cancer. N Engl J Med 2007;356(1):11–20.
49. Brock MV, Hooker CM, Ota-Machida E, et al. DNA methylation markers and early recurrence in stage I lung cancer. N Engl J Med 2008;358(11):1118–28.
50. Louie AV, Rodrigues G, Hannouf M, et al. Stereotactic body radiotherapy versus surgery for medically operable stage I non-small-cell lung cancer: a Markov model-based decision analysis. Int J Radiat Oncol Biol Phys 2011;81(4):964–73.

Surgeon's View
Is Palliative Resection of Lung Cancer Ever Justified?

Farid M. Shamji, MBBS, FRCS(C)[a,*],
Jean Deslauriers, MD, FRCS(C)[b]

KEYWORDS

• Surgery for lung cancer • Palliative resection for lung cancer • Palliative treatment • Chest wall pain • Massive hemoptysis • Syndrome of superior vena caval obstruction

KEY POINTS

- Clarification of terminology to avoid conceptual misunderstanding: complete resection, incomplete resection, and palliative resection of lung cancer.
- Recognize the indications of palliative resection of lung cancer in the past.
- Understand the pathogenesis and management of malignant pleural effusion accompanying lung cancer.
- Understand endobronchial complications of cancer in the main bronchi: obstruction with distal infected atelectasis and nonresolving sepsis, massive hemoptysis, wheezing, and stridor.
- Understanding complications of direct mediastinal invasion and mediastinal nodal metastases: superior vena cava obstruction, esophageal displacement and obstruction, compression and obstruction of trachea and main bronchi, phrenic nerve and recurrent laryngeal nerve palsies.

INTRODUCTION

The role of surgery in the management of patients with localized primary lung cancer of all histologic cell types, possibly with the exception of small cell lung cancer unless it is limited stage I disease, is to cure. The Lung Cancer Study Group was a multicentre initiative between 1977 and 1989 and had major influence on standardizing treatment of primary lung cancer and, for thoracic surgeons and the oncologists, it outlined guiding principles in the surgical management.

Of all patients with primary lung cancer, more than 50% are unsuitable for surgical management when first they are seen, because of clinical, radiographic, bronchoscopic, thoracoscopic, and mediastinoscopic evidence of metastases, in the form of either extrapulmonary intrathoracic spread or extrathoracic systemic dissemination. For this group of patients, primary treatment consisting of chemotherapy or radiation therapy sometimes works and survival is often limited to less than 6 months.

For primary lung cancer, like cancer that begins at other native sites, treatment is necessary for relief of symptoms. The treatment is surgical and curative for localized cancer, to prolong disease-free survival, or palliative for advanced cancer, to alleviate suffering for the duration of life.

DEFINITION OF RESECTIONS

Proper understanding and appropriate use of terminology in the types of surgical resection

[a] Division of Thoracic Surgery, Ottawa Hospital – General Campus, University of Ottawa, 501 Smyth Road, Room 6362, Box 708, Ottawa, Ontario K1H 8L6, Canada; [b] Division of Thoracic Surgery, Institut Universitaire de Cardiologie et de Pneumologie de Québec (IUCPQ), Laval University, 2725 chemin Sainte-Foy, L-3540, Quebec G1V 4G5, Canada
* Corresponding author.
E-mail address: fshamji@ottawahospital.on.ca

Thorac Surg Clin 23 (2013) 383–399
http://dx.doi.org/10.1016/j.thorsurg.2013.05.005
1547-4127/13/$ – see front matter

performed for primary lung cancer are necessary to avoid confusion and conceptual misunderstanding about the goal of resection and to evaluate the role of multimodality treatment regimens.[1,2]

First, there is the complete resection, which is the final aim of the surgical treatment of all types of localized non–small cell lung cancer and for stage I localized small cell cancer. Complete resection means that the primary tumor is completely removed, that there is no gross tumor left behind, that there is no microscopic residual disease in the resection margins, and that there is no metastatic tumor in the highest resected ipsilateral superior mediastinal node.[3–9] It is the only complete R0 resection that cures primary lung cancer.

Second, there is incomplete resection, when complete resection is unsuccessful and residual gross tumor is left behind at the margin of resection R2 or there is microscopic tumor present in the margin of resection R1. Incomplete resection does not cure in most instances. The higher the stage of the disease at surgical exploration, tumor (T) or node (N), or both descriptors, the greater is the likelihood for incomplete resection and the lower is the chance of cure. Incomplete resection must be distinguished from palliative resection; these are not synonymous terms and improper use of terminology has been a source of confusion in the published surgical literature and has misguided many novice chest surgeons.[1,4,8–13]

Third, there is palliative resection, when the resection of tumor-bearing lung, whole or part, is performed in the presence of known extrapulmonary intrathoracic spread or in the presence of distant metastases, when cure is not a goal and the aim is to relieve local symptoms. By definition, palliative resection is incomplete resection and gross tumor is left behind. Few patients are palliated by this type of resection; it is physiologically damaging, especially in the presence of inadvertent intraoperative injury or postoperative complications, both having an adverse impact on the duration and quality of life. With the advances made in radiation and chemotherapy in the last 4 decades, it is now preferable to use less invasive and less damaging methods of relieving local symptoms. In the remote past, palliative resection of primary lung cancer was performed on rare occasions in 4 clinical situations:

- To control septic complications in obstructive pneumonia
- To prevent asphyxiation in massive hemoptysis
- To palliate unstable vertebral body invasion and impending spinal cord compression
- To relieve severe pain from chest wall and thoracic spine invasion.

PALLIATION VERSUS SUFFERING

The expectations of palliative treatment need to be defined. According to the Concise Oxford English Dictionary, the word palliative means making the symptoms of a disease less severe without removing the cause; it is derived from the Latin lenimentum, meaning soothing. In order to consider palliative treatment to relieve suffering in selected cases of lung cancer, it is necessary first to understand the pathogenesis of certain clinical manifestations; the impact of each of these clinical manifestations on quality of life, as measured in length of survival and the general state of the patient during that period; when the local advanced extent of the growth is only manifest at operation; the benefit to be achieved by palliative treatment in the relief of suffering; and the effect of palliative treatment on the duration of terminal illness.

The duration of palliation to be expected by palliative treatment is hard to define but it must be longer than 9 months (because most patients with advanced lung cancer die within 6 months of the diagnosis), during which patients should be capable of caring for themselves, and the duration of terminal illness should be less than 1 month when patients are more or less incapable of caring for themselves and require the best supportive hospice care, supplemental oxygen, and narcotics.

Thoracic clinical manifestations for which palliative resection might be required:

1. Bronchopulmonary symptoms caused by the lung cancer arising proximally from the main or lobar bronchi (centrally located tumor) causing irritation, ulceration, or obstruction of the bronchus with distal lung atelectasis and nonresolving infection leading to septic complications.[4]

   Proximal involvement by tumor of both main bronchi and distal trachea constitutes oncologic emergency for urgent relief of acute airway obstruction

   Massive hemoptysis is life threatening, requiring urgent management to prevent fatality by asphyxiation

   Nonresolving distal pneumonia complicated by suppuration and formation of lung abscess in the infected lung, parapneumonic effusion, and rupture of lung abscess, resulting in pyopneumothorax

Diffuse mucinous lepidic adenocarcinoma in situ and bronchorrhea

2. Extrapulmonary intrathoracic symptoms caused by the lung cancer spreading by direct invasion into the adjacent structures or by metastasizing to the hilar and mediastinal lymph nodes.[4]

   Tumors arising from the true lung parenchyma (peripherally located tumors) may penetrate across the pleural surfaces into the chest wall causing severe pain or seed into the pleural space producing large pleural effusion and severe dyspnea.

   Metastatic spread to the mediastinal lymph nodes (often from centrally located tumors: small cell, squamous cell) may cause dysphagia by esophageal displacement and obstruction, plethoric facial swelling by obstructing superior vena cava, hoarseness by interrupting the recurrent laryngeal nerve, severe dyspnea from combined obstruction of main pulmonary artery and main bronchus, or stridor by invasion and ulceration of the main carina. On rare occasions, the metastatic malignant lymph node in the subcarinal space may invade both the main carina and esophagus, producing a fistulous connection and consequent aspiration pneumonia.[12]

   Direct invasion into the mediastinum (from centrally located tumors) on the right side can cause obstruction of the superior vena cava or interrupt the recurrent laryngeal nerve on the left side.

Factors to consider in the selection of palliative treatment:

1. In the planning of palliative treatment of unresectable and incurable primary lung cancer, it is vital in the pretreatment evaluation of the patient to measure the ability to undergo the planned treatment safely and still maintain adequate physiologic, psychological, and social functional capacity until the phase of terminal illness; presenting clinical manifestations caused by local complications from cancerous growth within the lung, or outside the lung but still inside the chest, and the impact on immediate threat to life or function and the quality of life; pretreatment evaluation of the primary tumor (T descriptor in tumor, node, metastasis [TNM] staging with increasing grade from T1 → T2 → T3 → T4) to determine the local extent of the growth and complications thereof; pretreatment evaluation of the local and regional lymph nodes (N descriptor with increasing grade from N0 → N1 → N2 → N3), which has a critical influence on the prognosis and on the selection of specific palliative treatment; accurate intraoperative evaluation for the extent of extrapulmonary intrathoracic spread during misguided surgical exploration of the chest (with increasing grade of lymph node metastases from N0 → N1 → N2, M1a pleura metastases with or without pleural effusion, T descriptor for direct invasion into the pericardium, chest wall, esophagus, thoracic aorta, and recurrent laryngeal nerve in the TNM staging); and evaluation of systemic spread (M descriptor, and the common sites of metastases are brain, bone, lung, liver, adrenal glands).[4,6,7,14,15]
2. Recognition of adverse extrapulmonary intrathoracic prognostic indicators for which palliative treatment is needed:
   - T4 and N2 descriptors, alone or in combination.[8,12,16]
   - Multiple mediastinal lymph node metastases on the ipsilateral side (N2 descriptor) affecting proximal airways, esophagus, superior vena cava, left recurrent laryngeal nerve.
   - One or more contralateral N3 descriptor discovered on positron emission tomography scan or by directed biopsy for confirmation.
   - Pleural metastases with or without pleural effusion (M1a descriptor).
   - Additional satellite malignant lesions in the same lobe T3, in the other lobes T4 on the same side.
   - Contralateral pulmonopulmonary metastases (M1b descriptor).
   - Presence of direct mediastinal invasion (T4 descriptor).
   - Deeper invasion of chest wall beyond the ribs into the overlying soft tissues (T3 or possibly T4 descriptor).
   - Inordinate delay in making the correct diagnosis of posterior superior sulcus tumor and therefore advanced disease when referred for diagnosis and treatment, and by this time the disease has progressed to a state that precludes effective relief of cancer pain, let alone a cure. The first symptom, often misdiagnosed, is steady localized pain in the shoulder and upper parascapular region; because the tumor extends by direct invasion, the clinical features typical of Pancoast syndrome appear with Horner syndrome (from invasion of sympathetic chain and stellate ganglion), worsening upper chest and shoulder pain (from invasion of intercostal nerves, upper 3 ribs, and possibly thoracic T1 and T2 vertebral body invasion),

pain radiating down from the shoulder along the ulnar surface of the forearm into small and ring fingers of the hand (from invasion of the lower brachial plexus C8 and T1), wasting of the small muscles of the hand (from T1 nerve root invasion), and neurologic complication from epidural spinal cord compression by central perineural extension of cancer through the spinal foramen (T3 or possibly T4 descriptors).[17–19]

- Inordinate delay in making the correct diagnosis of anterior superior sulcus tumor (not classic Pancoast tumor) invading anterior parts of first and second rib, subclavian vessels, and possibly lower trunk of the brachial plexus (T3 or possibly T4 descriptors)
- Primary lung cancer in the paravertebral gutter with direct invasion of the thoracic spine with complications of impending fracture and collapse leading to spinal cord compression (T3 or possibly T4 descriptors)
- Invasion of pericardium with or without pericardial effusion (T4 descriptor)
- Malignant esophagorespiratory fistula formation
- Diffuse form of mucinous adenocarcinoma in situ with lepidic pattern symptomatic with severe bronchorrhea

EFFECTIVE COMMUNICATION

When a decision for palliative resection or palliative treatment needs to be made knowing that the goal is alleviating suffering and not cure, it is the quality of communication with the patient and family members that directs the course of action. The communication should be both effective and supportive and not taken in haste. It is essential to allow adequate time for questions and to ensure privacy during discussion. It is expected that the patient will respond with emotional outpouring, shock, and anger. It is expected to be a difficult clinical situation and the surgeon will have to rely on experience and wisdom and to be prepared with a positive attitude and management plan to help the patient deal with these emotions. Ample time should be allowed for effective communication and discussion, answering all the questions to their satisfaction. The goals of the operation must be explained and the patient must be well informed. It is important to provide supportive care from skilled nurses, social workers, palliative care nurses, family doctors, and from the specialists. The surgeon should be well informed and honest in the discussion about different palliative treatment options and the duration and quality of life with or without palliative treatment.[20]

SPECIAL CLINICAL CONSIDERATIONS IN PALLIATIVE TREATMENT

Malignant Pleural Effusion

Malignant pleural effusion may be the first manifestation of primary lung cancer. If large, this often causes patients marked respiratory discomfort and incapacity, and interferes with their ability to lead an active and independent life for the limited survival time, which is often 6 months or less. Because palliation is so important to these patients, an understanding of the factors involved in the formation of malignant pleural effusion, as well as its diagnosis and management, is essential. Investigation by pleural fluid cytology and thoracoscopic pleural biopsy are valuable in confirming the diagnosis of malignant pleural effusion in 90% of patients when both procedures are used. Early palliation is cardinal and this is best obtained by complete evacuation of free pleural effusion to expand the lung and decrease respiratory distress. Once the pleural space has been evacuated and the diagnosis confirmed, bronchoscopy and noninvasive staging investigations are valuable in planning further treatment under interdisciplinary directive. Management is complicated when the pleural effusion is loculated, expansion of the lung is prevented by cancer, and coaptation of the pleural surfaces does not occur after drainage. Best palliation is obtained by insertion of PleurX catheter and systemic chemotherapy. There is no role for decortication pleurectomy or palliative pulmonary resection; both procedures are associated with higher morbidity and mortality, without survival advantage (no patient survives longer than 6 months), than standard local intrapleural therapy.[21–25]

Malignant Pleural Involvement Without Pleural Effusion

Malignant pleural involvement without pleural effusion may be discovered as an incidental finding of pleural metastases during pulmonary resection undertaken when operating on localized lung cancer for resection with curative intent. Such pleural metastases may be isolated or diffuse. Although pulmonary resection may technically be possible, it is ill-advised and pointless because survival longer than 6 months is rare.

In this manifestation of lung cancer, it is unclear whether there is a role for induction chemotherapy and radiotherapy and palliative extrapleural pneumonectomy using diffuse malignant mesothelioma as a model of care. More than 80% of patients with pleural metastases from primary lung cancer die within 6 months of diagnosis, which is significantly different from diffuse malignant mesothelioma, in which the median survival is 21 months with trimodality therapy (in most cases it is incurable). It may be reasonable to consider this type of palliative treatment in patients with lung cancer with pleural metastases who are otherwise young and fit, preferably less than 50 years of age, and without N2 nodal metastases and systemic spread. The author has performed the operation twice and obtained 24-month survival in 1 patient and 36-month survival in the second patient with good quality of life until terminal illness.

Patient 1: a 52-year-old man who presented with atypical left chest pain and was found to have non–small cell lung cancer in the lingula (**Fig. 1**). Surgical staging of the mediastinum was normal. Exploratory left thoracotomy for curative resection revealed multiple pleural metastases (stage IV, M1a); by definition an incurable disease. An aggressive surgical approach was chosen, to control the disease and not necessarily cure it, by giving induction chemotherapy and followed by extrapleural intrapericardial pneumonectomy. Final pathology was adenosquamous cell cancer. Although resection was thought to be complete by the absence of residual parietal pleural metastases, it was still found to be T4N0 disease. The patient died 3 years later from systemic relapse with brain metastases. Autopsy was not performed.

Patient 2: a 34-year-old woman presented with nonresolving pneumonia in right lung and was found to have adenocarcinoma in the right middle lobe, stage T2N0M0. After induction chemotherapy, surgical staging of the mediastinum revealed metastatic spread to R10 lymph node (N1). Right chest exploration undertaken for curative pulmonary resection revealed biopsy-proven multiple pleural metastatic tumor deposits, stage IV, M1a; talc poudrage was performed without pulmonary resection. For the next 6 months, further chemotherapy kept the disease under good control without manifestation of extrathoracic distant spread of cancer. Eight months after the initial operation, she underwent palliative right extrapleural pneumonectomy for persistent cancer to maximize optimal local control of the persistent cancer, and not necessarily a cure (**Fig. 2**). The patient died 2 years later of metastatic disease. Autopsy was not performed.

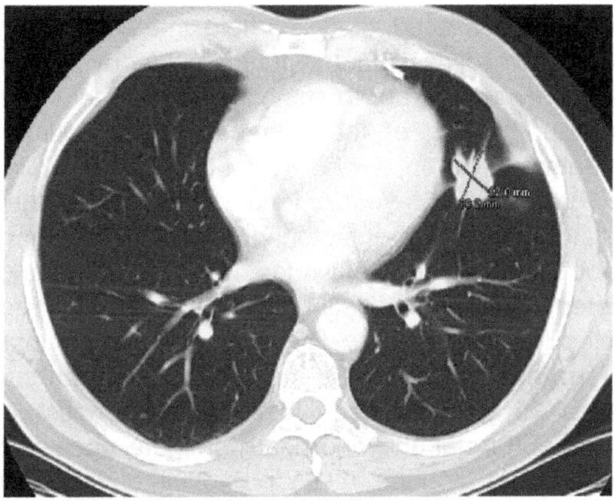

Fig. 1. Preoperative left lung cancer and pleural metastases: induction chemotherapy and left pneumonectomy.

Massive Hemoptysis

Massive hemoptysis is life-threatening hemoptysis, defined as expectoration of more than 600 mL of blood in 24 hours. It can be lethal within a matter of minutes as the result of ensuing asphyxiation. Massive hemoptysis should be distinguished from exsanguinating hemoptysis when copious airway bleeding continues and more than 1000 mL of blood are lost quickly at a rate of 150 mL or more per hour and the mortality approaches 100% because of the added effect of hypovolemia. Both massive and exsanguinating hemoptysis are life threatening and occur rarely in lung cancer. Often the cancer is in advanced stages when this complication manifests. It is most likely to occur when the cancer is arising in the main bronchi, causing both obstruction and infection in the distal collapsed lung. Another cause is cavitating lung cancer with superimposed infection resulting in the formation of malignant lung abscess or caused by erosion into major pulmonary arterial branch precipitated by radiation therapy. The volume of blood required to cause sudden death in massive hemoptysis by asphyxiation is 150 mL, which is just enough to fill the anatomic dead space and rapidly interfere with gas exchange; it can be lethal within a matter of minutes as the result of asphyxiation. The source of bleeding is from the bronchial artery 90% of

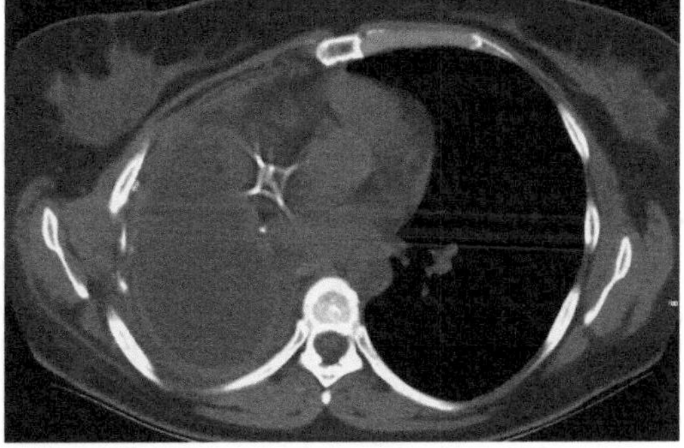

Fig. 2. Induction chemotherapy and after pneumonectomy, 3 months later.

the time; the increased demand for nutritive blood flow to the tumor and distal infected lung by bronchial arterial circulation is met by hyperplasia and hypertrophy of the bronchial artery with consequent increased risk of rupture of fragile blood vessels. In the presence of pleural adhesions developing because of pleural inflammation caused by infected atelectasis (which is frequently present), nonbronchial collateral arteries develop from the chest wall systemic arteries and also contribute to bleeding.[26–31]

Urgent pulmonary resection, most likely requiring pneumonectomy because of centrally located cancer, should be avoided at all costs for the following reasons:

1. Unacceptable high operative mortality of 15% to 20% when pulmonary resection is performed urgently for massive hemoptysis, and this increases to 33% in the presence of ongoing airway bleeding during resection.[32–34]
2. Lung cancer staging has not been performed to justify the operation.
3. Success with medical treatment of arresting bleeding in massive hemoptysis is now far superior than what was reported in 1968, with the availability of improved double-lumen endotracheal tubes for satisfactory lung separation, intubating flexible bronchoscopes for accurate placement of the double-lumen tube, bronchial irrigation with cold saline and dilute epinephrine solution, and expertise in interventional radiology for bronchial and nonbronchial arteriogram and embolization. Bronchial artery embolization, along with embolization of non bronchial collateral arteries (a search should always be made for these), produces immediate control of bleeding in more than 85% of patients.[26,35,36]
4. Advances in radiation therapy such as image-guided radiation treatment (IMRT) and stereotactic body radiation therapy (SBRT). After the life-threatening situation has been aborted by optimal medical management (described earlier), hemoptysis and cough, perhaps the most common distressing symptoms, are easily controlled by radiotherapy. Up to 75% of patients experience a significant degree of relief.

Patient 1: in the spring of 1983, when the first author was still in thoracic surgery residency training in Toronto, a man in his late 60s presented with massive airway hemorrhage (1000 mL) and the source of bleeding was centrally located primary cancer in the right lung. After urgent rigid bronchoscopy in the operating room to remove blood clots from the tracheobronchial tree and restore ventilation to the left lung, irrigation of the right bronchial tree with cold saline (normal saline at 4°C in 50-mL aliquots) and dilute epinephrine solution (0.2 mL of 1:1000 epinephrine added to 500 mL of normal saline in 5-mL to10-mL aliquots) the bleeding subsided. After confirming the diagnosis of non–small cell lung cancer on frozen section of the tumor biopsy, lung separation was obtained with left-sided double-lumen endotracheal tube. Because urgent bronchial artery angiogram and embolization were not available (this program was nonexistent at the hospital in 1983), the on-call surgeon, the late Dr Robert Ginsberg, advised the author to proceed with right thoracotomy and perform lung resection. The cancer was locally advanced and unresectable and the only option remaining was to divide the nutritive arterial blood flow to the right lung by circumcising the pericardium at the hilum of the lung, ligating the bronchial artery on the posterior wall of the right main bronchus, and dividing pleural adhesions and pulmonary ligament to interrupt contained nonbronchial collateral arterial circulation from systemic chest wall arteries (internal thoracic artery, acromiothoracic artery, intercostal artery, and lateral thoracic artery). Bleeding stopped almost immediately and further treatment was with palliative radiation. The best advice, after this experience, if faced with similar situation is that, unless it is exsanguinating hemoptysis, significant airway hemorrhage almost always stops with the current medical treatment, which is in the operating room with rigid bronchoscopy and irrigation with cold saline or dilute epinephrine solution followed by lung separation with double-lumen endotracheal tube to protect the good lung while maintaining the ability to continue with irrigation of the bleeding side, followed by urgent angiography and embolization. After bleeding has been arrested, there is ample time and opportunity to allow satisfactory functional recovery and leisurely investigate the fitness of the patient and proper staging of the lung cancer for specific treatment.

Patient 2: a 55-year-old woman with a 3-month history of cough, infected phlegm, chills, fever, nocturnal sweating episodes, left chest pain, and intermittent hemoptysis up to 1 cup of bright red blood each time and 6.8-kg (15-lb) weight loss (**Fig. 3**). She was treated for pulmonary tuberculosis 15 years earlier. Fiberoptic bronchoscopy was abnormal showing near-complete occlusion of left upper lobe (LUL) bronchial orifice with inflamed friable mucosa, and biopsy revealed squamous cell cancer. Reactivation of pulmonary tuberculosis was a concern in management.

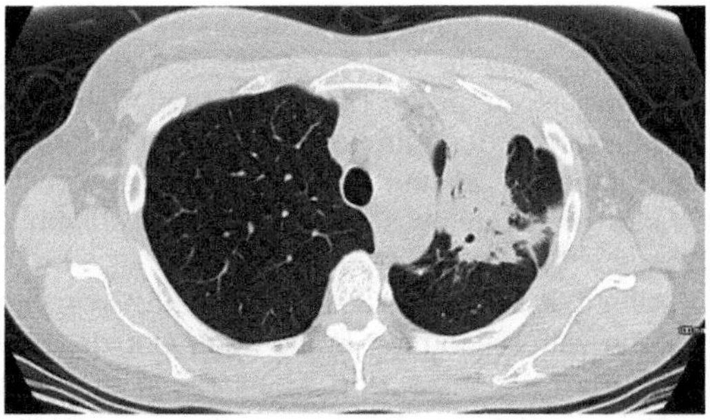

Fig. 3. Left upper lobe (LUL) mass suspected to be inflammatory distal to obstructed LUL bronchus and possible reactivation of pulmonary tuberculosis.

Surgical staging of the mediastinum was incomplete for N2 or N3 disease. Operation was performed, excising the left lung for locally advanced cancer measuring 8.5 cm, pT3 and extensive pN1 and obstructive distal pneumonitis. She remains well 6 weeks after surgery and a plan for adjuvant chemotherapy is under consideration.

Chest Wall Invasion

Chest wall invasion is caused by the peripherally located lung cancer penetrating across the pleural surfaces and then invading the chest wall (parietal pleura, costal periosteum, intercostal nerves, vertebral body, and the ribs). An accompanying pleural effusion is uncommon. The more extensive the involvement of the bony thoracic cage and surrounding soft tissues, the greater is the resulting chest wall pain and the more difficult is the management. Because en bloc pulmonary and chest wall resection is recommended with intent to cure after induction therapy for non–small cell lung cancer that is invading the chest wall in the confirmed absence of N2 mediastinal nodal metastases and systemic dissemination, palliative resection for chest wall pain in other situations is never needed because chest wall pain can be effectively treated with the state-of-art radiation therapy. Local pain caused by chest wall or rib involvement can be partially relieved in most patients, whereas pain caused by brachial plexus involvement in apical lesions is less responsive to radiation.[18,37]

Severe intractable chest pain and suffering from invading lung cancer, whatever its location, tends to be severe and worsening as it destroys more tissues and it impairs both physiologic and psychological well being of the affected patient. Physical deterioration results from sleep disturbance, loss of appetite, nausea, and vomiting, and often leads to excessive medication. This process leads to general fatigue and debility. The psychological effects of cancer pain are behavioral changes, depression, and emotional outbursts. The social effects of uncontrolled cancer pain manifest in deterioration of interpersonal relationships with family and friends, feeling of being useless, and loss of independence.[20]

Symptomatic relief of severe chest pain, for relief of suffering for those who cannot have the benefit of trimodality therapy, requires a combination of care with narcotic analgesics, radiation, chemotherapy, epidural spinal blocks, and possibly central nervous system stimulation for cancer pain.[20]

Chest wall invasion may be lateral or anterior and the patient complains of persistent severe pain, sometimes accompanied by an enlarging and painful tender chest wall mass caused by deeper invasion beyond eroded ribs. As the lung cancer invades deeply, it has the potential to gain access to the somatic chest wall lymphatic vessels and spread to the cervical and axillary lymph nodes, precluding the possibility of cure by resection with or without induction treatment. Because it is impossible to control the disease with deep invasion, the quality of life becomes important in management. It is reasonable to perform en bloc resection of the primary tumor and the involved chest wall after induction treatment for best and durable control of the disease for symptomatic relief.

Patient 1, anterior chest wall invasion: a 60-year-old man with persistent left anterior chest pain for 6 months and palpable enlarging mass was found to have locally advanced non–small cell lung cancer in the LUL with invasion into the mediastinal fat in the anterior superior mediastinum and extending through the eroded second rib into the overlying pectoral muscle (**Fig. 4**). Cancer staging was favorable and induction chemotherapy and radiotherapy were administered, producing only a partial response. Palliative en bloc resection

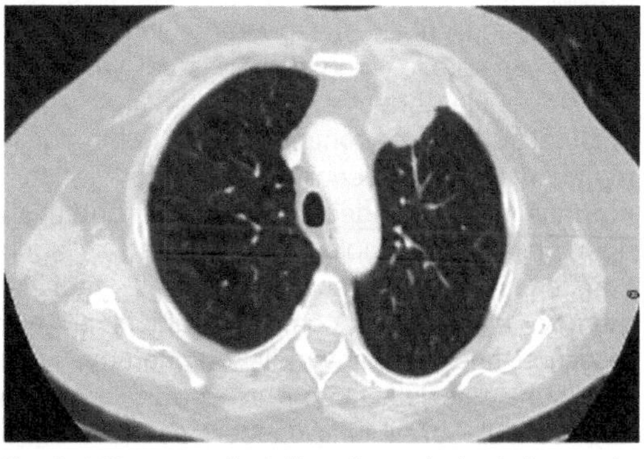

Fig. 4. LUL cancer invading through the left anterior chest wall into the overlying soft tissues.

was performed excising manubrium sternum and left anterior chest wall (pectoral muscle and left first to fourth ribs, segmental lingular-preserving left upper lobectomy, anterior pericardiectomy with sacrifice of left phrenic nerve because of suspected invasion by adherence, omentopexy, and latissimus dorsi myoplasty). Patient died 2 years later from systemic spread.

Apical chest wall invasion is by superior sulcus tumor. This condition is often it is a lung cancer arising in the extreme apex of the lung in the superior pulmonary sulcus (Pancoast tumor). It begins within the confines of the bony thoracic inlet where it often grows into the posterior parts of the first, second, and sometimes third ribs, sympathetic stellate ganglion, and the lower brachial plexus, causing severe neuropathic pain in the distribution of C8 and T1 dermatomes. Direct invasion of the adjoining thoracic vertebral bodies is also a frequent finding. It has specific clinical findings. All patients complain of severe upper chest wall and shoulder pain, worsening as the cancer progressively invades more adjoining structures, varying in duration from 2 to 18 months before the correct diagnosis is considered. By this time it is too late, and local invasion by the cancer is so advanced that effective relief of severe pain is impossible and there is no hope for a cure. Treatment becomes palliative at this stage for relief of severe neuropathic pain and to prevent invaded spine fracture and spinal cord compression. Along with severe upper chest wall and shoulder pain (starting with invasion of the upper chest wall and first, second, and maybe third ribs, and likely adjoining thoracic spine invasion at T1 and T2 vertebral bodies), patients usually complain of constant pain radiating down the ulnar side of the arm and have wasting of the small muscles of the hand with associated weakness and paresthesia (as the tumor progresses involving the lower brachial plexus: C8 and T1 roots, T2 nerve root, and intercostobrachial nerve), and Horner syndrome (from medial extension invading sympathetic chain and stellate ganglion). In the posterior location, this cancer can spread along the perineural lymphatics into the spinal foramina and eventually result in epidural spinal cord compression. The trimodality treatment of the superior sulcus tumor, which is now the recommended treatment of potentially operable and resectable tumor, consists of induction chemotherapy and concurrent radiation therapy, followed by complete radical en bloc resection and adjuvant radiation therapy. However, superior sulcus tumors are rare and represent less than 5% of all lung cancers seen. Because they are rare, the correct diagnosis is frequently made too late and, by the time diagnosis is considered, the disease is so advanced that effective relief of severe pain is impossible and there is no hope for a cure. Treatment then becomes palliative only for control of cancer pain, with radiation therapy, as the disease continues on its course of local invasion of bone and brachial plexus.[17,19,20,38]

Patient 2, superior sulcus tumor: a 52-year-old woman with discomfort in the right shoulder and axilla for 14 months, and weakness in the right hand for 6 months before the diagnosis of superior sulcus tumor was made (**Fig. 5**). There was wasting of the small muscles of the hand, satisfactory extension, but flexion of fingers impaired. There was a question of solitary brain metastases or infarct on head magnetic resonance imaging (MRI). Advice for management was sought from a neurosurgeon and neuroradiation oncologist and the decision was to proceed with Pancoast tumor resection. Brachial plexus MRI showed right Pancoast tumor invading T1 and T2 nerve roots and the lower trunk of brachial plexus, possibly involving C8 nerve root; tumor was encroaching onto the spinal foramina. Induction chemotherapy and radiotherapy was given. En bloc resection was performed: Dartevelle approach for exploration of brachial plexus, right posterior thoracotomy, chest wall resection of upper 3 ribs, spinal laminectomy T1 to T3, right hemivertebrectomy T1 and T2 and spinal instrumentation, division of T1 and T2 nerve

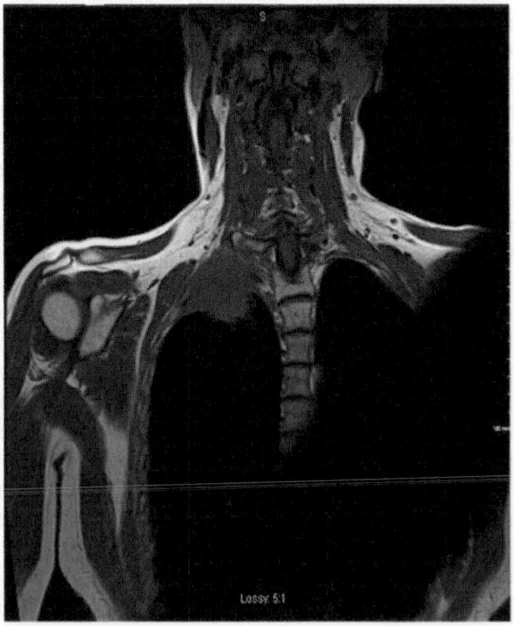

Fig. 5. Right superior sulcus tumor invading adjoining uppermost 3 ribs, T1 and T2 thoracic spine, sympathetic chain and stellate ganglion, and lower brachial plexus.

roots, and preserving portion of the lower trunk brachial plexus. Three months later, craniotomy for resection of solitary brain metastases was performed and now she is receiving chemotherapy for further recurrence of cancer in the abdomen; all within 3 to 4 months after undergoing resection of the superior sulcus tumor. This surgery was palliative resection for the sole purpose of obtaining best local control of invading cancer in the thoracic inlet, diagnosed 14 months late after onset of symptoms and expected to be locally advanced and beyond the realm of cure by multimodality treatment in the presence of possible brain metastases.

Posterior chest wall invasion is from peripheral lung cancer that begins in the paravertebral gutter and can eventually invade the adjoining thoracic spine causing severe pain and with the risk of spinal cord compression by epidural extension or pathologic fracture of the vertebral body and collapse. En bloc resection of the tumor-bearing lobe with spine resection and instrumental stabilization may be necessary for palliation after induction chemotherapy and radiotherapy.[37,39–41] Radiation therapy as an alternate treatment carries a risk of radiation myelitis and is to be avoided.

Patient 3, posterior chest wall and spine invasion: a 54-year-old woman with a 4-month history of worsening constant pain in the right upper anterior chest radiating into the right axilla. Investigations after abnormal chest radiograph revealed locally advanced right upper lobe non–small cell cancer invading thoracic spine at T2 to T3 and posterior second and third ribs (**Fig. 6**). At present, she is completing induction chemotherapy and radiation with the plan for palliative resection to prevent spinal cord compression.

Superior Vena Caval Obstruction Syndrome

Superior vena caval obstruction syndrome is a specific clinical entity that has many causes; the most common cause is malignant disease, particularly primary lung cancer situated in the right main or upper lobe bronchus, directly invading and encasing the vein or compressing it by enlarged bulky metastatic right paratracheal lymph nodes (**Figs. 7** and **8**). The specific clinical symptoms and signs, confined to the upper half of the body, are caused by fixed increased venous pressure. It occurs particularly in small cell lung cancers because of the propensity to extensive local dissemination. Twelve percent of patients with small cell lung cancer present with superior vena caval obstruction. Evidence of extrapulmonary intrathoracic and extrathoracic systemic dissemination of lung cancer other than superior vena caval obstruction is common in this group of patients.

The patient often complains of headaches and fullness in the face, exacerbated by bending forward. There is often facial swelling, particularly under the eyes, together with swelling of the upper limbs, and appearance of dilated collateral veins on the chest wall and a leash of tiny dilated purplish veins over the precordium. The patient may have stridor, dyspnea, and hoarseness secondary to edema of the tracheobronchial tree or larynx and possibly caused by bronchial obstruction by the underlying locally advanced lung cancer. There is a risk of central venous hypertension developing rapidly, before adequate collateral circulation has had time to establish, resulting in impaired cerebration or florid wet-brain syndrome. Survival depends on establishment of an adequate collateral circulation if blockage is complete.

Palliative treatment is urgent, requiring judicious use of diuretics and fluid restriction, radiation therapy, and chemotherapy. The syndrome of a superior vena cava obstruction can be relieved by radiotherapy and more than half the patients experience complete relief. Anticoagulation may help if complicating venous thrombosis is suspected. It is considered an oncologic emergency

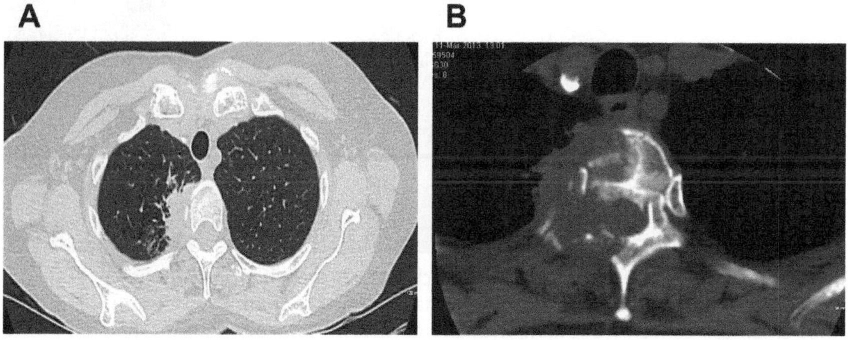

Fig. 6. (*A*) Right upper lobe (RUL) cancer with thoracic spine invasion. (*B*) RUL cancer showing progression on induction treatment; palliative resection now under consideration.

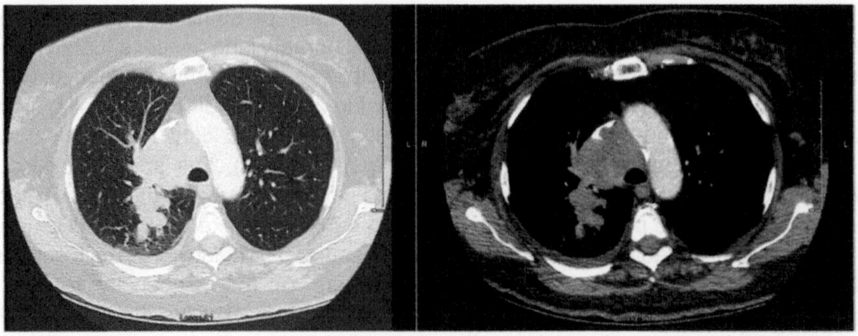

Fig. 7. A 70-year-old woman complaining of illness evolving over 4 weeks with worsening dyspnea, fullness in the face, fainting on coughing, and abdominal distension. Chest computed tomography (CT) scan confirmed superior vena cava obstruction (SVCO) from RUL mass with bulky mediastinal lymphadenopathy. Biopsy of multiple liver nodules confirmed small cell neuroendocrine carcinoma. Presence of ascites and left portal vein thrombosis was noted on CT scan.

that demands rapid palliation to ameliorate central venous hypertension by combined radiation therapy and chemotherapy. Rapid clinical improvement should be evident within days after starting treatment. If the objective of palliation is not achieved quickly as expected with treatment, it is important to administer systemic anticoagulation and thereafter plan for insertion of intravascular stent by an interventional radiologist and then to continue with radiation and chemotherapy for the specific cancer treatment (**Fig. 9**). There is a beneficial role for rapid palliation within days by intravascular stent insertion by interventional radiology and this expertise is much valued in the palliative care setting. Although palliative lung resection is contraindicated in most cases of superior vena cava syndrome secondary to locally advanced lung cancer, operative therapy is of benefit in some instances by performing venous bypass procedures using saphenous vein or prosthetic Gor-Tex or Dacron graft. This operation should be a rarity at the present time and likely only to be recommended if expertise in interventional radiology is not available.[42–44]

Delayed Resolution of Pneumonia

Delayed resolution of pneumonia is a clinical feature of malignant bronchial obstruction, partial or complete, by cancer arising in the main or lobar bronchi interfering with bronchial drainage and encouraging infection in the lung distal to the obstruction. The resulting lingering distal obstructive pneumonia often fails to respond favorably to antibiotics and the infection may progress rapidly to necrotizing suppuration with abscess formation. Pleural effusion or empyema may develop, or the lung abscess may rupture into the pleural space causing serious-looking pyopneumothorax and toxemia, or result in life-threatening profuse airway hemorrhage or death from rupture of mycotic cerebral aneurysm or metastatic brain abscess. Urgent treatment is necessary to relieve bronchial obstruction and attempts should be

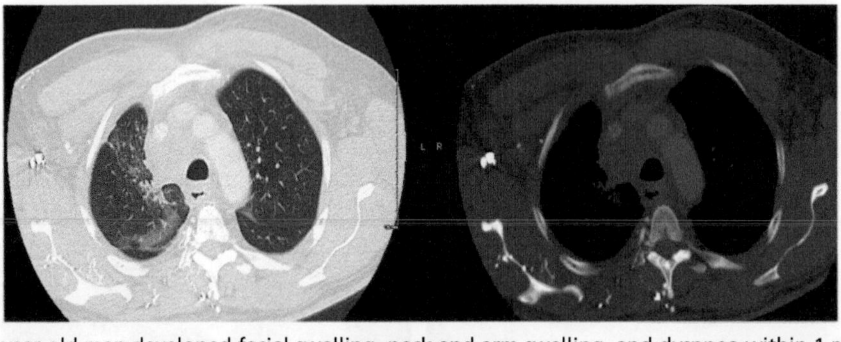

Fig. 8. A 52-year-old man developed facial swelling, neck and arm swelling, and dyspnea within 1 month. Chest CT scan showed SVCO from bulky right-sided mediastinal lymphadenopathy. Endobronchial ultrasound–guided biopsy confirmed small cell cancer. Treatment with chemotherapy and radiation therapy did not result in rapid palliation of SVCO and treatment planning was redesigned by giving urgent anticoagulation and insertion of intravascular stent before continuing with specific cancer treatment.

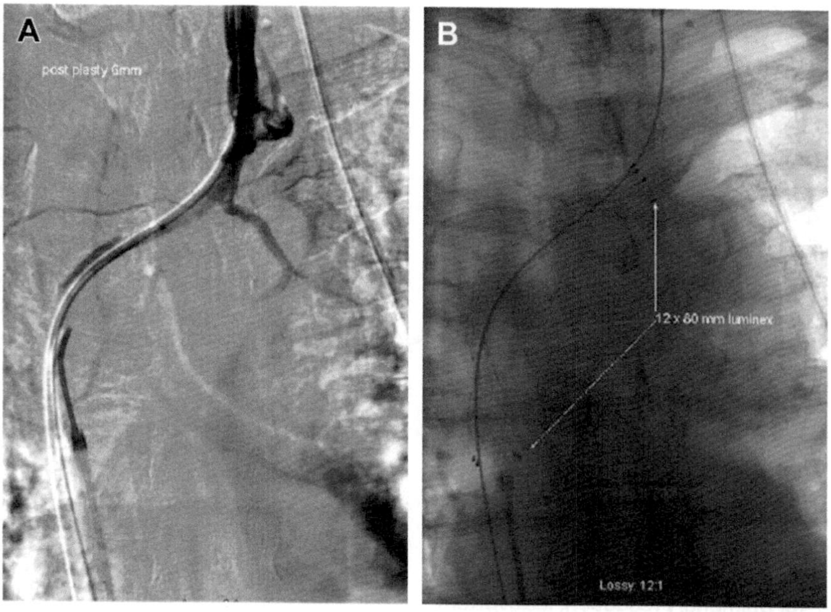

Fig. 9. (*A*) Venoplasty of superior vena cava from left arm access before stent insertion. (*B*) Intravascular stent deployed in good position.

made in the controlled environment of the operating room to restore patency in the obstructed bronchus by coring out tumor and debridement with rigid bronchoscope followed by application of laser treatment to achieve further debridement and coagulation (**Fig. 10**). Intercostal chest drainage is necessary for concomitant pleural effusion. This protocol for urgent treatment permits satisfactory early resolution of pulmonary sepsis by bronchial drainage and antibiotics. It allows time to establish accurate diagnosis of suspected bronchial cancer and the cell type, and

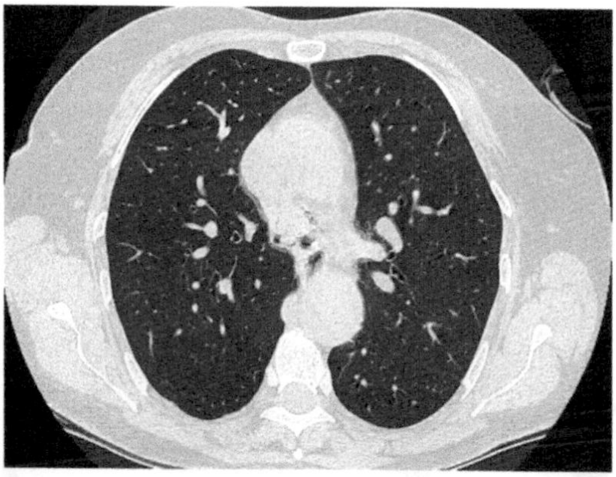

Fig. 10. Surgical bronchoscopic emergency therapy for high-grade airway obstruction of both proximal main bronchi caused by a large verrucous frondlike squamous cell cancerous mass arising from the main carina.

accurate staging of lung cancer and assessment of fitness of the patient for further definitive treatment. Although operative therapy for pulmonary resection is contraindicated in obstructive pneumonia because of locally advanced lung cancer, it is of benefit by restoring patency in the obstructed bronchus by the endobronchial therapy mentioned earlier, and further helped by insertion of bronchial stent.[45] Further palliative treatment with radiation and chemotherapy, although absolutely contraindicated in septic lung, is now possible after adequate bronchial drainage and resolution of pulmonary-pleural sepsis. Malignant bronchial obstruction can be improved in approximately half of patients with radiation therapy.[45]

On rare occasions of malignant bronchial obstruction and associated septic lung, palliative pulmonary resection may be necessary and beneficial when it is recognized that adequate patency of the airway cannot be restored by endobronchial therapy or because it is not available, and treatment with chemotherapy is contraindicated in the presence of pulmonary sepsis and radiation therapy is ill-advised.

Patient 1, obstructive pneumonia: a 79-year-old man with LUL non–small cell cancer obstructing LUL bronchus and distal infected atelectasis (**Fig. 11**). Preoperative mediastinal staging, in retrospect inadequate, was considered favorable but the patient was not a candidate for pneumonectomy because of limitation of respiratory function. Intraoperative finding revealed extensive

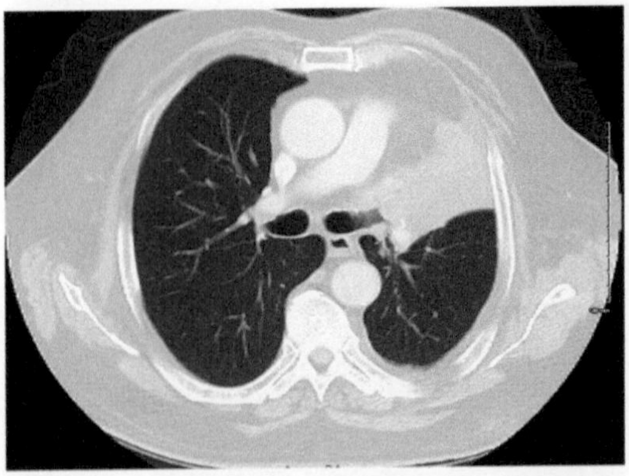

Fig. 11. LUL cancer with bronchial obstruction and distal infected atelectasis.

interlobar N1 lymph node metastases and N2 lymph node status not determined. The only option was to perform sleeve upper lobectomy and, in preparation for pulmonary resection, inadvertent pulmonary arterial injury occurred in the major fissure requiring repair and pulmonary resection could not be performed. Instead, the patient was referred for radiation therapy and chemotherapy as definitive treatment, which is when the first author assumed care of the patient. Complete bronchial obstruction and distal infected atelectasis contraindicated the requested treatment and extrapleural, intrapericardial pneumonectomy was then performed. Final pathology was squamous cell cancer pT2 pN2. Adjuvant chemotherapy was given and the patient remains alive and functioning well 5 years later.

The development of malignant lung abscess when the neoplasm undergoes central necrosis and cavitation and becomes secondarily infected is unusual. This condition is especially likely to occur in peripherally situated squamous cell carcinoma. The clinical picture is that of a patient with a large cavitating tumor mass in the lung that is producing a combination of persistent bronchopulmonary symptoms with severe cough, fever, significant hemoptysis, pleuritic chest, and febrile illness. Relief of symptoms is necessary. Radiation therapy and chemotherapy are not possible in the presence of sepsis, and there is a potential risk of erosion of major pulmonary arterial branch during the course of radiation and massive hemoptysis. The necessity for surgical intervention requiring pulmonary resection will be declared for palliation.

Patient 2, infected cavitating lung cancer (malignant lung abscess): a 48-year-old man with large cavitating right upper lobe (RUL) squamous cell was symptomatic with febrile illness with fever, chills, cough with greenish phlegm, sweating episodes, significant hemoptysis (60–90 mL [2 to 3 oz] daily) for 6 months before seeking medical care (**Fig. 12**). The patient had developed the serious complication of malignant lung abscess formation from the tumor undergoing central necrosis and becoming secondarily infected. Palliative resection was the only treatment option in this patient in whom chemotherapy and radiation therapy were absolutely contraindicated. Right extrapleural pneumonectomy was performed after preoperative embolization of bronchial and nonbronchial arteries to minimize intraoperative blood loss for pT4, pN2 cancer. Patient died 14 months later from systemic relapse of cancer.

Palliative Lung Resection

Palliative lung resection is undertaken in rare instances for recurrent cancer not controlled with chemotherapy. There are unusual cases of new ipsilateral multicentric primary lung cancer stable for extended periods but not curable by adjuvant chemotherapy after remote lobectomy for locally advanced but resectable non–small cell lung cancer. At present, when high-quality imaging with computed tomography (CT) scan of chest is readily available, the ability to detect asymptomatic lung cancer after pulmonary resection during follow-up has increased, with implications for the need to bring the new disease under effective control for the longest possible time This is a situation in which there is a need to change the philosophy in management of recurrent lung cancer and to treat it not as an incurable fatal disease but as a chronic disease; this has been seen in the treatment of human immunodeficiency virus-acquired immunodeficiency syndrome, breast cancer, lymphoma, germ cell tumors, and leukemia.

For a patient with delayed multicentric metachronous lung cancer, either recurrence or new disease, relying more on intuition and wisdom

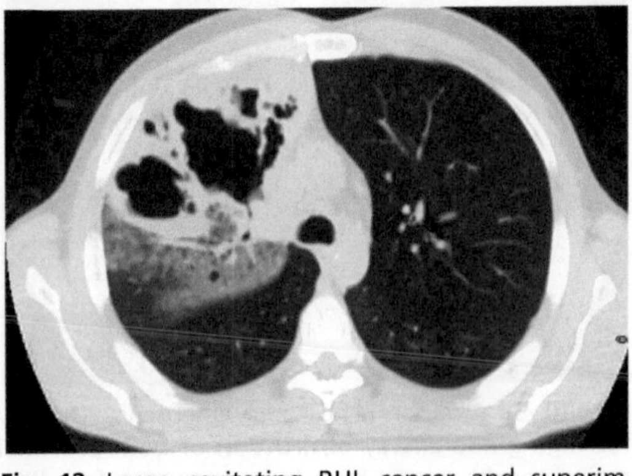

Fig. 12. Large cavitating RUL cancer and superimposed infection, symptomatic with persistent significant hemoptysis and febrile illness.

than on evidence-based medicine, treatment was undertaken with good long-term control of the disease. A 76-year-old man required sleeve RUL resection for stage IIIB, 9.5-cm RUL adenocarcinoma and in situ adenocarcinoma at the bronchial resection margin. Recommended adjuvant chemotherapy was completed. Multiple malignant lung nodules in the remaining right lung were noted 2 years after surgery and systemic chemotherapy was given (**Fig. 13**). Completion right pneumonectomy for stable disease was performed 18 months later. Final pathology was adenocarcinoma pT4 pN0 and he now has several discrete solid nodules, likely metastases, in the remaining left lung 3 years later. There is no doubt now that the completion pneumonectomy that was undertaken with intent to cure has proved to be palliative. Eradication of multiple nodular recurrent non–small cell cancer in his remaining right lung would have been extremely unlikely with chemotherapy, so pneumonectomy was performed for long-term control and palliation.

Multicentric Mucinous Adenocarcinoma and Bronchorrhea

Multicentric mucinous adenocarcinoma and bronchorrhea: disabling symptoms of drowning in excessive bronchial secretions from diffuse mucinous unilateral multicentric adenocarcinoma with microscopic lepidic pathologic features.

Within the atypical spectrum of adenomatous hyperplasia, adenocarcinoma in situ, invasive adenocarcinoma, a disabling clinical presentation is that caused by production of abundant, thin, and mucoid sputum resembling the respiratory fluid discharge in sheep infected with the Jaagsiekte sheep retrovirus. This condition is termed bronchorrhea because of overactive secretory functions of type-2 pneumocytes and Clara cells, and in the presence of pneumonic consolidation it is often confused as pneumonia and treated with several courses of antibiotics to no avail. The correct diagnosis is often overlooked for several months. When the diagnosis is eventually made, the treatment options are limited to relief of the dominant symptom and control of the disease. Resection alone by pneumonectomy or combined with single lung transplantation is an option but with the realization of universal failure.[46–48]

A 74-year-old woman, a known case of chronic myelogenous leukemia for 7 years, complained of cough productive of a large amount of thin mucus for 3 months. A diagnosis of well-differentiated adenocarcinoma with background of acute and chronic inflammation was made on CT scan showing large 8-cm airspace disease in RUL, multiple small areas of airspace disease in right middle lobe and left lower lobe (LLL). The radiologic diagnosis was multifocal adenocarcinoma (**Fig. 14**). Surgical staging was favorable and palliative right upper lobectomy was performed for well-differentiated invasive mucinous lepidic predominant adenocarcinoma and acute bronchopneumonia pT2b, PN0. She is alive 2 years later, without progression in ground-glass opacities.

Ectopic and Paraneoplastic Syndromes in Lung Cancer

Primary lung cancer of all histologic cell types, but mostly small cell, present with the various extrapulmonary nonmetastatic manifestations classified as endocrine and metabolic, neuromuscular, skeletal, dermatologic, and vascular. The incidence is higher than is often quoted (2%). In all cases, except for small cell lung cancer, resection with intent to cure is possible except when there is evidence of systemic spread or unresectable extrapulmonary intrathoracic spread of cancer.

Hypercalcemia caused by ectopic peptide parathyroid hormone secretion by advanced squamous cell cancer is effectively managed with medical therapy and clinicians should not be

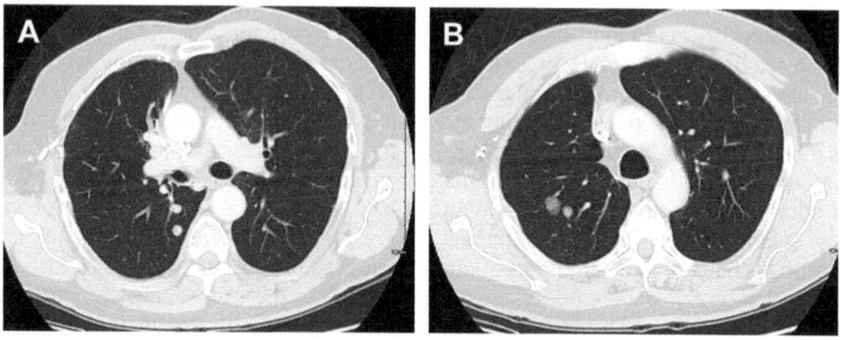

Fig. 13. (*A, B*) Right lower lobe (RLL) multiple malignant lung nodules.

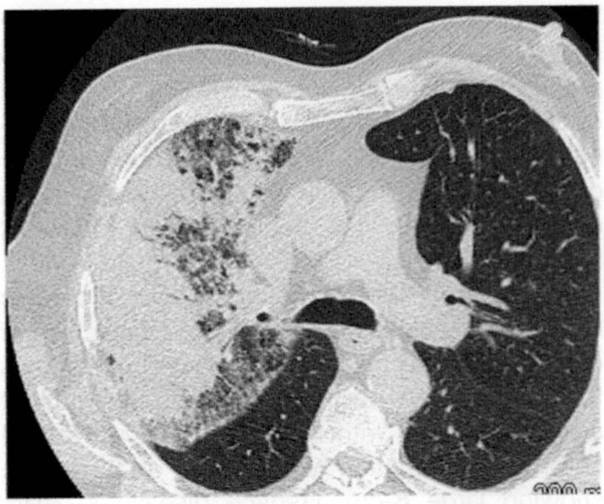

Fig. 14. Multifocal adenocarcinoma and bronchorrhea.

misled into performing unnecessary palliative lung resection.

Hypertrophic pulmonary osteoarthropathy, seen in all histologic cell types except possibly the small cell, responds favorably to radiation therapy to the primary tumor, if advanced and inoperable unresectable, or to ipsilateral video-assisted suprahilar vagotomy, avoiding the need for unnecessary palliative lung resection. It is manifested by painful clubbing of the digits, joint pain and swelling, painful periostitis, and arthralgia, and it may be the first clinical evidence of primary lung cancer.

Migratory thrombophlebitis may be seen in all cell types of lung cancer and sometimes with proximal extension from lower limbs with risk of pulmonary thromboembolism. Ready access to interventional radiology for insertion of temporary or permanent inferior vena cava filters has expedited nonsurgical care in the management of these difficult situations and helps avoid the attendant high risk of unnecessary palliative pulmonary resections.

Dysphagia

The proximity of the upper thoracic esophagus in the posterior superior mediastinum to the upper lobe of the right lung puts it at risk for direct invasion from RUL posterior-based lung cancer. The risk is similar for the lower thoracic esophagus with cancer arising from the lower lobe in the inferior posterior mediastinum. In both instances, dysphagia is more likely to be caused by esophageal displacement and direct compression by the tumor mass spreading directly outside the lung, and there is seldom evidence of esophageal mucosal invasion and disruption. A more frequent mechanism by which bronchial carcinoma causes dysphagia is by tumor spread to the subcarinal and inferior mediastinal nodes, which become enlarged and bulky, compressing the esophagus. Pulmonary resection may be considered an acceptable treatment, in the absence mediastinal nodal metastases, in the rare instances when extrinsic compression by the tumor is the reason for dysphagia. Otherwise, there is often no role for any type of palliative lung resection and mediastinal lymphadenectomy without intent to cure when the cause is esophageal compression by bulky mediastinal lymphadenopathy. The most effective short-term palliation is obtained by insertion of permanent or temporary esophageal stent and radiation therapy combined with chemotherapy. In cases in which mediastinal lymph node enlargement causes compression of the esophagus, the dysphagia can be relieved with radiation therapy in 80% of patients.

Survival is often limited to less than 6 months with stent alone in 28% of all cases; less than 12 months with added radiation therapy and chemotherapy in 35% of all cases; and less than 18 months with added treatment in 15% of all cases. It is only a few patients with favorable disease who respond well to the treatment and survive until the third year after multimodality palliative therapy that does not include palliative pulmonary resection.

Direct Intra-atrial Tumor Venous Extension

Direct intra-atrial tumor venous extension as a cord from malignant tumor in the lung is rarely seen in primary lung cancer, but occurs with pulmonary metastases from sarcoma and renal cell carcinoma, acting as a source of systemic tumor emboli and infarction, by extending through the pulmonary vein into the left atrium. Saddle tumor embolus in the distal aorta that manifested by bilateral acute lower limb ischemia in the recovery room soon after right lower lobectomy performed for sarcoma metastases was one such case that the author recalls from many years ago. It was unexpected and the intravenous cord of tumor extending from the centrally located tumor deposit in the right lower lobe embolized from the inferior pulmonary vein during manipulation for lobectomy. This occurrence was not recognized until the patient reached the recovery room, and it was a nurse who made the diagnosis and called for urgent assistance. Urgent embolectomy saved the surgeon's reputation and the patient's legs. After this experience as a resident in training, there were 2 cases (mentioned later) in which successful palliative lung resection was performed in the presence of tumor extending from the lung into the atrium through the pulmonary vein.

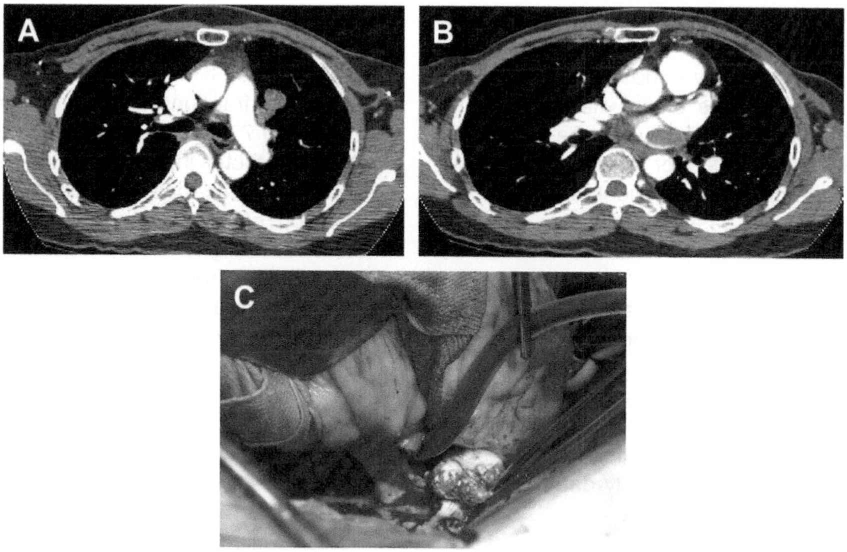

Fig. 15. (*A*) LUL tumor. (*B*) Intra-atrial extension from LUL tumor. (*C*) Atrial component of tumor removed under cardiopulmonary bypass.

Patient 1 presented with tumor embolus and stroke. A 55-year-old man, with past history of nephrectomy for renal cell cancer, developed hemiplegic stroke and was found to have tumor in the LLL with direct venous extension through the inferior pulmonary vein into the left atrium. It was thought that the stroke was caused by tumor embolus and the lung tumor was metastases from the previous renal cell cancer. Uneventful left lower lobectomy, without cardiopulmonary bypass, was completed after inflow and outflow vascular clamping of left main pulmonary artery and superior pulmonary vein and inferior pulmonary venotomy to extrude the tumor thrombus from the left atrium by controlled back bleeding. The operation was performed to palliate against further potential and serious neurologic complications of recurrent tumor emboli from the precarious intra-atrial tumor extension from the lower lobe. Patient died 5 months later from widespread metastatic disease.

Patient 2 presented with exertional dyspnea. A 45-year-old woman with past history of breast cancer treated 2 years previously with bilateral simple mastectomy and adjuvant chemotherapy developed progressive exertional dyspnea and was found to have a mass in the LUL on CT scan (**Fig. 15**A). Fine-needle aspiration confirmed non-small cell cancer of no specific type. CT scan indicated intra-atrial extension through the superior pulmonary vein and confirmed with transesophageal echocardiography (see **Fig. 15**B). Staging investigations were favorable. Cardiac CT ruled out coronary artery disease. Palliative operation was proposed for both symptomatic relief and to obviate the future risk for systemic tumor-thrombus embolization. A combined operation of, first, excision of intra-atrial tumor mass and reconstruction of atrium with bovine pericardium patch on cardiopulmonary bypass, followed by left upper lobectomy off bypass (see **Fig. 15**C). Final pathologic examination was multiple metastatic breast cancer nodules in LUL with venous extension into the left atrium. Patient remains well but with brain metastases 6 years later.

Pericardial Involvement

Pericardial involvement is by direct spread to the pericardium causing both pericarditis and a pericardial effusion. Palliation is only required for management of large symptomatic pericardial effusion with impending or actual cardiac tamponade. It is only when the cardiologist is unable to insert a catheter into the pericardial space (by the Seldinger technique) to relieve cardiac tamponade that the thoracic or cardiac surgeon is requested to perform subxiphoid pericardiostomy, which is safer under local anesthesia and with an anesthetist standing by in the operating room under controlled conditions. Palliative resection of lung cancer presenting with malignant pericardial effusion is to be avoided.

SUMMARY

Palliative operations (not necessarily pulmonary resection only) are for relief of symptoms that are disabling and reducing the quality of life; this benefit is more important than long-term survival and is not attainable by any other means, considering that a cure is unlikely in most instances. Palliative treatment must be given with the aim of minimum morbidity and inconvenience to the patient. In making a decision for resection for palliation it is important to consider the adverse prognostic indicators besides the primary cancer, the type and fitness of the patient who has the disease, the type of symptom or symptoms to be relieved, the type of operation required to achieve the objective, and the cost to the patient by incurring morbidity and mortality. It is crucial that intraoperative complications are avoided and that postoperative morbidity is low for patients to enjoy satisfactory postoperative palliation for the rest of their lives, which should be solely determined by the advanced stage of the cancer.

This article discusses the current treatment options for palliation in the inoperable unresectable lung cancer. Treatment options are no longer limited by lack of technology and nonsurgical specialties, and there are other options for palliation than chest exploration with attendant high complication and fatality rates. The treating physician can now take advantage of recent advances in the following areas:

1. Interventional radiology for angiography and embolization of bronchial and nonbronchial arterial collaterals to arrest life-threatening massive airway hemorrhage, and for insertion of intravascular stents for rapid symptomatic relief of superior vena caval obstruction syndrome.
2. Therapeutic rigid bronchoscopy for relief of acute major airway obstruction in the trachea or main bronchi by coring out obstructing tumor and using laser treatment to achieve coagulation and debridement, and stent insertion to maintain patent airway.
3. Thoracic anesthesia for expeditious airway management and lung separation techniques, expertise in high-frequency jet ventilation, and for intraoperative and postoperative acute chest pain control with epidural analgesia.
4. Various modes of radiation therapy (image-guided radiation treatment, IMRT, SBRT, and brachytherapy) for targeted less normal tissue damaging treatment for relief of severe chest wall pain, central venous hypertension from superior vena cava obstruction, and dysphagia from enlarged malignant mediastinal lymph nodes. Successful palliation of symptoms with radiation therapy is almost always caused by tumor regression and it is therefore necessary to use techniques and doses that reliably produce a tumor response. Numerous doses and fractionation schedules are in use; for example, 30 Gy in 10 fractions over 2 weeks, 20 Gy in 5 fractions over 1 week, and a single fraction of 7.5 to 10 Gy.
5. PleurX catheter insertion for the management of symptomatic malignant pleural effusion.
6. Insertion of endotracheal and/or esophageal stent for malignant esophagoairway fistula to prevent aspiration pneumonia.
7. Current availability of more effective targeted chemotherapy.

REFERENCES

1. Shields TW. The "incomplete resection". Ann Thorac Surg 1989;47:487–8.
2. Shields TW. The fate of patients after incomplete resection of bronchial carcinoma. Surg Gynecol Obstet 1974;139:569–71.
3. The Lung Cancer Study Group: final analysis. Chest 1994;106:279S–410S.
4. Le Roux BT. Bronchial carcinoma. Edinburgh (Scotland): E & S Livingstone; 1968.
5. Jensik RJ, Penfield Faber L, Milloy FJ, et al. Segmental resection for lung cancer: a fifteen-year experience. J Thorac Cardiovasc Surg 1973;66:563–72.
6. Mountain CF. Assessment of the role of surgery for control of lung cancer. Ann Thorac Surg 1977;24:365–73.
7. Pearson FG. Lung cancer. The past twenty-five years. Chest 1986;89:200S–5S.
8. Martini N, Flehinger BJ. The role of surgery in N2 lung cancer. Surg Clin North Am 1987;67:1037–49.
9. Martini N, Rusch VW, Bains MS, et al. Factors influencing ten-year survival in resected stages I to IIIA non-small cell lung cancer. J Thorac Cardiovasc Surg 1999;117:32–8.
10. Abbey Smith R. Cure of lung cancer from incomplete resection. Br Med J 1971;2:563–5.
11. Abbey Smith R. The results of raising the resectability rate in operations for lung carcinoma. Thorax 1957;12:79–86.
12. Burt ME, Pomerantz AH, Bains MS. Results of surgical treatment of stage III lung cancer invading the mediastinum. Surg Clin North Am 1987;67:987–1000.
13. Martini N, Yellin A, Ginsberg RJ, et al. Management of non-small cell lung cancer with direct mediastinal involvement. Ann Thorac Surg 1994;58:1447–51.
14. Overholt RH, Neptune WB, Ashraf MM. Primary cancer of the lung: a 42-year experience. Ann Thorac Surg 1975;20:511–9.
15. Paulson DL, Urschel HC. Selectivity in the surgical treatment of bronchogenic carcinoma. J Thorac Cardiovasc Surg 1971;62:554–62.

16. Martini N, Flehinger BJ, Zaman EJ, et al. Results of resection in non-oat cell carcinoma of the lung with mediastinal lymph node metastases. Ann Surg 1983;198:386–97.
17. Paulson DL. Management of superior sulcus carcinomas. In: Choi NC, Grillo HC, editors. Thoracic oncology. New York: Raven Press; 1983. p. 147–62.
18. Choi NC. Curative radiation therapy for unresectable non-small-cell carcinoma of the lung: indications, techniques, results. In: Choi NC, Grillo HC, editors. Thoracic oncology. New York: Raven Press; 1983. p. 163–99.
19. Paulson DL. Carcinomas in the superior pulmonary sulcus. J Thorac Cardiovasc Surg 1975;70:1095–104.
20. Bonica JJ, Ventafridda V, Pagni CA. Advances in pain research and therapy, vol. 4. New York: Raven Press; 1981.
21. Waller DA, Morritt GN, Forty J. Video-assisted thoracoscopic pleurectomy in the management of malignant pleural effusion. Chest 1995;107:1454–6.
22. Chen H, Brahmer J. Management of malignant pleural effusion. Curr Oncol Rep 2008;10:287–93.
23. Putnam JB. Malignant pleural effusions. Surg Clin North Am 2002;82:867–83.
24. Lee YC, Light RW. Management of malignant pleural effusions. Respirology 2004;9:148–56.
25. Bennett R, Maskell N. Management of malignant pleural effusions. Curr Opin Pulm Med 2005;11: 296–300.
26. Shamji FM, Vallieres E. Airway hemorrhage. Chest Surg Clin N Am 1991;1:255–89.
27. Shamji FM. Optimal management of massive hemoptysis. In: Franco KL, Putnam JB, editors. Advanced therapy in thoracic surgery. Hamilton, Ontario: BC Decker; 1998. p. 254–64.
28. Miller RR, McGregor DH. Hemorrhage from carcinoma of the lung. Cancer 1980;46:200–5.
29. Crocco JA, Rooney JJ, Fankushen DS. Massive hemoptysis. Arch Intern Med 1968;121:495–8.
30. Cudkowicz L. The blood supply of the lungs in pulmonary tuberculosis. Thorax 1952;7:270–6.
31. Muller KM, Meyer-Schwickerath M. Bronchial arteries in various stages of bronchogenic carcinoma. Pathol Res Pract 1978;163:34–46.
32. Garzon A, Gourin A. Surgical management of massive hemoptysis. Ann Surg 1978;187:267–71.
33. Garzon A, Cerruti M, Golding M. Exsanguinating hemoptysis. J Thorac Cardiovasc Surg 1982;84: 829–33.
34. Gourin A, Garzon AA. Operative treatment of massive hemoptysis. Ann Thorac Surg 1974;18:52–60.
35. Conlan AA, Hurwitz SS. Management of massive hemoptysis with the rigid bronchoscope and cold saline lavage. Thorax 1980;35:901–4.
36. Remy J, Arnaud A, Fardou H, et al. Treatment of hemoptysis by embolization of bronchial arteries. Radiology 1977;12:33–7.
37. Saito Y, Hayakawa K, Nakayama Y, et al. Radiation therapy for stage III non-small cell lung cancer invading chest wall. Lung Cancer 1997;18:171–8.
38. Komaki R, Roth JA, Walsh GL, et al. Outcome predictors for 143 patients with superior sulcus tumors treated by multidisciplinary approach at The University of Texas M.D. Anderson Cancer Center. Int J Radiat Oncol Biol Phys 2000;48:347–54.
39. Sundaresan N, Sachdev VP, Holland JF, et al. Surgical treatment of spinal cord compression from epidural metastasis. J Clin Oncol 1995;13:2330–5.
40. Young RF, Post EM, King GA. Treatment of spinal epidural metastases. J Neurosurg 1980;53:741–8.
41. Greenberg HS, Kim J, Posner JB. Epidural spinal cord compression from metastatic tumor: results with a new treatment protocol. Ann Neurol 1980;8: 361–6.
42. Avasthi RB, Moghissi K. Malignant obstruction of the superior vena cava and its palliation. J Thorac Cardiovasc Surg 1977;74:244–8.
43. Wilson P, Bezjak A, Asch M, et al. The difficulties of a randomized study in superior vena caval obstruction. J Thorac Oncol 2007;2:514–9.
44. Piccione W, Penfield Faber L, Warren WH. Superior vena caval reconstruction using autologous pericardium. Ann Thorac Surg 1990;50:417–9.
45. Kim JH, Shin JH, Song H, et al. Palliative treatment of inoperable malignant tracheobronchial obstruction: temporary stenting with radiation therapy and/or chemotherapy. AJR Am J Roentgenol 2009;193: W38–42.
46. Egan TM, Detterbeck FC. The ABCs of LTX for BAC. J Thorac Cardiovasc Surg 2003;125:20–2.
47. Gómez-Román JJ, Del Valle CE, Zarrabeitia MT, et al. Recurrence of bronchioloalveolar carcinoma in donor lung after lung transplantation: microsatellite analysis demonstrates a recipient origin. Pathol Int 2005;55:580–4.
48. Zorn GL, McGiffin DC, Young KR. Pulmonary transplantation for advanced bronchioloalveolar carcinoma. J Thorac Cardiovasc Surg 2003;125:45–8.

Current Status of Systemic Therapies

Adjuvant Chemotherapy After Pulmonary Resection for Lung Cancer

Celine Mascaux, MD, PhD, Frances A. Shepherd, MD, FRCPC*

KEYWORDS

- Non–small cell lung cancer • Adjuvant • Chemotherapy • Biomarkers • Targeted therapy

KEY POINTS

- Adjuvant chemotherapy using a cisplatin-based regimen currently is recommended for patients with stage II and III non–small cell lung cancer (NSCLC) after complete tumor resection.
- In Japanese patients with stage I NSCLC, uracil-tegafur may be administered as postoperative adjuvant chemotherapy.
- Adjuvant chemotherapy also has shown benefit in fit elderly patients.
- Efforts are ongoing to identify new treatments in the adjuvant setting.
- The era of personalized medicine to select patients for individualized treatment based on biomarkers is under development in the adjuvant setting.

ADJUVANT CHEMOTHERAPY IN SURGICALLY RESECTED NON–SMALL CELL LUNG CANCER

Early studies testing the role of postoperative adjuvant chemotherapy did not show significant survival benefit for patients with stage I to IIIA non–small cell lung cancer (NSCLC), and so until recently, surgery alone remained the standard of care. However, 5-year survival rates after surgery were less than 50% for stages II and III, leaving considerable room for improvement.[1] In 1995, the Medical Research Council (MRC) performed a large meta-analysis by pooling individualized data from randomized trials of adjuvant chemotherapy versus best supportive care and showed a trend for prolongation of overall survival (hazard ratio [HR] 0.87, $P = .08$) with adjuvant chemotherapy, particularly with platinum-based regimens.[2] As the differences were not statistically significant, adjuvant chemotherapy after complete surgical resection could not be recommended based on this meta-analysis. However, these results prompted several randomized trials testing adjuvant chemotherapy in completely resected NSCLC.

The study details and results of the meta-analyses and the prospective trials including more 150 patients published after the 1995 MRC meta-analyses are described in **Table 1**. The International Adjuvant Lung Cancer Trial (IALT), which included 1867 patients with stage I to III disease, was the first to show a survival benefit from postoperative cisplatin-based adjuvant chemotherapy (HR 0.86, $P<.03$).[3] Subsequently, the National Cancer Institute of Canada Clinical Trials Group JBR.10 (NCIC-CTG JBR.10) trial[4] (n = 482, stage IB and II only) and the Adjuvant Navelbine International Trialists Association (ANITA) study (n = 840, stage IB to IIIA) confirmed significant prolongation of survival (HR 0.69, $P = .04$ and HR 0.79, $P = .013$, respectively) with cisplatin/vinorelbine adjuvant chemotherapy.[5] However,

Princess Margaret Cancer Centre, University of Health Network, University of Toronto, Toronto, Ontario, Canada
* Corresponding author. Princess Margaret Cancer Centre, University of Health Network, 610 University Avenue, 5-103, Toronto, Ontario M5G 2M9, Canada.
E-mail address: frances.shepherd@uhn.ca

Thorac Surg Clin 23 (2013) 401–410
http://dx.doi.org/10.1016/j.thorsurg.2013.04.005
1547-4127/13/$ – see front matter

Table 1
After the 1995 MRC meta-analyses and randomized cisplatin-based adjuvant chemotherapy trials enrolling more than 150 patients

Meta-Analyses/ Trial Name	Stage	Number of Patients Assessed	Chemotherapy Regimen	Overall Survival With or Without Adjuvant Chemotherapy, HR (95% CI)	*P* Value
UFT meta-analyses[14]	I	2003	UFT	0.74 (0.61–0.88)	.001
UFT meta-analyses, subset analyses[15]	IA	1269	UFT		
	T1a	670		0.84 (0.58–1.23)	
	T1b	599		0.62 (0.42–0.90)	*P*-int = .30
MRC update[8]	Overall	8147	Multiple	0.88 (0.81–0.97)	.009
	I			NR	NR
	II				
	IIIA				
	IIIB				
LACE[7]	Overall	4584	Multiple	0.89 (0.82–0.96)	.005
	IA	387		1.40 (0.95–2.06)	*P*-trend = .04
	IB	1371		0.93 (0.78–1.10)	
	II	1616		0.83 (0.72–0.94)	
	III	1247		0.83 (0.72–0.94)	
ECOG 3590[50]	Overall	488	Cisplatin + etoposide	0.93 (0.74–1.18)	NR
	II	202		NS but values NR	NR
	IIIA	285		NS but values NR	NR
ALPI[51]	Overall	1088	Mitomycin + vindesine + cisplatin	0.96 (0.81–1.13)	.589
	I	423		0.97 (0.71–1.33)	*P*-trend = .728
	II	355		0.80 (0.60–1.06)	*P*-het = .624
	IIIA	310		1.06 (0.82–1.38)	
IALT[3]	Overall	1867	Cisplatin + etoposide or vinorebline or vindesine	0.86 (0.76–0.98)	.03
	I	681		0.95 (0.74–1.23)	*P*-int = .41
	II	452		0.93 (0.72–1.20)	*P*-trend = .21
	III	734		0.79 (0.66–0.95)	
NCIC-CTG JBR.10[4]	Overall	482	Cisplatin + vinorelbine	0.69 (0.52–0.91)	.04
	IB	219		0.79 (0.77–1.95)	*P*-int = .13 .79
	II	263		0.59 (0.42–0.85)	.004
CALBG 9633[6]	Overall	344	Paclitaxel + carboplatin	0.83 (0.64–1.08)	.12
	IB	344		0.83 (0.64–1.08)[a]	.12
ANITA[5]	Overall	829	Cisplatin + vinorelbine	0.80 (0.66–0.96)[a]	.017
	IB	301		1.10 (0.76–1.57)	*P*-int = .07
	II	203		0.71 (0.49–1.03)	
	IIIA	325		0.69 (0.53–0.90)	

Abbreviations: ALPI, Adjuvant Lung Project Italy; ANITA, Adjuvant Navelbine International Trial Association; CABG, Cancer and Leukemia Group B; CI, confidence interval; ECOG, Eastern Cooperative Oncology Group; HR, hazard ratio; IALT, International Adjuvant Lung Cancer Trial; LACE, Lung Adjuvant Cisplatin Evaluation; MRC, Medical Research Council; NA, nonapplicable; NCIC-CTG, National Cancer Institute of Canada Clinical Trials Group; NR, not reported; NS, not significant; *P*-het, *P* value for heterogeneity; *P*-int, interaction *P* value; *P*-trend, *P* value for trend.
[a] 90% CI.

the Cancer and Leukemia Group B (CALBG) 9633 trial (n = 344) failed to demonstrate a significant survival benefit (HR 0.83, *P* = .12) for paclitaxel/carboplatin adjuvant therapy in patients with stage IB NSCLC.[6] Nevertheless, this study was underpowered to demonstrate a significant difference of this magnitude. Thereafter, 2 meta-analyses confirmed that adjuvant chemotherapy increases survival in NSCLC. The LACE (Lung Adjuvant Cisplatin Evaluation), which pooled individual patient data from 5 trials, demonstrated an absolute decrease in lung cancer death of 6.9% and an absolute increase of 5.4% for overall survival at 5 years in patients with completely resected NSCLC.[7] An update of the 1995 MRC meta-analysis also confirmed a 5% increase in survival at 5 years.[8] Furthermore, the impact on survival outcome has been shown at the population level in Ontario, Canada. By comparing all patients undergoing surgery for NSCLC in 2001 to 2003 (before the introduction of adjuvant chemotherapy) and 2004 to 2006 (after the introduction of adjuvant chemotherapy), Booth and colleagues[9] showed that the proportion of patients receiving adjuvant chemotherapy increased significantly from 7% to 31% (P<.001) without an increase of the rate of hospitalization in the first 6 months after surgery. In addition, there was a significant absolute improvement in overall survival of 3.6% (P = .001) among all surgical patients in the province. These results indicate that the benefits observed in the clinical trials may be generalized to the entire population.

SELECTION OF PATIENTS FOR ADJUVANT CHEMOTHERAPY BASED ON STAGE

The evidence is strong to recommend adjuvant cisplatin-based chemotherapy for patients with completely resected stage II and stage IIIA NSCLC (see **Table 1**). The LACE pooled analysis,[7] ANITA,[5] and the NCIC-CTG JBR.10 trial[4] reported significant overall survival benefit for patients with stage II (pooled HR 0.83, 95% confidence interval [CI] 0.72–0.94, HR 0.83, 95% CI 0.73–0.95; HR 0.71, 95% CI 0.49–1.03; and HR 0.59, P = .004, respectively). In patients with stage IIIA NSCLC, the LACE meta-analysis found a significant benefit (pooled HR 0.83; CI 95% 0.72–0.94).[7] The ANITA[5] and IALT[3] trials also reported significant improvement in overall survival for adjuvant chemotherapy in stage IIIA disease (HR 0.69, 95% CI 0.53–0.90; HR 0.79, 95% CI 0.66–0.95, respectively).

In the Caucasian population, adjuvant chemotherapy cannot be recommended for stage I NSCLC, particularly in patients with stage IA resected NSCLC. Although few patients with stage IA were included in the studies that reported an advantage for adjuvant chemotherapy, the LACE meta-analyses showed a potential detrimental effect of adjuvant chemotherapy in the stage IA subgroup (HR 1.41, 95% CI 0.95–2.06).[7] However, 87% patients with stage IA disease did not receive regimens combining cisplatin and vinorelbine, the combination that was associated with the greatest benefit in the other stages.

The role of adjuvant chemotherapy in patients with stage IB resected NSCLC also is debated. The positive IALT, ANITA, NCIC-CTG JBR.10 trials and the meta-analyses showed a significant benefit in overall survival in stage IB resected NSCLC.[3–5] The CALBG 9633 trial, which was limited to stage IB alone, did not show an overall survival benefit with adjuvant chemotherapy paclitaxel/carboplatin (HR 0.83, P = .12).[6] However, in an unplanned subset analyses, significantly longer overall survival was found in patients with tumors of 4 cm diameter or more (HR 0.66, P = .04). In a survival update of JBR.10, Butts and colleagues[10] also showed that stage IB patients with tumors greater than 4 cm in diameter derived significant benefit from vinorelbine/cisplatin (HR 0.66, 95% CI 0.39–1.14, P = .13 and HR 1.73 95% CI 0.98–3.04, P = .06, interaction P = .02). Based on these results, adjuvant chemotherapy may be considered for patients with stage IB resected NSCLC of 4 cm diameter or more.[11–13]

In Japanese patients with stage I NSCLC, and particularly adenocarcinomas, there is evidence that the use of uracil-tegafur (UFT) as postoperative adjuvant chemotherapy improves survival. However, many trials of adjuvant therapy with UFT in patients with stage I NSCLC have been conducted and some have provided contradictory results. Six trials comparing surgery alone with surgery plus UFT were pooled in a meta-analysis including 2003 patients with NSCLC (adenocarcinomas in 1679 and squamous cell carcinomas in only 299).[14] This meta-analysis demonstrated a significant survival benefit with a pooled HR 0.74 (P = .001) and an improvement of 4.3% and 7% in survival rates at 5 and 7 years, respectively, when adding UFT to surgery compared with surgery alone.[14] Data from this meta-analysis were reanalyzed to evaluate the effectiveness of UFT in stage IA disease in 1269 patients, 670 with T1a tumors and 599 with T1b, respectively.[15] A significant survival benefit was demonstrated with adjuvant UFT compared with surgery alone in patients with stage T1b resected NSCLC (HR 0.62, CI 95% 0.42–0.90, P = .011) but not in those with stage T1a disease (HR 0.84, CI 95% 0.58–1.23), but this difference was not significant (interaction P = .30).[15] In addition, adjuvant chemotherapy combining cisplatin/vinorelbine/UFT demonstrated a survival benefit in Japanese patients with stage I NSCLC compared with surgery alone (87.9% vs 66.3% at 5 years), P = .045) with less effect for UFT alone (67.7% 5-year survival).[16]

SELECTION OF THE ADJUVANT CHEMOTHERAPY REGIMEN

Most of the published trials used cisplatin-based chemotherapy (see **Table 1**). NCIC-CTG JBR.10,

IALT, and ANITA trials achieved statistically and clinically significant survival benefits with vinorelbine/cisplatin.[3–5] The LACE meta-analysis also reported that the greatest overall survival benefit was associated with the cisplatin and vinorelbine combination (HR 0.80, P = .10), which was marginally better than that of other drug combinations when all regimens were considered separately and significantly better (P = .04) when other combinations were pooled.[7] However, the cisplatin/vinorelbine regimen used in both the NCIC-CTG JBR.10 and ANITA trials administrated vinorelbine weekly for 16 weeks (4 cycles). Analysis of compliance in the NCIC-CTG JBR.10 trial showed that the median administered dose of vinorelbine was only 52%. In addition, dose reduction and incomplete chemotherapy administration were more likely in patients who had undergone pneumonectomy, were older, or were female. For advanced NSCLC, a randomized trial demonstrated that a 3-week cycle of vinorelbine on days 1 and 8 and cisplatin on day 1 had better tolerance and similar efficacy to the less convenient weekly regimen administered in the adjuvant setting.[17] In situations where constraints preclude the use of the weekly schedule of administration, practitioners might prescribe the more convenient intravenous regimen tested for advanced disease or even oral vinorelbine for patients living far from the hospital.[18]

Carboplatin should not be administered routinely in the adjuvant setting because currently available data do not support it. The use of adjuvant chemotherapy involving alkylating agents is not recommended because the 1995 MRC meta-analysis found a statistically significant survival disadvantage when using adjuvant chemotherapy regimens involving alkylating agents.[2]

As reported in the previous paragraph, for Japanese patients with stage I NSCLC, and particularly adenocarcinomas, UFT may be administered as postoperative adjuvant chemotherapy.[14,15] This agent is not approved in North America.

ADJUVANT CHEMOTHERAPY IN THE ELDERLY

The median age of the patients in the studies showing a survival advantage for adjuvant chemotherapy was only 60 years, and this does not reflect the general population of patient with lung cancer for which the median age is estimated to be approximately 69 years. Furthermore, ~40% of patients diagnosed with lung cancer are more than 70 years of age. An unplanned analysis of results from patients in JBR.10 found an overall survival benefit for patients older than age 65 years (HR 0.61, P = .04), without an increase in treatment-related toxicity or hospitalization.[19] Individual patient data from the 5 trials of the LACE meta-analyses were pooled and analyzed in 3 groups: young (<65 years), mid-category (65–69 years), and elderly (≥70 years).[20] The results demonstrated that, despite the significantly lower total cisplatin dose that they received, elderly patients who met the eligibility criteria for trial enrollment achieved the same survival benefit from adjuvant chemotherapy as did younger patients with lung cancer (interaction P = .42), with no difference in toxicity or treatment-related deaths.[20] A population-based study in Ontario demonstrated that, after the introduction of adjuvant chemotherapy in 2004, the survival rate of surgical patients aged 70 years or more significantly increased by 2.8% (P = .01). Furthermore, there was no increase in hospitalization rates that would suggest increased severe toxicity in the elderly population.[21] Based on these different studies, adjuvant cisplatin-based chemotherapy should not be withheld from elderly patients with NSCLC purely because of age.

ROLE OF INDIVIDUAL BIOMARKERS TO PREDICT RESPONSE TO ADJUVANT CHEMOTHERAPY

The use of prognostic biomarkers in the adjuvant setting could identify patients who are likely to be cured with surgery alone, and for this group, it might be possible to avoid the toxicities of adjuvant chemotherapy. Conversely, prognostic biomarkers could identify patients who are highly likely to relapse and who might derive benefit from adjuvant treatment after surgical resection. This could be of particular importance for patients with stage I cancers for which adjuvant chemotherapy is not currently recommended. Predictive biomarkers may help to identify patients who may or may not respond to chemotherapy or other treatments. The translational research projects for JBR.10, the International Adjuvant Lung Cancer Trial Biologic Program (IALT-Bio), the Lung Adjuvant Cisplatin Evaluation Biologic Program (LACE-Bio) attempted to characterize and/or validate several biomarkers. Biomarkers are tested including individual proteins involved in DNA repair and DNA replication, regulation of the cell cycle, apoptosis, and mitosis or complex gene expression signatures. A summary of available data about biomarkers for the adjuvant setting is presented in **Table 2**.

High DNA repair capacity eliminates cisplatin-induced DNA adducts and thus leads to platinum resistance. Excision repair cross-complementing rodent repair deficiency, complementation group 1 (ERCC1), is a key protein involved in DNA repair. In

Table 2
Individuals biomarkers tested to predict outcome with adjuvant chemotherapy clinical trials by the JBR.10, IALT-Bio, and LACE-bio in NSCLC

Study	Biomarker	Assay	Marker Low or Absent, HR (95% CI)	*P* Value	Marker High or Present, HR (95% CI)	*P* Value	Interaction Test *P* Value
IALT-Bio[22]	ERCC1	IHC	0.65 (0.50–0.86)	.002	1.14 (0.84–1.55)	.40	.009
IALT-Bio[27]	MSH2	IHC	0.76 (0.59–0.97)	.03	1.12 (0.81–1.55)	.48	.06
IALT-Bio[31]	p27	IHC	0.66 (0.50–0.88)	.006	1.09 (0.82–1.45)	.54	.02
LACE-Bio[32]		IHC	0.87 (0.64–1.18)	.26	0.83 (0.59–1.15)	.37	.83
JBR.10[33]	p53	IHC	1.40 (0.78–2.52)	.26	0.54 (0.32–0.92)	.02	.02
LACE-Bio[34]		IHC	0.82 (NR)	.03	0.87 (NR)	.22	.64
JBR.10[33]		Mutation	0.67 (0.46–0.98)	.04	0.78 (0.46–1.32)	.35	.65
LACE-Bio[34]		Mutation	0.79 (0.63–0.98)	.03	1.03 (0.80–1.34)	.80	.12
IALT-Bio, JBR.10[35]	Bax	IHC	1.13 (0.89–1.45)	.31	0.72 (0.56–0.91)	.007	.009
JBR.10[36]	TUBB3	IHC	1.00 (0.57–1.75)	.99	0.64 (0.39–1.04)	.07	.25
LACE-Bio[37]		IHC	1.03 (0.81–1.30)	.82	0.83 (0.66–1.04)	.11	.81
JBR.10[38]	*EGFR*	Mutation	0.78 (0.57–1.06)	.11	0.44 (0.11–1.70)	.22	.50
JBR.10[33]	*KRAS*	Mutation	0.69 (0.49–0.97)	.03	0.95 (0.53–1.71)	.87	.29
LACE-Bio[40]		Mutation	0.89 (0.76–1.06)	.20	1.02 (0.73–1.41)	.91	.50

Abbreviations: CI, confidence interval; HR, hazard ratio; IALT, International Adjuvant Lung Cancer Trial; IHC, immunohistochemistry; LACE, Lung Adjuvant Cisplatin evaluation; NR, not reported.

IALT-Bio, high ERCC1 expression was found to be a favorable prognostic factor in patients who do not receive adjuvant chemotherapy. In the same study, the lack of ERCC1 expression predicted a longer overall survival with adjuvant cisplatin-based chemotherapy compared with observation alone (HR 0.65, *P* = .002 and HR 1.14, *P* = .40) for ERCC1 negative and positive tumors, respectively (interaction *P* = .009).[22] For advanced NSCLC, recent data suggest that this cisplatin efficacy might be limited to squamous cell carcinoma with low ERCC1 expression.[23] Unfortunately, these results could not be validated in LACE-Bio.[24] ERCC1 protein expression was assessed in the entire IALT cohort (589 samples) using 16 commercial ERCC1 antibodies. The results of the previously studied IALT samples with the 8F1 antibody could not be validated, indicating a lack of stability of the antibodies. More importantly, however, none of the 16 antibodies could distinguish the 4 ERCC1 protein isoforms although only 1 isoform was functional in terms of nucleotide excision repair (NER) and cisplatin resistance therapy.[24] Before the LACE-Bio results were known, several trials were initiated with stratification and randomization based on ERCC1 levels: the Tailored Post-Surgical Therapy in Early Stage NSCLC (TASTE), a phase II/III trial comparing adjuvant chemotherapy (cisplatin/pemetrexed) with customized adjuvant treatment based on epidermal growth factor receptor (*EGFR*) gene mutation status and ERCC1 immunohistochemistry (IHC) expression in stage II to IIIA nonsquamous NSCLC and the Southwest Oncology Group (SWOG)-0720, a phase II feasibility trial based on ERCC1/RMM1 expression in stage I NSCLC.

High thymidylate synthetase expression is a poor prognostic marker for survival in patients with resected NSCLC[25] and is associated with reduced efficacy of pemetrexed.[26] The predictive value of combined ERCC1 and thymidylate synthetase expression in the adjuvant setting is under assessment in the International Tailored Chemotherapy Adjuvant (ITACA) study, a randomized phase III trial comparing customized adjuvant chemotherapy based on ERCC1 and thymidylate synthase gene expression in stage II to IIIA NSCLC with standard chemotherapy.

The role of several other biomarkers related to DNA repair, including MutS homolog 2 (MSH2), Breast Cancer 1 (BRCA1), and ribonucleotide reductase M1 (RRM1) has also been assessed in the adjuvant setting. IALT-Bio[27] showed that low MSH2 expression was associated with a trend toward improved overall survival when using cisplatin-based adjuvant chemotherapy compared with observation (HR 0.76, *P* = .03), whereas no difference in overall survival was observed in the high MSH2 group (HR 1.12, *P* = .48, interaction *P* = .06). A high level of BRCA1 mRNA, which also plays a central role in DNA repair, is associated with shorter overall survival (HR = 1.98, P = .02).[28] In the phase II, nonrandomized, pilot Spanish Customized Adjuvant Treatment (pilot SCAT) trial, patients with high BRCA1 levels were treated with single-agent docetaxel without platinum, whereas those with low levels received cisplatin/gemcitibine.[29] No detrimental effect on survival was shown with treatment using single-agent docetaxel in BRCA1 high expression compared with cisplatin/gemcitabine in BRCA1 low expression. A validation, randomized, phase III Spanish Customized Adjuvant Treatment (validation SCAT) trial for resected stage II to III NSCLC is currently testing standard adjuvant chemotherapy (cisplatin/docetaxel) versus customized adjuvant chemotherapy based on BRCA1 mRNA expression.

High expression of RRM1 has been reported to be a good prognostic factor for overall survival in patients who have undergone resection for early-stage NSCLC.[30] Based on data published on advanced NSCLC, RRM1 may be a biomarker for gemcitabine chemotherapy. No data are available for the predictive role of RRM1 in the adjuvant chemotherapy setting but this currently is being evaluated in SWOG-0720.

Other proteins involved in cell cycle regulation or in apoptosis have also been shown to have prognostic or predictive roles in lung cancer. The lack of p27 expression was shown in IALT-Bio to predict a longer survival after chemotherapy compared with surgery alone (HR 0.66, P = .006 and HR 1.09, P = .54, for low p27 vs high p27, respectively; interaction test P = .02).[31] However, these results were not cross-validated in a pooled analysis within the LACE-Bio program (HR 0.87, P = .26 and HR 0.83, P = .37, for p27 negative and positive tumors, respectively; interaction P = .83).[32]

In JBR.10, p53 protein expression was a poor prognostic factor (HR 1.89, P = .03 in the observation arm) and predicted benefit from cisplatin/vinorelbine adjuvant therapy (HR 0.54, P = .02 and HR 1.4, P = .26 for p53 IHC positive vs negative tumors, respectively; interaction P = .02).[33] However, these results again could not be validated in LACE-Bio (HR 0.82, P = .03 and HR 0.87, P = .22, for p53 negative and positive patients, respectively; interaction P = .64).[34] *p53* mutation was not found to be a prognostic factor (JBR.10, HR 1.15, P = .45)[33] nor was it predictive of response to adjuvant chemotherapy in JBR.10 (HR 0.67, P = .04 and HR 0.78, P = .35, for patients with p53 wild type and mutated, respectively; interaction P = .65).[33] Similar results were found in LACE-Bio (HR 0.79, P = .03 and HR 1.03, P = .80, for patients with p53 wild type and mutated, respectively; interaction P = .12).[34]

In a pooled analysis of IALT-Bio and JBR.10, IHC protein expression of Bax, a proapoptotic factor that is activated by p53, significantly predicted survival benefit from adjuvant chemotherapy (HR 1.13, P = .31 and HR 0.72, P = .007, for Bax negative and positive patients, respectively; interaction P = .009).[35]

The class III β-tubulin (TUBB3) was assessed for its predictive role in trials using antitubulin agents. Although associated with a borderline better prognosis in the JBR.10 (P = .08), high TUBB3 expression was not found to predict response to adjuvant chemotherapy either in JBR.10 (interaction test P = .25)[36] or in LACE-Bio (interaction test P = .81).[37]

The role of *EGFR* also has been assessed in the adjuvant chemotherapy setting. *EGFR* mutation was associated with a potential but not significant survival benefit from adjuvant chemotherapy (HR 0.44, P = .22, interaction P = .50) in JBR.10.[38]

KRAS mutation is seen frequently in NSCLC, most often in adenocarcinoma, where approximately 30% of tumors may harbor a mutation. In JBR.10, where it was used as a stratification variable, *KRAS* mutation was not found to be a significant negative prognostic marker for survival.[33] Similar results were found in LACE-Bio, and in particular, there was no prognostic effect (HR 1.04, CI 0.77–1.40 vs HR 1.01, CI 0.47–2.17, for codon 12 and 13, respectively, compared with wild type).[39] Wild-type *KRAS* status was associated with a survival benefit from adjuvant chemotherapy compared with observation in JBR.10 (HR 0.69, P = .03 and HR 0.95, P = .87 for *KRAS* wild type vs mutated status), but the interaction test was not significant (interaction P = .29).[33] The LACE-Bio validation study also assessed the role of *KRAS* mutation and could not confirm its prognostic or predictive effect for adjuvant chemotherapy (HR 0.89, P = .15 and HR 1.05, P = .77, for *KRAS* wild type or mutated, respectively; interaction P = .37).[40] Analysis according to the subtype of mutation showed that codon 13 mutation was predictive of a deleterious effect of chemotherapy (HR 5.78, P = .001; interaction P = .002).[39] Recently, the LACE-Bio group assessed the role of *KRAS* in 426 patients with EGFR wild-type adenocarcinomas.[41] *KRAS* mutation did not have any prognostic effect on overall survival of *EGFR* wild-type adenocarcinomas (HR 1.00, P = .650) or predictive value for outcome with chemotherapy compared with observation (HR 1.22, P = .55). In the same study, the double *p53/KRAS* mutation status was not of prognostic value (HR 0.85, interaction P = .58) but, compared with double wild-type patients, those with a double mutation had a detrimental effect (HR 2.49, P = .003) from chemotherapy versus observation. However, comparison of the effects of chemotherapy among the 4 groups defined by *KRAS* and *TP53* mutations was not significant (P = .06).[41]

ROLE OF GENE SIGNATURES TO DETERMINE PROGNOSIS AND PREDICT RESPONSE TO ADJUVANT CHEMOTHERAPY

Panels of biomarkers or signatures may be used to predict prognosis or response to therapy. To date, however, all signatures lack sufficient validation to be implemented in clinical practice. Recently, Zhu and colleagues[42] identified a 15-gene signature derived from patients participating in JBR.10 that discriminates patients at high and low risk in the observation arm (HR 13.32, CI 2.86–62.11, P<.0001 and HR 13.47, CI 3.00–60.43, P<.0001), for patients with stage IB and stage II NSCLC, respectively). Furthermore, high-risk patients derived significant benefit from chemotherapy (HR 0.33, CI 0.17–0.63, P = .0005), whereas chemotherapy seemed to be detrimental compared with observation in low-risk patients (HR 3.67, CI 1.22–11.06, P = .0133; interaction P = .0001). As few randomized trials have frozen sample tumor banks, attempts to validate and translate the signature to paraffin-embedded samples are ongoing. Tang and colleagues[43] reported another signature of 12 genes that predicted survival benefit with adjuvant chemotherapy. The signature was identified on a cohort of 442 stage I to III NSCLC specimens and further validated in 2 independent data sets of 90 (University of Texas [UT] cohort) and 176 patients (JBR.10), respectively. The groups that were predicted to benefit from adjuvant chemotherapy had improved survival with adjuvant chemotherapy in both cohorts (HR = 0.34, P = .038 and HR = 0.91, P = .82, for UT and JBR.10, respectively), whereas the groups that were predicted not to benefit from adjuvant chemotherapy did not show any survival benefit after adjuvant chemotherapy (HR = 0.80, P = .70 and HR 0.91, P = .82, respectively).[43]

ROLE OF TARGETED THERAPY IN THE ADJUVANT SETTING OF NSCLC?

Targeted therapies that have demonstrated effect on advanced NSCLC are now being assessed in the adjuvant setting. In the BR.19 phase III randomized trial, the epidermal growth factor receptor tyrosine kinase inhibitor (EGFR TKI) gefitinib did not provide any survival benefit over placebo in unselected patients with completely resected stage IB to IIIA NSCLC (HR 1.24, P = .14 and 1.22, P = .15 for overall survival and disease-free survival, respectively) or even in the small subgroup of patients with *EGFR*-mutant tumors (HR for overall survival 1.58, P = .16).[44] The trial was closed prematurely. A retrospective study suggested a trend for improved outcome in terms of disease-free survival for patients with resected stages I to III lung adenocarcinomas harboring *EGFR* mutations who were treated with adjuvant therapy by EGFR TKIs (2-year disease-free survival and overall survival 89% vs 72%, HR 0.53, P = .06 and 96 vs 90%, HR 0.62, P = .296).[45] A phase III trial (C-TONG 1104, NCT01405079) is currently evaluating gefitinib versus vinorelbine/platinum as adjuvant treatment in stage II to IIIA (N1-N2) NSCLC with *EGFR* mutation. Erlotinib, another EGFR TKI, is under evaluation in the ongoing phase III Randomized Double-Blind Trial in Adjuvant NSCLC with erlotinib (RADIANT) study. Patients with resected stage IB to IIIA NSCLC who are EGFR positive by IHC and/or fluorescent in situ hybridization are randomized to erlotinib or placebo for 2 years after surgical resection and optional adjuvant chemotherapy. Accrual is complete and the final results are awaited. Another ongoing study, the phase II SELECT trial, is evaluating adjuvant erlotinib for 2 years in patients with resected, early-stage NSCLC (stage IA to IIIA) and confirmed mutations in *EGFR*.[46]

In stage II to IIIA (non-N2) resected nonsquamous NSCLC, the TASTE phase II/III randomized trial comparing a noncustomized standard adjuvant chemotherapy arm and a genotypic arm based on 2 different biomarkers for targeted therapy and for chemotherapy sensitivity is now closed for accrual. In the genotypic arm, *EGFR* activating mutation status determined the choice between erlotinib versus chemotherapy for *EGFR* mutated versus wild type, respectively, and the level of ERCC1 expression drove the choice of the chemotherapy regimen in patients with EGFR wild type (cisplatin/pemetrexed vs non–platinum-based chemotherapy for low and high ERCC1, respectively). Phase III will not proceed because of the recent results showing the absence of reliability of ERCC1 expression assessments.[24]

Bevacizumab is a recombinant humanized monoclonal antibody against vascular endothelial growth factor (VEGF) that inhibits angiogenesis.[47] The role of bevacizumab in the adjuvant setting of NSCLC currently is being evaluated in Eastern Cooperative Oncology Group (ECOG)-1505. Patients with resected stage IB (≥4 cm diameter) to stage IIIA NSCLC may receive 4 cycles of various cisplatin-based doublet chemotherapy combinations and they are randomized to receive bevacizumab every 3 weeks for 1 year or chemotherapy alone.

Recently, promising phase II results have been obtained with immunotherapy in the adjuvant setting of NSCLC. In particular, the antigen-specific melanoma-associated antigen 3 (MAGE-A3) vaccine (MAGE-A3 ASCI) is being tested in phase III trials in patients with early NSCLC (see **Table 2**). A pilot study showed a trend toward longer disease-free interval (HR 0.74, *P* = .107), disease-free survival (HR 0.73, *P* = .093), and overall survival (HR 0.66, *P* = .088) in stage IB/II MAGE-A3 NSCLC patients treated postoperatively with MAGE-A3 immunotherapy compared with placebo.[48] A large phase III placebo-controlled trial MAGRIT (MAGE-A3 as Adjuvant non–small cell lunG cancer ImmunoTherapy) has completed accrual and results are awaited.[49]

SUMMARY

Cisplatin-based adjuvant chemotherapy currently is recommended for patients with stage II and III NSCLC after complete tumor resection and may be considered for patients with stage IB NSCLC (≥4 cm diameter). In Japanese patients with stage I NSCLC, UFT may be administered as postoperative adjuvant chemotherapy. Adjuvant chemotherapy should not be withheld from elderly patients with NSCLC purely because of age. The population of patients who have undergone surgical resection of NSCLC is heterogeneous and there is still a relatively high risk of relapse even for early-stage NSCLC. It would, thus, be of great value to identify those patients who are cured by surgery alone and those who are at risk of relapse and therefore have the greatest potential to benefit from adjuvant therapy and to match these patients with biomarker-driven targeted therapy. Efforts are ongoing to select patients for individualized treatment based on biomarkers, but at this time, no biomarker can be recommended based on currently published data. Innovative molecularly targeted therapies and immunotherapy with vaccines have shown promising early results but the results of phase III trials must be awaited before these treatments can be recommended.

REFERENCES

1. Goldstraw P, Crowley J, Chansky K, et al. The IASLC Lung Cancer Staging Project: proposals for the revision of the TNM stage groupings in the forthcoming (seventh) edition of the TNM classification of malignant tumours. J Thorac Oncol 2007;2:706–14.
2. Chemotherapy in non-small cell lung cancer: a meta-analysis using updated data on individual patients from 52 randomised clinical trials. Non-small Cell Lung Cancer Collaborative Group. BMJ 1995;311:899–909.
3. Arriagada R, Bergman B, Dunant A, et al. Cisplatin-based adjuvant chemotherapy in patients with completely resected non-small-cell lung cancer. N Engl J Med 2004;350:351–60.
4. Winton T, Livingston R, Johnson D, et al. Vinorelbine plus cisplatin vs. observation in resected non-small-cell lung cancer. N Engl J Med 2005; 352:2589–97.
5. Douillard JY, Rosell R, De Lena M, et al. Adjuvant vinorelbine plus cisplatin versus observation in patients with completely resected stage IB-IIIA non-small-cell lung cancer (Adjuvant Navelbine International Trialist Association [ANITA]): a randomised controlled trial. Lancet Oncol 2006;7:719–27.
6. Strauss GM, Herndon JE 2nd, Maddaus MA, et al. Adjuvant paclitaxel plus carboplatin compared with observation in stage IB non-small-cell lung cancer: CALGB 9633 with the Cancer and Leukemia Group B, Radiation Therapy Oncology Group, and North Central Cancer Treatment Group Study Groups. J Clin Oncol 2008;26:5043–51.
7. Pignon JP, Tribodet H, Scagliotti GV, et al. Lung adjuvant cisplatin evaluation: a pooled analysis by the LACE Collaborative Group. J Clin Oncol 2008;26:3552–9.
8. Arriagada R, Auperin A, Burdett S, et al. Adjuvant chemotherapy, with or without postoperative radiotherapy, in operable non-small-cell lung cancer: two meta-analyses of individual patient data. Lancet 2010;375:1267–77.
9. Booth CM, Shepherd FA, Peng Y, et al. Adoption of adjuvant chemotherapy for non-small-cell lung cancer: a population-based outcomes study. J Clin Oncol 2010;28:3472–8.
10. Butts CA, Ding K, Seymour L, et al. Randomized phase III trial of vinorelbine plus cisplatin compared with observation in completely resected stage IB and II non-small-cell lung cancer: updated survival analysis of JBR-10. J Clin Oncol 2010;28:29–34.
11. Pisters KM, Evans WK, Azzoli CG, et al. Cancer Care Ontario and American Society of Clinical Oncology adjuvant chemotherapy and adjuvant radiation therapy for stages I-IIIA resectable non small-cell lung cancer guideline. J Clin Oncol 2007;25:5506–18.
12. Crino L, Weder W, van Meerbeeck J, et al. Early stage and locally advanced (non-metastatic) non-small-cell lung cancer: ESMO Clinical Practice Guidelines for diagnosis, treatment and follow-up. Ann Oncol 2010;21(Suppl 5):v103–15.
13. Brodowicz T, Ciuleanu T, Crawford J, et al. Third CECOG consensus on the systemic treatment of non-small-cell lung cancer. Ann Oncol 2012;23: 1223–9.

14. Hamada C, Tanaka F, Ohta M, et al. Meta-analysis of postoperative adjuvant chemotherapy with tegafur-uracil in non-small-cell lung cancer. J Clin Oncol 2005;23:4999–5006.
15. Hamada C, Tsuboi M, Ohta M, et al. Effect of postoperative adjuvant chemotherapy with tegafur-uracil on survival in patients with stage IA non-small cell lung cancer: an exploratory analysis from a meta-analysis of six randomized controlled trials. J Thorac Oncol 2009;4:1511–6.
16. Imaizumi M. Postoperative adjuvant cisplatin, vindesine, plus uracil-tegafur chemotherapy increased survival of patients with completely resected p-stage I non-small cell lung cancer. Lung Cancer 2005;49:85–94.
17. Gebbia V, Galetta D, Lorusso V, et al. Cisplatin plus weekly vinorelbine versus cisplatin plus vinorelbine on days 1 and 8 in advanced non-small cell lung cancer: a prospective randomized phase III trial of the G.O.I.M. (Gruppo Oncologico Italia Meridionale). Lung Cancer 2008;61:369–77.
18. Gralla RJ, Gatzemeier U, Gebbia V, et al. Oral vinorelbine in the treatment of non-small cell lung cancer: rationale and implications for patient management. Drugs 2007;67:1403–10.
19. Pepe C, Hasan B, Winton TL, et al. Adjuvant vinorelbine and cisplatin in elderly patients: National Cancer Institute of Canada and Intergroup Study JBR.10. J Clin Oncol 2007;25:1553–61.
20. Fruh M, Rolland E, Pignon JP, et al. Pooled analysis of the effect of age on adjuvant cisplatin-based chemotherapy for completely resected non-small-cell lung cancer. J Clin Oncol 2008;26:3573–81.
21. Cuffe S, Booth CM, Peng Y, et al. Adjuvant chemotherapy for non-small-cell lung cancer in the elderly: a population-based study in Ontario, Canada. J Clin Oncol 2012;30:1813–21.
22. Olaussen KA, Dunant A, Fouret P, et al. DNA repair by ERCC1 in non-small-cell lung cancer and cisplatin-based adjuvant chemotherapy. N Engl J Med 2006;355:983–91.
23. Pierceall WE, Olaussen KA, Rousseau V, et al. Cisplatin benefit is predicted by immunohistochemical analysis of DNA repair proteins in squamous cell carcinoma but not adenocarcinoma: theranostic modeling by NSCLC constituent histological subclasses. Ann Oncol 2012;23:2245–52.
24. Friboulet L, Olaussen KA, Pignon JP, et al. Nonfunctional isoforms confound the proper evaluation of ERCC1 in non-small cell lung cancer. N Engl J Med 2013;368:1101–10.
25. Grimminger PP, Schneider PM, Metzger R, et al. Low thymidylate synthase, thymidine phosphorylase, and dihydropyrimidine dehydrogenase mRNA expression correlate with prolonged survival in resected non-small-cell lung cancer. Clin Lung Cancer 2010;11:328–34.
26. Giovannetti E, Mey V, Nannizzi S, et al. Cellular and pharmacogenetics foundation of synergistic interaction of pemetrexed and gemcitabine in human non-small-cell lung cancer cells. Mol Pharmacol 2005;68:110–8.
27. Kamal NS, Soria JC, Mendiboure J, et al. MutS homologue 2 and the long-term benefit of adjuvant chemotherapy in lung cancer. Clin Cancer Res 2010;16:1206–15.
28. Rosell R, Skrzypski M, Jassem E, et al. BRCA1: a novel prognostic factor in resected non-small-cell lung cancer. PLoS One 2007;2:e1129.
29. Cobo M, Massuti B, Moran T, et al. Spanish customized adjuvant trial (SCAT) based on BRCA1 mRNA levels. J Clin Oncol 2008;26:7533.
30. Bepler G, Sharma S, Cantor A, et al. RRM1 and PTEN as prognostic parameters for overall and disease-free survival in patients with non-small-cell lung cancer. J Clin Oncol 2004;22:1878–85.
31. Filipits M, Pirker R, Dunant A, et al. Cell cycle regulators and outcome of adjuvant cisplatin-based chemotherapy in completely resected non-small-cell lung cancer: the International Adjuvant Lung Cancer Trial Biologic Program. J Clin Oncol 2007;25:2735–40.
32. Pirker R, Rousseau V, Paris E, et al. LACE-Bio: cross-validation and pooled analyses of the putative prognostic/predictive biomarkers p27, p16 and cyclin E in IALT, ANITA, JBR10 and CALBG 9633. J Thorac Oncol 2010;5:S503.
33. Tsao MS, Aviel-Ronen S, Ding K, et al. Prognostic and predictive importance of p53 and RAS for adjuvant chemotherapy in non small-cell lung cancer. J Clin Oncol 2007;25:5240–7.
34. Graziano SL, Paris E, Ma X. LACE-Bio pooled analysis of the prognostic and predictive value of p53 mutations and expression by immunohistochemistry (iHC) in patients with resected non-small cell lung cancer (NSCLC). Ann Oncol 2012;21:VIII130.
35. Brambilla E, Bourredjem A, Lantuejoul S, et al. Bax expression as a predictive marker of survival benefit in non-small cell lung carcinoma treated by adjuvant cisplatin-based chemotherapy. J Thorac Oncol 2010;5:S503–4.
36. Seve P, Lai R, Ding K, et al. Class III beta-tubulin expression and benefit from adjuvant cisplatin/vinorelbine chemotherapy in operable non-small cell lung cancer: analysis of NCIC JBR.10. Clin Cancer Res 2007;13:994–9.
37. Reiman T, Lai R, Veillard AS, et al. Cross-validation study of class III beta-tubulin as a predictive marker for benefit from adjuvant chemotherapy in resected non-small-cell lung cancer: analysis of four randomized trials. Ann Oncol 2012;23:86–93.
38. Tsao MS, Sakurada A, Ding K, et al. Prognostic and predictive value of epidermal growth factor

receptor tyrosine kinase domain mutation status and gene copy number for adjuvant chemotherapy in non-small cell lung cancer. J Thorac Oncol 2011; 6:139–47.
39. Shepherd FA, Domerg C, Hainaut P, et al. A pooled analysis of the prognostic and predictive effects of KRAS mutation status and KRAS mutation subtype in early stage resected non-small cell lung cancer in four trials of adjuvant chemotherapy. J Clin Oncol 2013;31(17):2173–81.
40. Tsao MS, Hainaut P, Bourredjem A. LACE-Bio pooled analysis of the prognostic and predictive value of KRAS mutation in completely resected non-small cell lung cancer. Ann Oncol 2010;21: viii63–77.
41. Janne PA, Shepherd FA, Domerg C, et al. Prognostic and predictive value of KRAS in EGFR-based subgroups and combined with p53 in completely resected non-small cell lung cancer (NSCLC): a LACE-Bio study. Ann Oncol 2012; 23(Suppl 9):xi74 [abstract 1700].
42. Zhu CQ, Ding K, Strumpf D, et al. Prognostic and predictive gene signature for adjuvant chemotherapy in resected non-small-cell lung cancer. J Clin Oncol 2010;28:4417–24.
43. Tang H, Xiao G, Behrens C, et al. A 12-gene set predicts survival benefits from adjuvant chemotherapy in non-small-cell lung cancer patients. Clin Cancer Res 2013;19(6):1577–86.
44. Goss GD, Tsao MS, O'Callagan CJ, et al. A phase III randomized, double-blind, placebo-controlled trial of the epidermal growth factor receptor inhibitor gefitinib in completely resected stage IB-IIIA non-small cell lung cancer (NSCLC): NCIC CTG BR.19. J Clin Oncol 2010;28:18s, LBA7005.
45. Janjigian YY, Park BJ, Zakowski MF, et al. Impact on disease-free survival of adjuvant erlotinib or gefitinib in patients with resected lung adenocarcinomas that harbor EGFR mutations. J Thorac Oncol 2011;6:569–75.
46. Pennell NA, Neal JW, Govindan R, et al. The SELECT trial: a multicenter phase II trial of adjuvant erlotinib (E) in patients with resected, early-stage non-small cell lung cancer (NSCLC) and confirmed mutations in the epidermal growth factor receptor (EGFR). J Clin Oncol 2011;29 [Suppl; abstract TPS209].
47. Ferrara N, Hillan KJ, Gerber HP, et al. Discovery and development of bevacizumab, an anti-VEGF antibody for treating cancer. Nat Rev Drug Discov 2004;3:391–400.
48. Vansteenkiste J, Zielinski CC, Linder A. Final results of a multi-center, double-blind, randomized, placebo-controlled phase II study to assess the efficacy of MAGE-A3 immunotherapy as adjuvant therapy in stage IB/II non-small cell lung cancer (NSCLC). J Clin Oncol 2007;25(18S):7554.
49. Tyagi P, Mirakhur B. MAGRIT: the largest-ever phase III lung cancer trial aims to establish a novel tumor-specific approach to therapy. Clin Lung Cancer 2009;10:371–4.
50. Keller SM, Adak S, Wagner H, et al. A randomized trial of postoperative adjuvant therapy in patients with completely resected stage II or IIIA non-small-cell lung cancer. Eastern Cooperative Oncology Group. N Engl J Med 2000;343:1217–22.
51. Scagliotti GV, Fossati R, Torri V, et al. Randomized study of adjuvant chemotherapy for completely resected stage I, II, or IIIA non-small-cell lung cancer. J Natl Cancer Inst 2003;95:1453–61.

Targeted Therapy and New Anticancer Drugs in Advanced Disease

Shobha Silva, MBBS, MRCP,
Sarah Danson, BMedSci, BMBS, MSc, PhD, FRCP*

KEYWORDS

• Targeted agents • Non–small cell lung cancer • Advanced lung cancer • Small cell lung cancer

KEY POINTS

- Conventional chemotherapy in lung cancer has reached a plateau in terms of efficacy and tolerability.
- Several molecular abnormalities have been identified, and various agents that target these abnormalities have been developed.
- Targeted therapies are improving clinical outcomes in non–small cell lung cancer.

INTRODUCTION

The treatment of lung cancer has seen significant advances in the last decade. A greater understanding of the biology of tumors, and the development of advanced molecular techniques, has resulted in various targeted agents being identified, some of which have significantly changed the natural history of lung cancer, a scenario that had not been achieved with cytotoxic therapy.

In the mid-1990s, conventional chemotherapy (using a platinum-based combination) was established as being superior to best supportive care in the first-line treatment of advanced non–small cell lung cancer (NSCLC), improving the median survival from 6 to 8 months, with a 10% absolute improvement in 1-year survival.[1] Various platinum combinations with third-generation cytotoxic agents have been compared and found to be roughly equivalent,[2] the caveat to this being the improved efficacy of cisplatin/pemetrexed over cisplatin/gemcitabine in the nonsquamous subtype. Platinum chemotherapy can improve symptoms and quality of life. Second-line treatment with docetaxel or pemetrexed provides modest survival benefit. The introduction of targeted agents has improved the options available to patients with NSCLC, and is enabling more personalized management. Several molecular abnormalities have been identified, each abnormality offering the prospect of a therapeutic target. The success with targeted therapies has been mainly confined to NSCLC. This article begins by looking at agents used in this group.

EPIDERMAL GROWTH FACTOR RECEPTOR TARGETING THERAPIES

The epidermal growth factor receptor (EGFR) is one of a family of four ErbB transmembrane receptors. After extracellular ligand binding, dimerization of EGFR receptors occurs, resulting in complex cascades of intracellular downstream signaling by various tyrosine kinase (TK) pathways, resulting in tumor growth, proliferation, and invasion. Thus, targeting EGFR has been identified as a useful oncologic therapeutic strategy. Overexpression of EGF is found in up to 80% of NSCLC, but not every overexpresser responds to EGFR inhibitors. Rather, activating mutations in EGFR seems to be responsible for sensitivity to EGFR inhibitors. Agents that target EGFR can be largely

Department of Oncology, Weston Park Hospital, Whitham Road, Sheffield S10 2SJ, UK
* Corresponding author.
E-mail address: s.danson@sheffield.ac.uk

Thorac Surg Clin 23 (2013) 411–419
http://dx.doi.org/10.1016/j.thorsurg.2013.05.008

divided into small-molecule inhibitors or monoclonal inhibitors.

Erlotinib

This small-molecule inhibitor reversibly inhibits EGFR TK. The BR.21 trial, in which unselected patients with NSCLC were randomized to either erlotinib or placebo as second- or third-line therapy, showed an improvement in progression-free survival (PFS) and overall survival (OS; 6.7 vs 4.7 months; hazard ratio [HR], 0.7; P = .001).[3] Subset analyses showed significantly better response rates in patients who had never smoked (HR, 0.42), whereas nonsmokers who were EGFR-positive had even greater survival benefit (HR, 0.27).[4] Erlotinib was thus approved as a therapeutic option in advanced NSCLC for patients who have previously received at least one line of chemotherapy.

The EURTAC trial compared erlotinib with standard chemotherapy in patients with EGFR mutation–positive NSCLC. A preplanned interim analysis showed an improvement in PFS from 5.2 to 9.7 months in the erlotinib arm (P<.0001).[5] There was no significant overall survival benefit, but more than three-quarters of patients in the chemotherapy arm went on to receive erlotinib on progression. The main toxicities are rash and diarrhea, and rarely interstitial pneumonitis. Erlotinib has been shown to be more tolerable than conventional chemotherapy in the previously mentioned trials.

The use of erlotinib concurrently with platinum-doublet chemotherapy has been studied in the TRIBUTE and TALENT first-line trials. These failed to show any OS benefit.[6,7] The SATURN study assessed the use of erlotinib as maintenance treatment after four cycles of platinum-based chemotherapy. There was a statistically significant (albeit clinically modest) prolongation in PFS (11.1–12.3 months) in the erlotinib arm compared with placebo (HR, 0.71; 95% confidence interval [CI], 0.62–0.82; P = .000003). Those with EGFR mutations had greatest benefit (HR, 0.10; 95% CI, 0.04–0.25; P<.0001).[8]

Gefitinib

This is another EGFR TK inhibitor (TKI). The IPASS trial demonstrated its superiority over standard platinum-doublet chemotherapy as first-line treatment in a select population of Asian, never/light smokers with adenocarcinoma. These clinical characteristics (adenocarcinoma histology, Asian ethnicity, female gender, never/light smoking history) have come to be recognized as surrogate markers for the presence of EGFR TK mutations.[9,10]

The improvement in 1-year PFS was 25% versus 7% in the gefitinib arm compared with the chemotherapy arm. In those patients with an EGFR mutation, PFS improved from 6.3 in the chemotherapy arm to 9.5 months in the gefitinib arm (HR, 0.48). No survival benefit was demonstrated (although most patients in the chemotherapy arm went on to receive an EGFR TKI as second-line therapy).[11] The ISEL study also failed to show any survival benefit from gefitinib compared with placebo. Like erlotinib, gefitinib has been shown to have a more tolerable toxicity profile than chemotherapy, with the commonest toxicities being rash and diarrhea.

Cetuximab

This is a chimeric monoclonal IgG_1 antibody that specifically inhibits the function of EGFR by blocking the binding of EGF ligands. Addition of cetuximab to vinorelbine/cisplatin in the first-line treatment of EGFR-positive patients with NSCLC (FLEX phase III study) provided no improvement in PFS, with a small improvement in OS (11.3 vs 10.1 months; P = .044).[12] Given this modest clinical benefit, and the cost and increased toxicity (mainly rash) of cetuximab, the first-line treatment for EGFR mutant NSCLC remains gefitinib or erlotinib.

Afatinib

This is an irreversible inhibitor of EGFR TK. In the LUX-Lung 3 trial, afatinib was compared with cisplatin plus pemetrexed as first-line therapy for patients with EGFR-mutated NSCLC.[13] PFS was increased (median, 11 vs 7 months; HR, 0.58; P = .0004) in the afatinib arm compared with chemotherapy. Afatinib-associated toxicities included diarrhea, rash, and paronychia.

In the LUX-Lung 1 trial, 585 patients with stage 3b/4 adenocarcinoma who had previously received one or two lines of chemotherapy and had progressed after at least 12 weeks of gefitinib or erlotinib were randomized to either afatinib or placebo (2:1). Median PFS was 3.3 months in the afatinib arm, versus 1.1 months in the placebo arm (HR, 0.38; P<.0001).[14]

INHIBITORS OF ANAPLASTIC LYMPHOMA KINASE FUSION GENE

Anaplastic lymphoma kinase (ALK)–positive tumors constitute a clinically and pathologically significant subset of NSCLC. These tumors contain the EML4-ALK (echinoderm microtubule-associated protein-like 4–anaplastic lymphoma kinase) fusion oncogene, which has been demonstrated to be a useful therapeutic target. The oncogene can be identified in tumor specimens by fluorescence in situ hybridization (gold standard).

Certain features are associated with tumors that contain the ALK fusion oncogene: younger age of onset[15]; never or light smoking history[14,16]; and adenocarcinoma histology,[14] with higher likelihood of having signet ring cells.[17]

Although the overall incidence of the ALK fusion oncogene in unselected NSCLC populations is relatively small (4%[18–20]), one study showed that when patients were selected for never/light smoking status and adenocarcinoma histology, among those in this cohort who were negative for the EGFR mutation, the frequency of the ALK fusion oncogene was as high as 33%.[21]

Crizotinib

This orally administered small-molecule ALK inhibitor was originally developed as a c-MET inhibitor, and it also inhibits ROS 1. In an early study, 82 ALK-positive patients were identified (out of 1500 patients with NSCLC screened), most of whom had received prior chemotherapy. The overall response rate was 57%.[22] In a similar phase I study involving 143 ALK-positive patients, the objective response rate was 61%, with a median time to objective response of 8 weeks, and a median PFS of 9.7 months.[23] The results from a phase III study comparing crizotinib with single-agent chemotherapy (pemetrexed or docetaxel) in ALK-positive patients who had previously received platinum-based chemotherapy confirmed an improvement in PFS (median, 7.7 vs 3 months; HR, 0.49). No significant survival benefit was observed, but a significant proportion of patients in the chemotherapy arm (64%) had crossed over to crizotinib.[24] The results of an ongoing phase II trial comparing crizotinib as first-line therapy with standard platinum-based chemotherapy in patients who are ALK-positive (NCT01154140) will be interesting to see. Crizotinib is reasonably well tolerated, with the main toxicities being grade 1 to 2 visual disturbances (mainly associated with transition from light to dark); gastrointestinal symptoms; and transaminitis.

INHIBITORS OF ANGIOGENESIS

New blood vessel formation (angiogenesis) is one of the key mechanisms in sustaining cancer growth and involves complex interactions between proangiogenic and antiangiogenic factors.[25] This key role it plays in cancer growth makes angiogenesis a useful therapeutic target.

Two main therapeutic strategies are used in targeting angiogenesis: inhibition of proangiogenic factors (eg, anti–vascular endothelial growth factor [VEGF] antibodies, small molecule VEGF receptor inhibitors); and use of agents that promote antiangiogenic factors (eg, matrix-metalloproteinases, endostatin).

Bevacizumab

This is a recombinant anti-VEGF monoclonal antibody administered as an intravenous infusion. Apart from inhibiting new vessel formation, it also interferes with and normalizes existing tumor vasculature, thus impeding tumor growth. Important serious side effects associated with its use include thrombosis, hypertension, and tumor-associated hemorrhage.

Major pulmonary hemorrhage was seen in an initial phase II study,[26] with squamous cell histology identified as a statistically significant variable correlating with bleeding. Thus, squamous histology subset was excluded from subsequent trials investigating bevacizumab.

In the E4599 trial,[27] patients with locally advanced, metastatic, or recurrent NSCLC (apart from squamous histology) were randomized to six cycles of paclitaxel/carboplatin in combination with bevacizumab versus paclitaxel/carboplatin alone. On completion of chemotherapy, those in the experimental arm continued to receive three-weekly bevacizumab until progression. PFS was improved significantly (from 4.8 to 6.4 months in the bevacizumab arm; HR, 0.65; $P<.0001$). Median survival was also improved significantly (from 10.3 to 12.3 months in the experimental arm; HR, 0.80; $P = .003$). Overall response rate was 13% in the standard arm and 29% in the bevacizumab arm.

The BO17704 (AVAiL)[28] study randomized patients into cisplatin/gemcitabine with placebo versus cisplatin/gemcitabine plus either 7.5 mg/kg or 15 mg/kg bevacizumab. This study also demonstrated an improvement in PFS, but no significant OS benefit in the bevacizumab-containing arms. Bevacizumab is used in first-line treatment (in combination with chemotherapy) in certain countries (eg, United States and European Union), but has not been approved in the United Kingdom.

Vandetanib

This orally available small-molecule inhibitor of VEGFR-2 and EGFR was compared with erlotinib in patients with NSCLC after failure of at least one chemotherapy regimen. No improvement in PFS or OS was seen.[29] Side effects include diarrhea, rash, nausea, hypertension, and headache. Vandetanib was studied in a placebo-controlled trial involving patients with advanced NSCLC who had previously been treated with an EGFR TKI and one or two chemotherapy regimens. No significant OS benefit was seen (8.5 vs 7.5 months in the vandetanib and placebo arms, respectively; HR, 0.95; P = .527).[30] A recent meta-analysis of four randomized controlled trials comparing chemotherapy plus vandetanib with chemotherapy alone in advanced NSCLC showed no survival benefit (HR, 0.91; 95% CI, 0.79–1.03), although the vandetanib-containing arms showed improvement in PFS (HR, 0.79; 95% CI, 0.71–0.87) and overall response rate (relative risk, 1.96; 95% CI, 1.53–2.52).[31]

Thalidomide

This drug possesses anti-inflammatory and antiangiogenic properties. In a phase III trial, thalidomide in combination with gemcitabine/carboplatin chemotherapy did not show any survival benefit.[32] The main toxicities were rash and neuropathy.

RAS/RAF/MEK INHIBITORS

Ras refers to a group of GTPase proteins involved in cellular signal transduction. Activation of Ras results in a cascade of events resulting ultimately in the turning on of genes involved in cell proliferation and survival. Three Ras genes have been identified (KRAS, HRAS, and NRAS), mutations of which can result in uncontrolled cell growth and survival.

The frequency of KRAS mutations in all NSCLC is around 17% (rarely seen in squamous subtype, up to 34% in nonsquamous NSCLC),[33,34] and this mutation is generally associated with a smoking history.[35] KRAS mutation is thought to confer a poorer prognosis in terms of survival (HR, 1.21; P = .048), in comparison with EGFR mutation (HR, 0.6; P<.001), according to a retrospective series of more than 1000 patients.[36]

The use of inhibitors targeting KRAS specifically (eg, farnesyl protein transferase, farnesylthiosalicylic acid) has been largely unsuccessful.[37,38] Targeting alternative downstream targets (eg, mTOR, MEK, MET, and MAPK) in KRAS-mutant populations is being studied in various phase II studies. One such approach that looks promising is reflected in the phase II trial comparing docetaxel alone with docetaxel plus selumetinib (an oral MEK inhibitor) in previously treated KRAS-mutant patients with NSCLC.[39] Median PFS was improved in the selumetenib group compared with the control arm (5.3 vs 2.1 months; HR, 0.58; P = .014), with an objective response rate of 37% in the selumetinib arm compared with 0% in the docetaxel-only arm. There was also an improvement in OS, although it was not statistically significant (9.4 vs 5.2 months; HR, 0.80; 80% CI, 0.56–1.14). Side effects include rash, diarrhea, fatigue, and peripheral edema.

BRAF is activated further downstream to KRAS, and it in turn activates MAPK. The frequency of BRAF mutations is between 1% and 3%. A phase II study is currently looking at the efficacy and safety of dabrafenib, a selective inhibitor of BRAF kinase in advanced NSCLC.

Sorafenib inhibits multiple kinases, including RAF. It was combined with standard chemotherapy as first-line treatment of advanced NSCLC (ESCAPE trial), and showed no improvement (in PFS or OS)[40] compared with chemotherapy alone. The squamous histology subset actually did worse in the experimental arm. Similarly, the NExUS trial failed to show any survival benefit when sorafenib was added to standard gemcitabine/cisplatin first-line therapy for advanced NSCLC.

INHIBITORS OF PI3K/AKT/PTEN PATHWAY

This pathway plays an important part in regulating various cellular signaling processes including apoptosis, cell proliferation, and cell growth. Different alterations in the pathway have been identified (including gain-of-function mutations in PI3K/AKT1 and loss-of-function of PTEN).[41] These oncologic alterations result in maintenance of cancer cell survival. The clinical usefulness of these alterations as therapeutic targets is being studied (using small-molecule inhibitors), although because there is considerable overlap in the pathway, the efficacy of any agent against a particular alteration remains to be determined.

MTOR INHIBITORS

mTOR belongs to a family of kinases known as PI3K-related kinases. Its activity is downstream to PI3K, where it orchestrates various signaling pathways in response to growth factors and nutrient availability.

Temsirolimus (an intravenous mTOR inhibitor) was shown in a phase II study of 55 previously untreated patients with NSCLC to have a partial response rate of 8% and stable disease rate of 30%. Median PFS was 2.3 months, and OS 6.6 months.[42]

Evorilimus, which is an oral mTOR inhibitor, was studied in a two-arm phase II study, with arm 1 containing patients with NSCLC who had progressed after less than or equal to two platinum-based chemotherapy regimens, and arm 2 containing those who had progressed after less than or equal to two chemotherapy and EGFR TKI regimens.[43] Median PFS was 11.3 and 9.7 weeks in arms 1 and 2, respectively. Combination therapy with everolimus and erlotinib was studied in a phase II study of patients with NSCLC who had progressed after less than or equal to two chemotherapy regimens.[44] The combination arm showed an improved disease control rate (39% vs 28%) compared with the erlotinib-only arm. PFS was also improved (2.9 vs 2 months).

Side effects of mTOR inhibitors include skin and gastrointestinal toxicity, hypertension, fatigue, bone marrow toxicity, and interstitial pneumonitis.

MET INHIBITORS

The MET-gene encodes for hepatocyte growth factor receptor kinase and its amplification is found in up to 75% of NSCLC[45] (squamous and nonsquamous). MET amplification is associated with a poorer prognosis[46] and it is also thought to be a mechanism that contributes to EGFR TKI resistance.[47] A phase III trial is currently underway comparing combination therapy with tivantinib (a MET inhibitor) and erlotinib with erlotinib alone in patients with NSCLC who have received one or two previous systemic therapies. Another phase III trial is comparing erlotinib alone with erlotinib and onartuzumab in c-MET–positive previously treated patients with NSCLC.

CYCLOOXYGENASE-2 INHIBITORS

Cyclooxygenase (COX)-2 is an enzyme responsible for the production of prostanoids, which are biologic mediators involved in various processes including inflammation and pain. COX-2–dependent mechanisms are known to influence carcinogenesis and neoplastic cell multiplication. Two phase III trials (NVALT-4, CYCLUS) investigating the addition of a COX-2 inhibitor (celecoxib) to palliative chemotherapy in advanced NSCLC failed to show any survival benefit.[48,49] The NVALT-4 study also showed that COX-2 expression did not independently predict survival. Concerns about the cardiotoxicity of COX inhibitors have limited its development.

HISTONE DEACETYLASE INHIBITORS

Histone deacetylase (HDAC) is a class of enzymes that influence gene expression by allowing increased DNA transcription. Increased expression of tumor-suppressor genes is a mechanism for survival of cancer cells, and so targeting HDAC was thought to be a useful therapeutic strategy. Vorinostat (an HDAC inhibitor) was found to improve the efficacy of platinum-based chemotherapy in NSCLC (response rate of 34% with vorinostat vs 12.5% with placebo).[50] No significant improvement was seen in PFS or OS.

PROTEASOME INHIBITORS

The ubiquitin-proteasome mechanism is another vital pathway in the proliferation and survival of cancer cells, making it an attractive therapeutic target. Bortezomib, a selective proteasome inhibitor, showed no objective response when used in chemonaive patients with NSCLC in a phase II study.[51] Several phase II studies have shown modest benefit, at best, when used in combination with chemotherapy.[52–54] A phase II study comparing erlotinib alone and in combination with bortezomib in previously treated NSCLC was terminated because of lack of clinical activity seen in the experimental arm.[55]

IMMUNOTHERAPIES

It is becoming increasingly evident that inducing or potentiating the body's immune system could be a viable therapeutic approach in treating cancer. The immune system has been manipulated for therapeutic purposes in two main ways.[56] The first is nonspecific stimulation of the innate immune system (eg, bacille Calmette-Guérin, interferons and interleukins, PF 3512676 [an agonist of toll-like receptor 9]). None of these have been found to be useful. Ipilimumab, a CTLA4 monoclonal antibody, was shown to improve PFS (when given either concurrently or sequentially with platinum-based chemotherapy) in a phase II randomized study of advanced NSCLC. Phase III studies are currently underway. The second is specific priming of the immune system, using vaccines that effectively act by enlisting T cytotoxic lymphocytes. Examples of vaccines that have had promising results in phase II studies include belagenpumatucel-L (an allogeneic cell vaccine); CimaVax (an EGF vaccine); and TG4010 (which targets the MUC1 antigen, a cell-surface glycoprotein). Following on from the impressive outcome of phase II studies, they are currently being studied in phase IIb/III studies.

Vaccines are also currently being studied in early NSCLC in phase III trials, such as the MAGRIT study (evaluating the MAGE-A3 vaccine in the adjuvant setting) and START trial (investigating L-BLP25, which targets MUC-1, for patients with stable disease or objective response after first-line chemotherapy for locally advanced NSCLC).

SMALL CELL LUNG CANCER

No targeted therapies have been approved for use in SCLC, and the use of targeted therapies in this group remain largely experimental. Signaling pathways and biologic markers have been identified and are being authenticated, and novel agents have been investigated with no great success. The following is a summary of agents that have been tried:

- EGFR inhibitors: Gefitinib failed to show any benefit when used in a small phase II study of chemosensitive and chemorefractory patients with SCLC.[57] The EGFR mutation is rare in SCLC, and where present, is more likely to be found in the histologic subset where SCLC is combined with adenocarcinoma.[58]
- Angiogenesis inhibitors: Bevacizumab improved PFS (but not OS) when used in the first-line setting in SCLC, in combination with chemotherapy, in phase II studies.[59,60] Its addition to chemotherapy in the setting of relapsed SCLC, however, did not show an improvement in outcomes.[61] Vandetanib did not have any benefit when used as maintenance treatment after first-line chemotherapy.[62] Thalidomide has been shown in phase III trials to have no significant survival benefit.[63,64] The oral angiogenesis inhibitors sunitinib, sorafenib, and cediranib have not shown much promise.
- Apoptotic inducers: Obatoclax, a BCl-2 inhibitor, demonstrated a trend for improved survival in a phase II study in combination with chemotherapy in extensive disease SCLC patients, and is currently being studied in a phase III study.[65] Oblimersen, an oligonucleotide that suppresses Bcl-2 levels, did not improve outcomes when combined with chemotherapy.[66] Phase II trials looking at other novel Bcl-2 inhibitors (AT-101 and ABT-263) are ongoing.
- Insulin-like growth factor-1R inhibitors: insulin-like growth factor-1 receptor has been identified as a pathway for mitogenic activity in SCLC lines.[67] Inhibitors currently undergoing phase II trials include linsitinib (a small-molecule inhibitor) and cixitumumab (a monoclonal antibody).
- c-kit inhibitors: Mutations of c-kit have been identified in SCLC, although in very small frequency. Imatinib has not demonstrated efficacy even in patients with c-kit expression.[57]
- Immunotherapy: A randomized phase II study in which ipilimumab was given either concurrently or sequentially with chemotherapy in chemonaive patients with SCLC showed improved PFS and a trend for improved OS in the sequential arm.[68] A phase III trial is ongoing.

Summary of targeted agents

Therapies in current clinical use
Erlotinib
Gefitinib
Cetuximab
Crizotinib
Bevacizumab

Therapies under review
Afatinib

Therapies in development
Selemutenib
Dabrafenib
Everolimus
Temsirolimus
Tivantinib
Onartuzumab
Ipilimumab
Belagenpumatucel-L
CimaVax
TG4010

Therapies with negative results
Vandetanib
Thalidomide
Farnesyl protein transferase
Farnesylthiosalicylic acid
Celecoxib
Voinostat
Bacille Calmette-Guérin
Interferon
Interleukins

REFERENCES

1. Chemotherapy in non-small cell lung cancer: a meta-analysis using updated data on individual patients from 52 randomised clinical trials. Non-small Cell Lung Cancer Collaborative Group. BMJ 1995;311(7010):899–909.
2. Schiller JH, Harrington D, Chandra PB, et al. Comparison of four chemotherapy regimens for advanced non-small-cell lung cancer. N Engl J Med 2002;346:92–8.
3. Shepherd FA, Rodrigues Pereira J, Ciuleanu T, et al. Erlotinib in previously treated non-small-cell lung cancer. N Engl J Med 2005;353:123–32.

4. Clark GM, Zborowski DM, Santabarbara P, et al. Smoking history and epidermal growth factor receptor expression as predictors of survival benefit from erlotinib for patients with non-small-cell lung cancer in the National Cancer Institute of Canada Clinical Trials Group study BR.21. Clin Lung Cancer 2006;7:389–94.
5. Rosell R, Carcereny E, Gervais R, et al. Erlotinib versus standard chemotherapy as first-line treatment for European patients with advanced EGFR mutation-positive non-small-cell lung cancer (EURTAC): a multicentre, open-label, randomised phase 3 trial. Lancet Oncol 2012;13(3):239–46.
6. Herbst RS, Prager D, Hermann R, et al. TRIBUTE: a phase III trial of erlotinib hydrochloride (OSI-774) combined with carboplatin and paclitaxel chemotherapy in advanced non-small-cell lung cancer. J Clin Oncol 2005;23:5892–9.
7. Gatzemeier U, Pluzanska A, Szczesna A, et al. Phase III study of erlotinib in combination with cisplatin and gemcitabine in advanced non-small-cell lung cancer: The Tarceva Lung Cancer Investigation Trial. J Clin Oncol 2007;25:1545–52.
8. Cappuzzo F, Ciuleanu T, Stelmakh L, et al. SATURN: a double-blind, randomized, phase III study of maintenance erlotinib versus placebo following nonprogression with first-line platinumbased chemotherapy in patients with advanced NSCLC. J Clin Oncol 2009;27(Suppl):S15.
9. Lynch TJ, Bell DW, Sordella R, et al. Activating mutations in the epidermal growth factor receptor underlying responsiveness of non-small-cell lung cancer to gefitinib. N Engl J Med 2004;350:2129.
10. Pao W, Miller V, Zakowski M, et al. EGF receptor gene mutations are common in lung cancers from "never smokers" and are associated with sensitivity of tumours to gefitinib and erlotinib. Proc Natl Acad Sci U S A 2004;101:13306.
11. Fukuoka M, Wu YL, Thongprasert S, et al. Biomarker analysis and final overall survival results from a phase III, randomised, open label, first line study of gefitinib versus carboplatin/paclitaxel in clinically selected patients with advanced non-small-cell lung cancer in Asia (IPASS). J Clin Oncol 2011;29:2866.
12. Pirker R, Pereira JR, Szczesna A, et al. Cetuximab plus chemotherapy in patients with advanced non-small-cell lung cancer (FLEX): an open-label randomized phase III trial. Lancet 2009;373: 1525–31.
13. Yang JC, Schuler MH, Yamamoto M, et al. LUX-Lung 3: a randomised, open-label, phase III study of afatinib versus pemetrexed and cisplatin as first-line treatment for patients with advanced adenocarcinoma of the lung harbouring EGFR activating mutations. [abstract LBA7500]. J Clin Oncol 2012; 30(Suppl).
14. Miller VA, Hirsh V, Cadranel J, et al. Afatinib versus placebo for patients with advanced, metastatic non-small-cell lung cancer after failure of erlotinib, gefitinib, or both, and one or two lines of chemotherapy (LUX-Lung 1): a phase 2b/3 randomised trial. Lancet Oncol 2012;13(5):528–38.
15. Food and Drug Administration. Available at: http://www.accessdata.fda.gov/drugsatfda_docs/label/2011/20270s000lbl.pdf. Accessed January, 2013.
16. Shaw AT, Solomon B. Targeting anaplastic lymphoma kinase in lung cancer. Clin Cancer Res 2011;17:2081.
17. Rodig SJ, Mino-Kenudson M, Docic S, et al. Unique clinicopathologic features characterise ALK-rearranged lung adenocarcinoma in the western population. Clin Cancer Res 2009;15:5216.
18. Soda M, Choi YL, Enomoto M, et al. Identification of the EML4-ALK fusion gene in non-small-cell lung cancer. Nature 2007;448:561.
19. Inamura K, Takeuchi K, Togashi Y, et al. EML4-ALK fusion is linked to histological characteristics in a subset of lung cancers. J Thorac Oncol 2008;3:13.
20. Martelli MP, Sozzi G, Hernandez L, et al. Anaplastic lymphoma kinase immunoreactivity correlates with ALK gene rearrangement and transcriptional up-regulation in non-small cell lung carcinomas. Hum Pathol 2009;40:1152.
21. Shaw AT, Yeap BY, Mino-Kenudson M, et al. Clinical features and outcome of patients with non-small-cell lung cancer who harbour EML4-ALK. J Clin Oncol 2009;27:4247–53.
22. Kwak EL, Bang YJ, Camidge DR, et al. Anaplastic lymphoma kinase inhibition in non-small-cell lung cancer. N Engl J Med 2010;363:1693.
23. Camidge DR, Bang Y, Kwak EL, et al. Activity and safety of crizotinib in patients with ALK positive non-small-cell lung cancer: updated results from a phase I study. Lancet Oncol 2012;13(10):1011–9.
24. Shaw AT, Kim DW, Nakagawa K, et al. Phase III study of crizotinnib versus pemetrexed or docetaxel chemotherapy in patients with advanced ALK-positive non-small-cell lung cancer [abstract LBA1 PR]. Presented at the 37th Congress of the European Society of Medical Oncology(ESMO), Vienna, Austria, September 28- October 2, 2012.
25. Danson S. Targeted therapy in non-small cell lung cancer. In: Manegold C, editor. Non-small cell lung cancer therapy. 2nd edition. Bremen (Germany): UniMedScience; 2010. p. 143–50.
26. Johnson DH, Fehrenbacher L, Novotny WF, et al. Randomized phase II trial comparing bevacizumab plus carboplatin and paclitaxel with carboplatin and paclitaxel alone in previously untreated locally advanced or metastatic non-small-cell lung cancer. Clin Oncol 2004;22(11):2184–91.
27. Sandler AB, Gray R, Brahmer J, et al. Paclitaxel-carboplatin alone or with bevacizumab for non-

small cell lung cancer (NSCLC). N Engl J Med 2006;355:2542–50.
28. Reck M, von Pawel J, Zatloukal P, et al. Phase III trial of cisplatin plus gemcitabine with either placebo or bevacizumab as first-line therapy for nonsquamous non-small-cell lung cancer: AVAiL. J Clin Oncol 2009;27:1227–34.
29. Natale RB, Thongprasert S, Greco A, et al. Vandetanib versus erlotinib in patients with advanced non-small cell lung cancer (NSCLC) after failure of at least one prior cytotoxic chemotherapy: a randomized, double-blind phase III trial (ZEST) [abstract 8009]. J Clin Oncol 2009;27(Suppl):15s.
30. Lee JS, Hirsh V, Park K, et al. Vandetanib versus placebo in patients with advanced non–small-cell lung cancer after prior therapy with an epidermal growth factor receptor tyrosine kinase inhibitor: a randomized, double-blind phase III trial (ZEPHYR). J Clin Oncol 2012;30(10):1114–21.
31. Xiao YY, Zhan P, Yuan DM. Chemotherapy plus vandetanib or chemotherapy alone in advanced non-small cell lung cancer: a meta-analysis of four randomised controlled trials. Clin Oncol (R Coll Radiol) 2013;25(1):e7–15. http://dx.doi.org/10.1016/j.clon.2012.09.005.
32. Lee SM, Rudd R, Woll PJ, et al. Randomized double-blind placebo-controlled trial of thalidomide in combination with gemcitabine and carboplatin in advanced non-small-cell lung cancer. J Clin Oncol 2009;27(31):5248–54.
33. Suzuki Y, Orita M, Shiraishi M, et al. Detection of ras gene mutations in human lung cancers by single-strand conformation polymorphism analysis of polymerase chain reaction products. Oncogene 1990;5(7):1037–43.
34. Schiller JH, Adak S, Feins RH, et al. Lack of prognostic significance of p53 and K-ras mutations in primary resected non–small-cell lung cancer on E4592: a laboratory ancillary study on an Eastern Cooperative Oncology Group prospective randomized trial of postoperative adjuvant therapy. J Clin Oncol 2001;19(2):448–57.
35. Ahrendt SA, Decker PA, Alawi EA. Cigarette smoking is strongly associated with mutation of the K-ras gene in patients with primary adenocarcinoma of the lung. Cancer 2001;92(6):1525.
36. Johnson ML, Sima CS, Chaft J, et al. Association of KRAS and EGFR mutations with survival in patients with advanced lung adenocarcinomas. Cancer 2013;119(2):356–62.
37. Appels NM, Beijnen JH, Schellens JH. Development of farnesyl transferase inhibitors: a review. Oncologist 2005;10(8):565–78.
38. Riely GJ, Johnson ML, Medina C, et al. A phase II trial of salirasib in patients with lung adenocarcinomas with KRAS mutations. J Thorac Oncol 2011;6(8):1435–7.
39. Janne PA, Shaw AT, Rodrigues Pereira J, et al. Selumetinib plus docetaxel for KRAS-mutant advanced non-small-cell lung cancer: a randomised, multicentre, placebo-controlled, phase 2 study. Lancet Oncol 2013;14(1):38–47.
40. Scagliotti G, Novello S, von PJ, et al. Phase III study of carboplatin and paclitaxel alone or with sorafenib in advanced non-small cell lung cancer. J Clin Oncol 2010;28(11):1835–42.
41. Liu P, Cheng H, Roberts TM, et al. Targeting the phosphoinositide 3-kinase pathway in cancer. Nat Rev Drug Discov 2009;8(8):627–44.
42. Molina JR, Mandrekar SJ, Rowland KR. A phase II NCCTG "window of opportunity front-line" study of the mTOR inhibitor, CCI-779 (temsirolimus) given as a single agent in patients with advanced NSCLC. J Thorac Oncol 2007;2(Suppl 4):S413.
43. Papadimitrakopoulou V, Adjei AA. The Akt/mTOR and mitogen-activated protein kinase pathways in lung cancer therapy. J Thorac Oncol 2006;1:749–51.
44. Leighl NB, Soria J, Bennouna J, et al. Phase II study of everolimus plus erlotinib in previously treated patients with advanced non-small cell lung cancer (NSCLC) [abstract 7524]. J Clin Oncol 2010;28(Suppl):15s.
45. Nakamura Y, Niki T, Goto A, et al. c-Met activation in lung adenocarcinoma tissues: an immunohistochemical analysis. Cancer Sci 2007;98(7):1006–13.
46. Ichimura E, Maeshima A, Nakajima T, et al. Expression of c-met/HGF receptor in human non-small cell lung carcinomas in vitro and in vivo and its prognostic significance. Jpn J Cancer Res 1996;87(10):1063.
47. Engelman JA, Zejnullahu K, Mitsudomi T, et al. MET amplification leads to gefitinib resistance in lung cancer by activating ERBB3 signaling. Science 2007;316:1039–43.
48. Groen HJ, Sietsma H, Vincent A, et al. Randomized, placebo-controlled phase III study of docetaxel plus carboplatin with celecoxib and cyclooxygenase-2 expression as a biomarker for patients with advanced non-small-cell lung cancer: the NVALT-4 study. J Clin Oncol 2011;29(32):4320–6.
49. Koch A, Bergman B, Holmberg E, et al. Effect of celecoxib on survival in patients with advanced non-small cell lung cancer: a double blind randomised clinical phase III trial (CYCLUS study) by the Swedish Lung Cancer Study Group. Eur J Cancer 2011;47(10):1546–55.
50. Ramalingam SS, Maitland ML, Frankel P, et al. Carboplatin and paclitaxel in combination with either vorinostat or placebo for first-line therapy of advanced non-small-cell lung cancer. J Clin Oncol 2010;28(1):56–62.

51. Besse B, Planchard D, Veillard AS, et al. Phase 2 study of frontline bortezomib in patients with advanced non-small cell lung cancer. Lung Cancer 2012;76(1):78–83.
52. Fanucchi MP, Fossella FV, Belt R, et al. Randomized phase II study of bortezomib alone and bortezomib in combination with docetaxel in previously treated advanced non-small-cell lung cancer. J Clin Oncol 2006;24(31):5025–33.
53. Davies AM, Chansky K, Lara PN Jr, et al. Bortezomib plus gemcitabine/carboplatin as first-line treatment of advanced non-small cell lung cancer: a phase II southwest oncology group study (S0339). J Thorac Oncol 2009;4(1):87–92.
54. Scagliotti GV, Germonpré P, Bosquée L, et al. A randomized phase II study of bortezomib and pemetrexed, in combination or alone, in patients with previously treated advanced non-small-cell lung cancer. Lung Cancer 2010;68(3):420–6.
55. Lynch TJ, Fenton D, Hirsh V, et al. A randomized phase 2 study of erlotinib alone and in combination with bortezomib in previously treated advanced non-small cell lung cancer. J Thorac Oncol 2009; 4(8):1002–9.
56. Decoster L, Wauters I, Vansteenkiste JF. Vaccination therapy for non-small-cell lung cancer: review of agents in phase III development. Ann Oncol 2012;23:1387–93.
57. Moore AM, Einhorn LH, Estes D, et al. Gefitinib in patients with chemo-sensitive and chemo-refractory relapsed small cell cancers: a Hoosier Oncology Group phase II trial. Lung Cancer 2006;52:93–7.
58. Lu HY, Wang XJ, Mao WM. Targeted therapies in small cell lung cancer. Oncol Lett 2013;5(1):3–11.
59. Horn L, Dahlberg SE, Sandler AB, et al. Phase II study of cisplatin plus etoposide and bevacizumab for previously untreated, extensive-stage small-cell lung cancer: Eastern Cooperative Oncology Group Study E3501. J Clin Oncol 2009;27(35):6006–11.
60. Spigel DR, Townley PM, Waterhouse DM, et al. Randomized phase II study of bevacizumab in combination with chemotherapy in previously untreated extensive-stage small-cell lung cancer: results from the SALUTE trial. J Clin Oncol 2011;29:2215–22.
61. Jalal S, Bedano P, Einhorn L, et al. Paclitaxel plus bevacizumab in patients with chemosensitive relapsed small cell lung cancer: a safety, feasibility, and efficacy study from the Hoosier Oncology Group. J Thorac Oncol 2010;5:2008–11.
62. Arnold AM, Seymour L, Smylie M, et al. Phase II study of vandetanib or placebo in small-cell lung cancer patients after complete or partial response to induction chemotherapy with or without radiation therapy: National Cancer Institute of Canada Clinical Trials Group Study BR.20. J Clin Oncol 2007; 25(27):4278.
63. Lee SM, Woll PJ, Rudd R, et al. Anti-angiogenic therapy using thalidomide combined with chemotherapy in small cell lung cancer: a randomized, double-blind, placebo-controlled trial. J Natl Cancer Inst 2009;101(15):1049.
64. Pujol JL, Breton JL, Gervais R, et al. Phase III double-blind, placebo-controlled study of thalidomide in extensive-disease small-cell lung cancer after response to chemotherapy: an intergroup study FNCLCC cleo04 IFCT 00-01. J Clin Oncol 2007;25(25):3945.
65. Langer CJ, Albert I, Kovacs P, et al. A randomized phase II study of carboplatin (C) and etoposide (E) with or without pan-BCL-2 antagonist obatoclax (Ob) in extensive-stage small cell lung cancer (ES-SCLC). J Clin Oncol 2011;29(Suppl) [abstract 7001].
66. Rudin CM, Salgia R, Wang X, et al. Randomized phase II study of carboplatin and etoposide with or without the bcl-2 antisense oligonucleotide oblimersen for extensive-stage small-cell lung cancer: CALGB 30103. J Clin Oncol 2008;26:870–6.
67. Nakanishi Y, Mulshine JL, Kasprzyk PG, et al. Insulin-like growth factor-I can mediate autocrine proliferation of human small cell lung cancer cell lines in vitro. J Clin Invest 1988;82(1):354.
68. Reck M, Bondarenko I, Luft A, et al. Ipilimumab in combination with paclitaxel and carboplatin as first-line therapy in extensive-disease-small-cell lung cancer: results from a randomized, double-blind, multicenter phase 2 trial. Ann Oncol 2013; 24(1):75–83.

Biologic Approaches to Drug Selection and Targeted Therapy
Hype or Clinical Reality?

Dennis A. Wigle, MD, PhD

KEYWORDS

- Targeted therapy • Individualized medicine • EGFR mutation • ALK translocation
- Tumor genome sequencing

KEY POINTS

- NSCLC is many different diseases with evolving differences in treatment approach.
- Targeted therapeutics are drugs directed against molecular drivers of cancer, with EGFR mutation and ALK translocation prominent examples in lung adenocarcinoma.
- Targeted therapy is advancing beyond initial use in stage IV disease to potential applications in locally advanced stage IIIA disease and as adjuvant therapy for stage II disease.
- Mutation analysis by genome sequencing is being rapidly adopted for clinical use in cancer care.
- Surgeons need to stay abreast of developments in the field and participate in the design and accrual of clinical trials evaluating the roles of targeted therapeutics in multimodality treatment regimens involving surgery.

OVERVIEW

Oncology remains at the forefront of the application of individualized or genomics-driven approaches to cancer care. In simplest terms, this approach acknowledges cancer as a genetic disease, driven by alterations in oncogenes and tumor suppressors, with the strategy of using this information to guide therapy based on therapeutics capable of targeting specific alterations. Leveraging such an approach involves many challenges. Although the grizzled skeptic might observe this as the latest iteration of undeliverable hype in cancer treatment, recent advances do suggest a changing landscape in how clinicians approach management decisions for the patient with non–small cell lung cancer (NSCLC). An expanding and functionally useful toolbox of novel targeted agents and biomarkers to drive therapeutic choices is beginning to impact patient care. Key advances are reviewed, with commentary and perspective as to what this all means for the practicing thoracic surgical oncologist.

INDIVIDUALIZING PATIENT CARE: TODAY'S NEWS OR OLD NEWS?

The concept of tailoring treatment or individualizing therapy for a specific patient is not a new idea to thoracic surgeons. They face these decisions every day in the clinic in the process of managing patients with NSCLC. Will this patient tolerate anatomic surgical resection? Is the tumor resectable? Are they a better candidate for stereotactic body radiation therapy? Should they have rehabilitation before surgery? Who should have a more detailed cardiopulmonary work-up? The questions can be endless. Although many published guidelines and expert commentaries strive to subclassify and guide patient management, the patient never fails to fall outside some established criteria. Individualizing treatment often

Thoracic Surgery, Mayo Clinic, 200 First Street, Southwest, Rochester, MN 55905, USA
E-mail address: wigle.dennis@mayo.edu

Thorac Surg Clin 23 (2013) 421–428
http://dx.doi.org/10.1016/j.thorsurg.2013.05.003
1547-4127/13/$ – see front matter

requires the judgment hailed as the "art" of medicine and surgery to supersede what is described in the latest expert panel guideline.

The concepts that have served well for many years to guide treatment of NSCLC continue to be widely clinically applied. TNM staging remains the major determinant of tumor classification and patient treatment. Despite recent revisions, it has remained largely unchanged for more than 25 years.[1,2] Imaging continues to improve the ability to classify patients based on TNM stage, further decreasing what used to be the not-so-infrequent exploratory or unnecessary thoracotomy for what turned out to be an unresectable tumor. The emergence of adjuvant platinum-based chemotherapy and minimally invasive surgical techniques notwithstanding, the surgical management of patients with early stage I and II disease has not really changed in decades. Surgery for locally advanced disease continues to be controversial, despite publication of results from the intergroup 0139 study.[3,4] Stage IV disease is basically managed by someone else.

So why all the recent hype? Molecular staging? Targeted agents? Biomarker-directed therapy? Is the world really all that different? Fortunately for patients and their physicians, yes it is different. Agents being tested and optimized in advanced disease are being integrated into clinical algorithms and trial protocols for resectable tumors. Although the current clinically applicable individualized therapies for NSCLC are small in number, the literature underpinning their use is increasingly complicated and difficult to stay abreast of. This will be more so going forward. The challenge for thoracic surgeons is to stay engaged and involved in these new directions and not delegate this emerging field to colleagues in other disciplines. Future developments will not only provide new treatment options, but will also change how clinicians apply those they currently know and with which they are familiar.

MOLECULAR HETEROGENEITY: NSCLC AS MANY DISEASES

Worldwide, lung cancer remains the leading cause of cancer-related death in men and the second leading cause of cancer-related deaths in women.[5–7] The American Cancer Society estimates an incidence of 221,130 new cases of lung cancer for 2011 with 156,940 deaths. NSCLC currently makes up approximately 85% of all lung cancers, with adenocarcinoma and squamous cell carcinoma (SqCC) each accounting for approximately 30% to 50%. Despite these histologic subclassifications, NSCLC has historically been treated as a single disease with a one-size-fits-all approach. Until recently, treatment strategies were determined by disease stage, with either surgery or platinum-based doublet chemotherapy comprising first-line treatment depending on stage. Despite roughly similar survival curves for adenocarcinoma and SqCC with these treatment approaches, emerging data clearly show the effect of histology on treatment response. Mutations in the epidermal growth factor receptor (EGFR) gene are found in approximately 15% of NSCLCs in North American patients and are associated with adenocarcinoma histology almost exclusively.[8] Overexpression of EGFR can be common in SqCC, but mutations are rarely found.[9] Mutations in KRAS are commonly found in adenocarcinoma but rarely in SqCC.[10] The echinoderm microtubule-associated protein-like 4 (EML4)/anaplastic lymphoma kinase (ALK) fusion oncogene defines a molecular subset of adenocarcinomas that is sensitive to the ALK inhibitor crizotinib.[11] Other agents with potential differences in efficacy based on histology include bevacizumab, where it is contraindicated for proximal SqCC because of an increased incidence of hemoptysis.[12] Pemetrexed does not seem to have significant benefit in squamous cell histology.[13] Erlotinib (Tarceva) and gefitinib (Iressa) are directed against activating mutations in the EGFR gene and as a consequence are best effective in adenocarcinomas in which these mutations are present.[14] Sorafenib, a vascular endothelial growth factor inhibitor, has poorer overall clinical outcomes in squamous cell histology compared with platinum-based chemotherapy alone, again as a result of issues with hemoptysis.[15]

The molecular heterogeneity of NSCLC is further exemplified by accumulating high-throughput genomic data. In a short time period, this information has exponentially multiplied what is known about molecular alterations in NSCLC. Genomic alterations in lung SqCC have recently been comprehensively characterized as part of The Cancer Genome Atlas (TCGA) project.[14] This benchmark paper has provided a rich resource of recurrent alterations present in this disease. This comprehensive assessment of genomic alterations present in invasive lung SqCC profiled 178 lung SqCCs using a combination of array and sequencing technologies to provide a comprehensive landscape of genomic and epigenomic alterations. Whole genome sequencing was also performed in 19 tumors. It was demonstrated that lung SqCC is characterized by complex genomic alterations, with a mean of 360 exonic mutations, 165 genomic rearrangements, and 323 segments of copy number alteration per tumor. Several recurrent alterations not previously associated with lung

SqCC were identified, and a potential therapeutic target was identified in most tumors studied, offering new approaches to the treatment of invasive lung SqCC. The index paper for lung adenocarcinoma from the TCGA project remains in preparation at the time of this article, but will have a focus on "driver negative" tumors, or those without well-characterized oncogenic drivers, among other areas of interest from the results of exome sequencing in more than 200 tumors. Recent publications from Govindan and colleagues (2012)[16] and Imilenski and colleagues (2012)[17] over the past year have highlighted the genomic diversity of lung adenocarcinoma observed through exome and whole genome sequencing. Although the molecular subtypes that continue to be discovered represent a smaller and smaller fraction of patients with the disease overall, many of them, such as ROS translocations, which are sensitive to crizotinib, are clinically relevant.

As a result of these emerging data, the potential for novel drug targets, targeted therapies, and biomarkers for stratification of prognosis and treatment response has never been brighter. The clinical heterogeneity in outcomes within TNM stages suggests that further patient subclassification based on molecular diagnosis is possible.[18] Biomarkers of treatment response, with EGFR mutation the most prominent example, are being used increasingly for therapeutic decision-making in clinical practice. Many different forms of genomic data, including mRNA expression, microRNA expression, single nucleotide polymorphism genotyping, and methylation status, have all shown potential correlation with clinical outcome and have suggested the possibility for molecular staging of NSCLC.

Despite these advances, however, there is still not a validated, biomarker-based molecular diagnostic for predicting NSCLC prognosis that influences patient management.[19] Although the opportunities for molecular substaging of NSCLC are numerous, it is unclear what form of genomic data will provide the most useful information for clinical translation. How such information would be incorporated into existing TNM systems is also unclear. Two obvious opportunities for the use of molecular substaging in NSCLC exist at the edges of the TNM classification system.[18] In the case of early stage disease with N1 level nodal spread (stage II NSCLC), the emerging standard of care for adjuvant chemotherapy likely overgeneralizes patients who are likely to benefit. Examples from other tumor types suggest the potential for molecular subtypes that would benefit from adjuvant chemotherapy, even for stage IA disease, in contrast with those who might not benefit or be harmed by such treatment approaches. In advanced NSCLC, there exists the possibility that molecular subtypes of stage III or even stage IV disease might have appropriate biology to be candidates for aggressive multimodality approaches to treatment that are not currently widely used. These and other questions are important research priorities for treatment algorithms involving surgical resection and reflect the potential for genomic information to individualize and improve patient care for NSCLC.

THE MODERN CONCEPT OF INDIVIDUALIZED OR GENOMICS-DRIVEN TREATMENT OF NSCLC

The increasing recognition of clinically relevant heterogeneity in NSCLC is similar to the evolution of the understanding of the biology for many solid tumors. Several examples illustrate the power of a rational drug development process and the impact of targeted therapies in molecularly selected patients. The impressive improvements seen with imatinib in advanced gastrointestinal stromal tumors and trastuzumab in metastatic breast cancer have led to thoughtful development of these drugs not only in advanced-stage disease but also in early stage disease to improve cure rates. Postoperative trastuzumab improves overall survival by nearly 50% in patients with resected HER2-positive breast cancer.[20] Adjuvant imatinib after resection of gastrointestinal stromal tumors leads to significant improvement in disease-free survival.[21] Although it is worth remembering that to date, targeted therapies have not cured a single patient with NSCLC, clearly this is only the tip of the iceberg with respect to further developments and the potential to impact treatment and survival.

In simplest terms, the idea that some form of mutation testing would be performed in a "reflex" or automatic manner for all if not specific clinical subsets of NSCLC to direct therapy is rapidly approaching standard of care in many leading cancer centers throughout the world. Although many challenges remain, the case for incorporating genomics-driven cancer care into standard treatment protocols is compelling. How to do this in a way that improves clinical outcomes in a cost-effective manner is unclear at present.

EGFR MUTATIONS: A SUCCESS STORY FOR TARGETED THERAPY IN NSCLC

EGFR-directed therapy in NSCLC remains the poster child for targeted agents in lung cancer. The underlying biology and therapeutic potential was revealed through investigations on the variability in response rates of patients to gefitinib, a tyrosine kinase inhibitor (TKI) targeting EGFR. Exploring potential underlying molecular mechanisms, Lynch and colleagues[22] found mutations in the EGFR gene leading to enhanced tyrosine kinase activity in EGFR, which was associated with clinical responsiveness to gefitinib. In a similar approach, Paez and colleagues[23] investigated the potential significance of somatic genetic alterations in the EGF receptor by using samples of a mixed cohort consisting of Japanese and US patients. Through sequencing the activation domain from numerous tyrosine kinase receptors in the human genome in NSCLC tumor specimens, they discovered mutations in EGFR that seemed to correlate with response to gefitinib. Their results were similar to those reported by Lynch and colleagues.[22] Furthermore, the authors found remarkable differences in frequency of EGFR mutation between geographic groups corresponding to observed differences in treatment response. Data from many studies have now shown superior response rates to TKIs in patients who carry an EGFR mutation (approximately 70% response rate), compared with those with wild-type EGFR (10% response).[24] Rational screening for mutations of the EGFR gene can facilitate the identification of patients who will respond to a TKI.

TKIs, such as erlotinib and gefitinib, have been studied extensively in several large international clinical trials. The BR-21 study, a randomized, double-blind trial conducted by the National Cancer Institute of Canada Clinical Trials Group, compared erlotinib with placebo after failure of first-line, standard chemotherapy for NSCLC. Overall, 731 patients with advanced NSCLC (stage IIIB/IV) were enrolled. The trial reported significantly improved survival for patients treated with erlotinib when compared with placebo.[25,26] Direct evidence confirming these findings evolved from two subsequent randomized studies comparing first-line erlotinib with standard chemotherapy. The OPTIMAL trial was an open label, phase III study comparing first-line erlotinib versus carboplatin plus gemcitabine in Chinese patients with advanced/metastatic NSCLC with EGFR activating mutations. This was the first prospective randomized study that has demonstrated the efficacy of erlotinib as first-line treatment in this subgroup of patients. The Iressa Pan-Asia Study was the first and largest randomized phase III study that compared gefitinib with paclitaxel/carboplatin in an Asian nonsmoker or light smoker population with adenocarcinoma. Tumor samples were available from 437 patients for EGFR mutation analysis and 261 (60%) were positive. Tumor response rates for gefitinib and chemotherapy in the mutation-positive population were 71% and 47%, respectively, and progression-free survival was significantly prolonged to 9.8 months in the gefitinib group with hazard ratio of 0.48.[3,18] Further phase III studies have also been supportive of the benefit for EGFR–TKI over standard chemotherapy.[19–21]

EML4-ALK FUSIONS AND TARGETED THERAPY

In 2007, Soda and colleagues[27] described EML4-ALK fusions as a novel candidate biomarker and potential therapeutic target in NSCLC. The authors found that an inversion within chromosome 2p leads to the formation of a fusion gene comprising portions of the EML4 gene and the ALK gene. This ALK rearrangement is relatively rare, with a frequency ranging between 3% and 5%; it is more frequent in adenocarcinomas and typically in never-smokers or light smokers. The rearrangement seems to be mutually exclusive with EGFR or KRAS mutations.[27–30] Data suggest that patients who harbor this mutation do not benefit from treatment with EGFR-kinase inhibitors.[30]

Experimental data in human cell line and animal models subsequently showed that targeted therapeutic approaches might be feasible by ALK inhibition.[5,31] Soda and colleagues[31] showed a reduction of tumor burden in EML4/ALK transgenic mice treated with an ALK inhibitor compared with control animals. Phase I study data showed promising clinical activity of the ALK inhibitor PF02341066 in ALK-positive NSCLC.[11] Recently, a nonrandomized, open label, phase II study (Study NCT00932451) opened accrual to study safety and efficacy of PF-02341066 in patients with ALK-positive advanced NSCLC. Based on this trial, patients from a phase III trial who received standard of care chemotherapy (Study A8081007) will be treated with PF-02341066 to compare the oral ALK inhibitor PF-02341066 with standard of care chemotherapy in patients with ALK-positive advanced NSCLC progressing on platinum-based prior chemotherapy. Results from these trials in NSCLC are awaited.

THE COMING AVALANCHE OF TUMOR GENOME SEQUENCING DATA

Mutations identified to date have largely come from candidate gene sequencing studies, with relatively low coverage of the NSCLC tumor genome. A convergence of the ongoing rapid decrease in cost combined with increases in throughput for massively parallel sequencing technologies has set the stage for an exponential increase in the amount of detailed tumor sequencing data available. The case for NSCLC is no exception. Conservative estimates suggest more than 100 fully sequenced NSCLC cancer whole genomes, and more than 500 exomes, might be available by the end of 2013. One would expect several novel mutations to be described and an emerging view of what constitutes the core mutations present in human lung cancer. Further results from the National Cancer Institute–sponsored TCGA project in addition to other large-scale sequencing efforts for NSCLC will no doubt shed light on recurring mutations in NSCLC and relevant molecular subtypes. Although the genomic alterations being recently described represent smaller and more unique patient subsets, there will soon be a comprehensive view of the mutation spectrum in common forms of human lung cancer. How to best clinically apply this information is the next challenge.

HOW TUMOR GENOME SEQUENCING DATA MAY BE USED FOR PATIENT CARE: NEW STRATEGIES FOR CANCER DRUG TARGET DISCOVERY

Beyond the obvious potential for prognostic biomarker discovery by correlating genomic alterations with clinical outcomes, further opportunities exist in the process of drug and target discovery itself. Modern drug discovery for cancer remains frustratingly difficult. Creating drugs that selectively kill cancer cells without harming normal cells is problematic for several reasons. First, oncogenes that are overexpressed in cancer cells are usually identical to or mutated in ways that make them only subtly different from their normal counterparts. Therefore, the development of treatment specifically targeting oncogenes in tumors is difficult. Furthermore, the products of tumor-suppressor genes with low or absent activity in tumors because of mutation are elusive targets because it is hard to restore an absent activity pharmacologically.

Given these challenges, synthetic lethality has been suggested as an exciting new avenue to disrupt cancer cells for targeted treatment.[32] Two genes are said to be synthetic lethal if a mutation in either gene alone is not lethal, but mutations in both cause the death of the cell. In applying synthetic lethality to the discovery of cancer drugs, the goal is to identify a target gene that, when mutated or chemically inhibited, kills cells that harbor a specific cancer-related alteration, such as a mutated tumor-suppressor gene or an activated oncogene but spares otherwise identical cells lacking the cancer-related alteration. Such a gene would be a promising candidate for an anticancer drug target.

The recent description of the successful use of poly (adenosine diphosphate ribose) polymerase (PARP) inhibitors in breast cancer has validated this novel approach to cancer drug discovery. This concept was originally introduced in 2005 in two articles showing how synthetic lethality could be applied to cells that are deficient in a DNA-repair pathway. These reports built on the observation that loss of activity of the enzyme PARP1 in normal cells induces high levels of DNA damage repair through the homologous-recombination pathway. It was hypothesized that deficient homologous recombination would be lethal to a cell lacking PARP1. BRCA1 and BRCA2 are tumor-suppressor genes that underlie high-penetrance, hereditary breast and ovarian carcinomas. The corresponding proteins are key participants in homologous recombination. As predicted by the hypothesis, small-molecule inhibitors of PARP1 are toxic to cells deficient in BRCA1 or BRCA2, whereas cells in which BRCA1 or BRCA2 had been restored were less sensitive to the inhibitors by several orders of magnitude. The recent article by Fong and colleagues[33–35] demonstrated stabilization or regression of BRCA1- or BRCA2-defective breast, ovarian, and prostate cancers in response to an oral PARP inhibitor, without observed activity outside of BRCA1- or BRCA2-defective tumors.

The success of PARP1 inhibitors has fueled interest in the area of synthetic lethal screens in the context of mammalian systems, and indeed more candidates have largely focused on a limited number of candidate genes and typically produce one or a small number of synthetic lethal candidates. Ideally, one would extend these synthetic lethal genetic analyses to include a broader set of cancer-associated mutations and an unbiased set of candidate target mutations. Detailed sequencing data for NSCLC will only enhance the potential of this approach.

Further opportunities exist in the realm of effective combination therapies. Estimates suggest that the number of oncogenic drivers in an individual cancer may be up to five or six. Responses to single-agent targeted therapy are almost always transient until the development of chemoresistance sets in. It is unclear how many driver genes or nodes in a driver pathway must be targeted simultaneously to eradicate all malignant cells within a tumor.

The multiplicity of genetic aberrations and the presence of resistant cell clones is a longstanding explanation for the improved efficacy of combination therapy with more than one chemotherapeutic agent administered simultaneously. As suggested for the treatment of tuberculosis, treatment with three or more targeted agents may be required to achieve durable clinical responses and minimize the potential for chemoresistance. Although the potential permutations and combinations seem bewildering, the use of mutation data and cellular network analysis to guide the use of combinations that may be efficacious holds promise.

TECHNOLOGIES FOR MUTATION ANALYSIS IN NSCLC

Disruptive advances in DNA sequencing technologies over the past several years have dramatically altered what is feasible for clinical applications in molecular oncology. Although traditional Sanger sequencing is still considered the gold standard molecular diagnostic technology for identifying mutations, it has several limitations, including being insensitive to alterations that occur at an allele frequency lower than approximately 20% (a phenomenon that may reflect low tumor content in a specimen), limited clinical scalability beyond a few genes, and being unable to detect structural rearrangements or DNA copy number changes. Next-generation or massively parallel sequencing technologies have several advantages over conventional techniques. First, they provide an exponential decrease in the cost of sequencing. This economic disruption has effectively democratized the genome sequencing arena, rendering the technology available to individual laboratories and point-of-care testing. Second, the development of massively parallel sequencing has enabled significant increases in the sensitivity and scalability of sequencing, thus rendering an analysis of thousands of genes in a single sequencing lane. In 2013, it is possible to sequence more than 10 human genomes in a single day by using an Illumina HiSeq sequencer (Illumina Inc, San Diego, CA, USA). Third, these technologies provide the capability to detect multiple types of cancer genome alterations (base mutations, indels, copy number alterations, and rearrangements).

To leverage advantages in cost and throughput, many centers have advocated for the use of targeted mutation panels consisting of tens to hundreds of genes for analysis. This approach facilitates interrogation of genes likely to have therapeutic impact if altered, in a manner many fold more sensitive and specific than performing whole genome or whole exome sequencing. Recent advances have also adapted such approaches to paraffin-embedded tissue to eliminate the requirement of fresh frozen biopsies in volumes often requiring surgical biopsy. These assays will likely proliferate in the short term given the current cost and complexity of whole genome or whole exome sequencing. Many challenges remain, including standardization of analyses, reporting of results, regulatory oversight, and decision support tools for applying results to therapeutic choices. How best to provide adequate tissue for subsequent sequencing analysis also remains an evolving challenge. Current requirements for whole exome or whole genome sequencing typically involve using fresh frozen tissue in volumes only attainable through surgically resected specimens or excisional biopsies. Concerns regarding tumor heterogeneity, tumor nuclear content, and the allele frequency of specific mutations are not yet resolved.

INTELLIGENT CLINICAL TRIAL DESIGN IN THE GENOMIC ERA

Demonstrating the efficacy of targeted therapies that may only be effective in a subset of patients harboring a specific mutation within a tumor presents several unique challenges for clinical trial design. As an example, trastuzumab is only active in the setting of HER2-expressing breast cancer. In patients with HER2-positive tumors, the combination of trastuzumab with chemotherapy improved time-to-progression over chemotherapy alone with a hazard ratio of 0.51 (95% confidence interval, 0.41–0.63).[2] This study was done in a total of 469 patients with HER2-overexpressing disease, which comprises approximately 15% to 20% of all breast cancers. If this study had been performed in a population unselected for HER2 overexpression, and if one assumes that trastuzumab has no effect in patients whose tumors do not overexpress HER2, the effect in the targeted population would have been diluted, and an average hazard ratio close to 0.90 (as opposed to 0.51) would result for the primary outcome. To power such a trial at 90% would require at least 2500 patients for a small effect. In a situation in which HER2 expression and HER2 amplification were not known as predictive markers for trastuzumab, the drug would have been likely to fail in an unselected population. This example points to the importance of understanding the biologic mechanism and biomarkers of treatment response in smaller studies before large, phase III trials, and to the potential for specific subpopulations identified by a predictive or prognostic biomarker making up most true responders.

These examples create unique problems in the setting of studying adjuvant targeted therapy for lung adenocarcinoma. The frequency of EGFR mutation is only 10% to 15% in white populations, and ALK translocation less at approximately 5%. To address this issue, the concept of "master protocols" for mutation testing, under which individual smaller trials can be run in an iterative manner for patients harboring specific mutations, has been proposed. This concept of nested trials within a larger trial is one example of the requirement for innovative clinical trial design to accommodate appropriate matching of the right drug for the right tumor in the right patient.

WHAT DOES ALL THIS MEAN FOR SURGEONS CARING FOR PATIENTS WITH LUNG CANCER?

As early as 10 years ago, one of the most frequently cited papers in NSCLC concluded that four different chemotherapeutic regimens performed equally poorly in stage IV lung cancer, summarizing an era of therapeutic nihilism. It is now known that patients with EGFR-mutant lung adenocarcinoma have a mean survival of more than 2 years,[2,3] a dramatic improvement when compared with the 12 months of survival seen in these prior chemotherapy studies. The ALK/ROS inhibitor, crizotinib, induces regressions in lung tumors bearing ALK and ROS rearrangements, and many new therapeutic regimens are being explored in genetically defined lung adenocarcinomas.[9–14] In a short decade, lung cancer has emerged from such therapeutic nihilism to become the prototype for genomics-driven targeted cancer therapy.

Although at risk of being obsolete by the time this article is printed, existing algorithms for individualized targeted therapy in NSCLC look similar to the following:

1. Test whether there is presence of an EGFR mutation that would provide sensitivity to EGFR TKIs. If present, consider EGFR TKIs as a treatment option. Testing for activating KRAS mutations can be an inexpensive and efficient way to rule out the potential for EGFR mutations, because both are rarely present concurrently.
2. Test for EML4-ALK rearrangements. If present, consider crizotinib as a treatment option.
3. If neither are present, consider histology as part of the assessment for further treatment options, such as pemetrexed, bevacuzimab, or others as part of combination therapy with cisplatin or as maintenance therapy.

Although these algorithms are largely based on studies from advanced stage IV disease, adjuvant treatment of earlier stages is progressing rapidly and large adjuvant trials will soon be underway. The future for personalized treatment of NSCLC is bright, but surgeons have to stay knowledgeable to be active participants in integrated, multimodal approaches to lung cancer management. These care pathways will be ever more complicated, and it will be an ongoing struggle to keep up with the literature and with standard of care. That being said, incorporating genomics into clinical care is clearly a team sport, requiring input from molecular geneticists, bioinformaticians, pathologists, ethicists and genetic counselors, and others as an adjunct to the clinical team. There is a need for surgeons to stay engaged or risk relegation to the sidelines in treating these patients if they do not stay current and participate in the development of evolving care paradigms.

REFERENCES

1. Mountain CF. A new international staging system for lung cancer. Chest 1986;89(Suppl):225S–33S.
2. Goldstraw P, Crowley J, Chansky K, et al. The IASLC Lung Cancer Staging Project: proposals for the revision of the TNM stage groupings in the forthcoming (seventh) edition of the TNM Classification of malignant tumours. J Thorac Oncol 2007;2:706–14.
3. Albain KS, Swann RS, Rusch VW, et al. Radiotherapy plus chemotherapy with or without surgical resection for stage III non-small-cell lung cancer: a phase III randomised controlled trial. Lancet 2009; 1:379–86.
4. American Cancer Society. Cancer facts and figures 2010. Atlanta (GA): American Cancer Society; 2010.
5. McDermott U, Iafrate AJ, Gray NS, et al. Genomic alterations of anaplastic lymphoma kinase may sensitize tumors to anaplastic lymphoma kinase inhibitors. Cancer Res 2008;68:3389–95.
6. Ding L, Getz G, Wheeler DA, et al. Somatic mutations affect key pathways in lung adenocarcinoma. Nature 2008;455:1069–75.
7. Weir BA, Woo MS, Getz G, et al. Characterizing the cancer genome in lung adenocarcinoma. Nature 2007;450:893–8.
8. Eberhard DA, Johnson BE, Amler LC, et al. Mutations in the epidermal growth factor receptor and in KRAS are predictive and prognostic indicators in patients with non-small-cell lung cancer treated with chemotherapy alone and in combination with erlotinib. J Clin Oncol 2005;23:5900–9.
9. Hirsch FR, Varella-Garcia M, Bunn PA Jr, et al. Epidermal growth factor receptor in non-small-cell lung carcinomas: correlation between gene copy number and protein expression and impact on prognosis. J Clin Oncol 2003;21:3798–807.
10. Massarelli E, Varella-Garcia M, Tang X, et al. KRAS mutation is an important predictor of resistance to therapy with epidermal growth factor receptor tyrosine kinase inhibitors in non-small-cell lung cancer. Clin Cancer Res 2007;13:2890–6.

11. Kwak EL, Bang YJ, Camidge DR, et al. Anaplastic lymphoma kinase inhibition in non-small-cell lung cancer. N Engl J Med 2010;363:1693–703.
12. Johnson DH, Fehrenbacher L, Novotny WF, et al. Randomized phase II trial comparing bevacizumab plus carboplatin and paclitaxel with carboplatin and paclitaxel alone in previously untreated locally advanced or metastatic non-small-cell lung cancer. J Clin Oncol 2004;22:2184–91.
13. Scagliotti GV, Parikh P, von Pawel J, et al. Phase III study comparing cisplatin plus gemcitabine with cisplatin plus pemetrexed in chemotherapy-naive patients with advanced-stage non-small-cell lung cancer. J Clin Oncol 2008;26:3543–51.
14. Mok TS, Wu YL, Thongprasert S, et al. Gefitinib or carboplatin-paclitaxel in pulmonary adenocarcinoma. N Engl J Med 2009;361:947–57.
15. Blumenschein GR Jr, Gatzemeier U, Fossella F, et al. Phase II, multicenter, uncontrolled trial of single-agent sorafenib in patients with relapsed or refractory, advanced non-small cell lung cancer. J Clin Oncol 2009;27:4274–80.
16. Govindan R, Ding L, Griffith M, et al. Genomic landscape of non-small cell lung cancer in smokers and never-smokers. Cell 2012;150(6):1121–34.
17. Imielinski M, Berger AH, Hammerman PS, et al. Mapping the hallmarks of lung adenocarcinoma with massively parallel sequencing. Cell 2012; 150(6):1107–20.
18. Tomaszek SC, Huebner M, Wigle DA. Prospects for molecular staging of non-small-cell lung cancer from genomic alterations. Expert Rev Respir Med 2010;4: 499–508.
19. Subramanian J, Simon R. Gene expression-based prognostic signatures in lung cancer: ready for clinical use? J Natl Cancer Inst 2010;102:464–74.
20. Romond EH, Perez EA, Bryant J, et al. Trastuzumab plus adjuvant chemotherapy for operable HER2-positive breast cancer. N Engl J Med 2005;353: 1673–84.
21. Dematteo RP, Ballman KV, Antonescu CR, et al. Adjuvant imatinib mesylate after resection of localised, primary gastrointestinal stromal tumour: a randomised, double-blind, placebo-controlled trial. Lancet 2009;373:1097–104.
22. Lynch TJ, Bell DW, Sordella R, et al. Activating mutations in the epidermal growth factor receptor underlying responsiveness of non-small-cell lung cancer to gefitinib. N Engl J Med 2004;350:2129–39.
23. Paez JG, Jänne PA, Lee JC, et al. EGFR mutations in lung cancer: correlation with clinical response to gefitinib therapy. Science 2004;304:1497–500.
24. Mitsudomi T, Yatabe Y. Mutations of the epidermal growth factor receptor gene and related genes as determinants of epidermal growth factor receptor tyrosine kinase inhibitors sensitivity in lung cancer. Cancer Sci 2007;98:1817–24.
25. Shepherd FA, Rodrigues Pereira J, Ciuleanu T, et al. Erlotinib in previously treated non-small-cell lung cancer. N Engl J Med 2005;353:123–32.
26. Mitsudomi T, Morita S, Yatabe Y, et al. Gefitinib versus cisplatin plus docetaxel in patients with non-small-cell lung cancer harbouring mutations of the epidermal growth factor receptor (WJTOG3405): an open label randomised phase 3 trial. Lancet Oncol 2010;11:121–8.
27. Soda M, Choi YL, Enomoto M, et al. Identification of the transforming EML4-ALK fusion gene in non-small cell lung cancer. Nature 2007;448:561–6.
28. Choi YL, Takeuchi K, Soda M, et al. Identification of novel isoforms of the EML4-ALK transforming gene in non-small cell lung cancer. Cancer Res 2008;68: 4971–6.
29. Koivunen JP, Mermel C, Zejnullahu K, et al. EML4-ALK fusion gene and efficacy of an ALK kinase inhibitor in lung cancer. Clin Cancer Res 2008;14: 4275–83.
30. Shaw AT, Yeap BY, Mino-Kenudson M, et al. Clinical features and outcome of patients with non-small-cell lung cancer who harbor EML4-ALK. J Clin Oncol 2009;27:4247–53.
31. Soda M, Takada S, Takeuchi K, et al. A mouse model for EML4-ALK-positive lung cancer. Proc Natl Acad Sci U S A 2008;105:19893–7.
32. Hartwell LH, Szankasi P, Roberts CJ, et al. Integrating genetic approaches into the discovery of anticancer drugs. Science 1997;278:1064–8.
33. Fong PC, Boss DS, Yap TA, et al. Inhibition of poly(ADP-ribose) polymerase in tumors from BRCA mutation carriers. N Engl J Med 2009;361:123–34.
34. Luo J, Emanuele MJ, Li D, et al. A genome-wide RNAi screen identifies multiple synthetic lethal interactions with the Ras oncogene. Cell 2009;137: 835–48.
35. Scholl C, Frohling S, Dunn IF, et al. Synthetic lethal interaction between oncogenic KRAS dependency and STK33 suppression in human cancer cells. Cell 2009;137:821–34.

Follow-up After Surgery and Palliative Care

What is the Most Practical, Optimal, and Cost Effective Method for Performing Follow-up After Lung Cancer Surgery, and by Whom Should It be Done?

Lise Tremblay, MD, FRCPC[a,*], Jean Deslauriers, MD, FRCS(C)[b]

KEYWORDS

• Follow-up • Lung cancer • Surgery • Imaging modality • Guidelines

KEY POINTS

- Most current recommendations suggest that clinical and radiological follow-up should be done in patients who have had previous surgery for lung cancer.
- Follow-up should be more intensive during the first 2 postoperative years.
- The thoracic surgeon or the family physician may do the long-term follow-up.
- There is little evidence supporting the use of structured postoperative monitoring programs to improve survival.

INTRODUCTION

Lung cancer is among the most commonly diagnosed malignant neoplasms and is currently the leading cause of cancer deaths worldwide.[1] Unfortunately, only 20% of new cases will present with localized disease amenable to surgical resection,[2] and of these cases, approximately 60% will eventually relapse either locally or at distant sites. By themselves, these figures should justify the organization of structured follow-up clinics aimed at improving overall and disease-free survival through early detection and treatment of recurrences and second primaries. However, there are no available validated follow-up programs, and each physician or institution basically establishes his or her own follow-up protocol[3] based on his or her experience, costs, and availability of human and physical resources.

This article reviews the literature with regards to the usefulness of follow-up clinics to monitor patients with resected lung cancer either for the detection of late postoperative events or for early diagnosis of recurrences and second primaries.

DIAGNOSIS OF TREATMENT-RELATED COMPLICATIONS

One of the important objectives of follow-up programs is to give the surgeon an opportunity to diagnose and manage late complications that may arise after pulmonary resection. These

Disclosure: The authors declare no conflicts of interest.
[a] Multidisciplinary Department of Pulmonology and Thoracic Surgery, Institut universitaire de cardiologie et de pneumologie de Québec (IUCPQ), 2725 chemin Sainte-Foy, L-3540, Quebec City, Quebec G1V 4G5, Canada; [b] Division of Thoracic Surgery, Institut universitaire de cardiologie et de pneumologie de Québec (IUCPQ), 2725 chemin Sainte-Foy, L-3540, Quebec City, Quebec G1V 4G5, Canada
* Corresponding author.
E-mail address: lise.tremblay@cricupq.ulaval.ca

Thorac Surg Clin 23 (2013) 429–436
http://dx.doi.org/10.1016/j.thorsurg.2013.05.010

complications, which can occur as late as 1 year postoperatively, are usually cardiopulmonary or infectious in nature (empyemas with or without bronchopleural fistula). In an interesting paper, Handy and colleagues[4] reported that close to 20% of patients discharged after pulmonary resection had to be readmitted within 90 days, mostly for pulmonary problems, postsurgical infections, or cardiac complications. Other uncommon but sometimes significant problems that can present late after pulmonary resection include postlobectomy infected spaces, postpneumonectomy syndromes,[5] where the main bronchus to the remaining lung is compressed between the aorta, the pulmonary artery, and the spine, and the platypnea–orthodeoxia syndrome, which relates to a right-to-left intra-atrial shunt through the reopening of a patent foramen ovale.

A loss of lung function, generally proportional to the amount of parenchyma that has been resected, is also expected to occur postoperatively (**Table 1**).[6] This functional loss reaches its peak 6 months after surgery, but patients often return to their preoperative status within a year of the operation, especially if they have stopped smoking. In an interesting study, Korst and colleagues[7] from the Memorial Sloan-Kettering Cancer Center in New York, have shown that patients with a very low preoperative forced expiratory volume in 1 second (FEV_1) were less likely to lose ventilatory function after lobectomy and that they may actually improve on it. According to the authors, such gain in function is probably related to the relief of hyperinflation with improvement of elastic recoil in the residual lung. In another study of 100 patients evaluated 5 or more years after pneumonectomy done for lung cancer,[8] the loss of expiratory lung volumes (FEV_1, forced vital capacity [FVC]) was in the range of 15% to 30% (**Table 2**), with a proportionally greater loss after right pneumonectomy than after left pneumonectomy. That study also showed that more compensatory hyperinflation of the remaining lung correlated with better FEV_1, (P<.01) and thus had a beneficial effect on postoperative lung function. Follow-up in a well-organized clinic with availability of physiotherapists, rehabilitation experts, and consultants in pulmonary medicine is the ideal place to monitor loss of pulmonary function and manage it when necessary.

Table 1
Approximate loss of lung function after pulmonary resection

	Type of Resection	
Parameter	**Lobectomy**	**Pneumonectomy**
FEV_1	10%–15%	25%–30%
Exercise tolerance	10%	20%

The true incidence of post-thoracotomy pain syndrome (PTPS), defined by the International Association for the Study of Pain as pain that recurs or persists along a thoracotomy incision for at least 2 months after the surgical procedure,[9] is difficult to state, as widely varying rates have been reported. In the authors' experience, less than 5% of patients will have chronic PTPS lasting for more than 2 years for which no singularly effective therapy can be successful. This incidence may currently be even lower, because modern techniques of pre-emptive analgesia abolish the neurochemical cascade that leads to chronic pain.[10,11]

To improve locoregional control as well as survival, strategies of multimodality therapies have become standard of care for patients undergoing pulmonary resection for lung cancer. Unfortunately, toxicities are often associated with such multimodality regimens, especially when chemotherapy is administered either preoperatively (induction therapy) or more commonly postoperatively (adjuvant therapy). Peripheral neuropathies, for instance, are a common chemotherapy-related toxicity usually associated with the use of platinum salts and vincristine alkaloids.[12] Although there is no effective treatment for this condition, most patients will improve over time, although recovery may be incomplete.

DIAGNOSIS OF CANCER RECURRENCES AND SECOND PRIMARIES

Terminology

The currently used terminology defining recurrences and second primaries is based on the recommendations made by Martini 40 years ago.[13] Unfortunately, Martini's definitions are difficult to apply to the ever-increasing multifocal synchronous or metachronous malignant lung nodules that are currently being seen. Essentially, Martini stated that the diagnosis of a second primary was most convincing if it occurred 2 or more years after the original resection, if it was located in the contralateral lung, and if it was of a different histology than that of the primary tumor. Arguments in favor of a recurrence (local or regional) were that if the new lesion occurred within 2 years of the initial operation, if it was located in the same lobe or lung, and if it had the same histology as the primary. A suggested easily applicable terminology for the definitions of synchronous and metachronous lung cancer is shown in **Box 1**.

Table 2
Effect of pneumonectomy on expiratory lung volumes and diffusing capacity

	Preoperative	Postoperative	Relative Change
FEV_1 (L)	2.47 ± 0.65	1.46 ± 0.39	
FEV_1 (% predicted)	86 ± 18	58 ± 16	−30 ± −22
FVC (L)	3.48 ± 0.99	2.28 ± 0.66	
FVC (% predicted)	86 ± 19	71 ± 20	−14 ± 30
DLCO (ML/mm Hg/min)	21 ± 6	14 ± 4	
DLCO (% predicted)	87 ± 20	58 ± 12	−33 ± 18

Abbreviations: DLCO, diffusing capacity for carbon monoxide; FEV_1, forced expiratory volume in 1 second; FVC, forced vital capacity.

Data from Deslauriers J, Ugalde P, Miro S, et al. Long-term physiologic consequences of pneumonectomy. Semin Thorac Cardiovasc Surg 2011;23:196–202.

A local recurrence is usually defined as tumor occurring at the resection margins, while a regional recurrence is defined as a recurrence occurring anywhere in the ipsilateral hemithorax, including the mediastinum and, for most people, the ipsilateral cervical lymph nodes. Distant recurrences occur in extrathoracic sites.

Box 1
Suggested terminology for the definition of synchronous or metachronous lung cancer

Synchronous lung cancer

Concurrent, separate tumors of different histologies

Concurrent, separate tumors of same histologies if:

- Arise in different location (lobe/lung)
- Origin from carcinoma in situ can be demonstrated
- No tumor in lymphatics common to both tumors
- No evidence of extrapulmonary metastases

Metachronous lung cancer

Nonconcurrent, separate tumors of different histologies

Nonconcurrent, separate tumors of same histologies if:

- Arise in different location (lobe/lung)
- Free interval greater than 2 years
- Origin from carcinoma in situ can be demonstrated
- No tumor in lymphatics common to both tumors
- No evidence of extrathoracic metastases

Although it is generally agreed that most recurrences (local or distant) will develop within 2 years of surgery, they can also happen several years later. In a recent study of 1294 consecutive patients with completely resected early-stage non-small cell lung cancer who were followed with CT, Lou and colleagues[14] showed that the risk of recurrence persisted during the first 4 years after resection before it began to decline. Unfortunately, most recurrences occur at distant sites where curative treatment is no longer possible.[15] Even local recurrences have an ominous prognosis, because most are unresectable.[16]

The incidence of second primary lung cancer is estimated to be 1% to 4% per patient per year, and this risk remains the same for up to 20 years after surgery, especially in patients who do not quit smoking. Smokers are also at high risk of developing second primaries in the otolaryngologic sphere or in the upper digestive tract.[17]

Frequency of Follow-up and Who Should do It

The first postoperative visit should be within 1 month of hospital discharge, the main purpose being to diagnose complications that may have arisen after the patient has left the hospital. After that, there are no clear guidelines as to what should be the frequency of follow-up visits, although the National Comprehensive Cancer Network recommends monitoring, including a history and physical examination every 4 months for the first 2 years and every 6 months thereafter.[18]

The discrepancies in conclusions among some of the published series (**Table 3**)[19–22] illustrate not only the problem of bias in the selection of patients included in the study (most studies are retrospective) and calculation of results, but also that of the nonstandardized terminologies used to define recurrences or second primaries. A meta analysis

Table 3
Results of follow-up programs for patients with completely resected NSCLC

Author (Country, Reference)	Study Design (Number of Patients)	% Recurrences Over Time	Conclusion
Westeel et al (France[19])	Prospective (N = 192)	71%	Intensive follow-up feasible May improve survival
Walsh et al (United States[20])	Retrospective (N = 358)	38%	Frequent follow-up probably unnecessary
Younes et al (Brazil[21])	Retrospective (N = 130)	25%	Routine imaging follow-up of questionable value
Gilbert et al (Canada[22])	Retrospective (N = 245)	45%	Follow-up can be done by family physician

and systematic review of survival benefits from the follow-up of patients with previously resected lung cancer done by Calman and colleagues[23] in 2011 showed no clear-cut benefit to intensive follow-up in 1669 patients with regards to survival (hazard ratio: 0.83; P = .13; confidence interval: 0.66–1.05). One possible explanation for these findings is that, when compared with other neoplasms, the period of time when a lung cancer recurrence remains asymptomatic is usually much shorter.

Although it is well recognized that the surgeon should do the follow-up for the first several months after surgery, it is less clear as who should do it over the long term. In 2002, Moore and colleagues[24] reported the results of a prospective study comparing follow-up done by a nurse practitioner versus regular medical follow-up, and they noted that progression of disease based on symptoms was often discovered earlier by nurses. In another study, Gilbert and colleagues[22] showed that long-term follow-up after resection of limited-stage nonsmall cell lung cancer could possibly be done by family doctors without compromising survival, and with significant cost savings. A study reported by thoracic surgeons from St. Louis[25] highlighted their motivation to carry out follow-ups by themselves. They felt that patients were more satisfied with this approach that also allowed them to maintain standards of good practice and positively impact on patients' quality of life.

From the patient's perspective, regular follow-ups are appreciated,[26] but they prefer that they be done in a hospital setting by specialists. Surveillance by phone or by family doctors is less popular. Follow-ups done through TeleHealth Systems are becoming more and more popular, because they are associated with lower costs. They also improve patient satisfaction, because patients no longer have to travel back and forth to the treatment center.

One other advantage of systematic follow-up within a structured program is that the system will be able to detect patients who are missing their prearranged visit. In such cases, a phone call is automatically made to inquire as to why the patient was unable to attend the clinic and the patient will be rescheduled.

Last but not least, the costs associated with structured follow-up programs are not negligible, and in one study,[27] it was estimated that intensive follow-ups with CT had a net cost of $47,676.00 per quality-adjusted life-year gained, suggesting, according to the authors, cost-effectiveness.

Follow-up Guidelines

Although cancer agencies are not unanimous with regards to follow-up guidelines and intensity of monitoring programs (**Table 4**),[28–31] all agree that patients should have a careful clinical history, a limited regional physical examination, and a standard chest radiograph at regular intervals. Signs and symptoms suggesting local recurrences or second primaries are listed in **Box 2**, and among them, hemoptysis, weight loss, and fatigue are perhaps the most important.

Radiographic signs suggesting recurrences (**Box 3**) include the demonstration of new densities or the presence of a pleural effusion not present before. In many cases, serial comparison of chest films will detect subtle changes that may not otherwise be obvious. This is the case, for instance, of hemoclips that have been used during the operation and have become distracted or displaced over time by local recurrent disease. Other tests often done at follow-up visits include liver function studies and hematological blood work.

The value of specific screening studies such as sputum cytology, bronchoscopy, and CT for follow-up is still unknown, although most agencies recommend follow-up CT at least annually. The

Table 4
Summary of recommendations by lung cancer agencies with regards to follow-up after curative resection of primary lung cancer

Agency (Year, Reference)	Year 1–2	Year 3–5	Long-Term	Other Recommendations
ACCC (2000[28])	Every 3 m: CH, PE, chest radiograph	Every 6 m: CH, PE, chest radiograph	Every 12 m: CH, PE, chest radiograph	
ACCP (2007[29])	Every 6 m: CH, PE, chest radiograph	Every 12 m: CH, EP, CT	Same as year 3–5	
ESMO (2010[30])	Every 6 m: CH, PE, chest radiograph	Every 12 m: CH, PE, CT	Same as year 3–5	Smoking cessation Patients to be warned about symptoms of recurrence
NCCN (2013[31])	Every 6–12 m: CH, PE, CCT	Every 12 m: CH, PE, CCT	Same as year 3–5	Smoking cessation

Abbreviations: ACCC, Association of Community Cancer Centers; ACCP, American College of Chest Physicians; CCT, contrast computed tomography; CH, clinical history; CT, computed tomography; ESMO, European Society for Medical Oncology; NCCN, National Comprehensive Cancer Network; PE, physical examination.

main criticism of screening CT is that it is unable to discriminate benign from malignant nodules and that this inability is magnified in postoperative patients, in whom inflammatory and fibrotic changes and anatomic distortion are always present. The identification of more and more patients with metachronous multifocal lung cancers, mostly of the adenocarcinoma type, is, however, likely to make CT an important imaging modality to be done at regular intervals in patients involved in structured follow-up programs.

Although there are no reports of systematic surveillance of lung cancer resection patients by sputum cytology, large studies of unresected but high-risk patients have shown that early diagnosis by cytology screening is not beneficial in terms of decreasing the number of cancer-related deaths.[32] These techniques may also have some potential to be harmful through false-positive cytologic reports (0%–1%/year) and chances of incorrect cancer diagnosis (0%–1%/y).[33,34] Similarly, biomarkers for lung cancer (immunostaining of sputum cytology specimens) are not specific (a positive result means that the patient has lung cancer) or sensitive (a negative test result means that the patient has no tumor) enough to justify their routine use. Newly discovered biomarkers[35,36] may, however, be more effective for early detection of lung cancer, but their role in the context of follow-up programs needs to be further evaluated. Screening patients by flexible bronchoscopy has enormous disadvantages in terms of costs as well as human and physical resources, while the role of autofluorescence bronchoscopy has yet to be determined.[37]

Given the relatively common occurrence of brain metastasis during the follow-up period, one could question the use of brain CT on a regular basis at least during the first 2 to 3 postoperative years. In an interesting study done in Japan, Yokoi and colleagues[38] looked at the value of intensive

Box 2
Signs and symptoms suggesting a locoregional recurrence or a new primary

Clinical symptoms

Hemoptysis or changes in cough habits

Chest pain not present before

Hoarseness not present space

Weight loss, fatigue, anorexia

Physical signs

Palpable cervical nodes

Superior vena cava obstruction

Box 3
Radiographic signs suggesting a locoregional recurrence or a new primary

New pulmonary lesion or atelectasis

New pleural effusion

Widening of mediastinum

Displacement of hemoclips that had been in stable position before

Further elevation of hemidiaphragm

follow-up with brain CT in 128 patients who had resected lung cancer. In that cohort, brain CT was done regularly during the first 2 postoperative years, and it allowed for the detection of 7 patients with asymptomatic brain metastases, 3 of whom had access to curative treatment. These results are interesting given the important advances that have occurred over the past 10 or 15 years in the management of brain metastases.

Positron emission tomography (PET) is now indispensable in the investigation of lung cancer patients, and it may soon become invaluable in follow-up programs, especially for patients at high risk of recurrence. The main advantage of PET over CT scanning is that it allows for distinguishing between recurrent cancers and surgical scars or anatomic postoperative distortion. Unfortunately, costs and accessibility of PET scanners are issues that have not yet been addressed. Despite these problems, sensitivity of PET is estimated to be of 96%, with a specificity of 84% and negative predictive value of 99%[39] in suspected recurrences of surgically treated nonsmall cell lung cancer. In a prospective study done on 241 patients who had undergone potentially curative surgery for NSCLC in Japan,[40] PET scanning helped to correctly identify 34 of 35 recurrences.

It is finally well documented that smoking cessation is associated with reduced smoking-related second primaries,[41] and pharmacologic help and behavior therapies should be offered to all patients who have had pulmonary resection for lung cancer. In the authors' experience, approximately 90% of individuals who were smokers before surgery will stop after the operation.

ADVANTAGES OF CANCER SURVEILLANCE PROGRAMS

Approximately 60% of patients with completely resected lung cancers will recur within 5 years of surgery, and patients who survive 5 years also have a 6% to 10% chance of developing a second primary. For those individuals, early detection of disease may translate into earlier initiation of therapy and improvement in outcomes such as survival. Similarly, patients with early discovered solitary sites of distant metastasis, such as those in the brain, the contralateral lung, or the adrenal, are more likely to benefit from multimodality therapies including surgical resection.

For patients, secondary benefits include easier accessibility to specialized services, such as antismoking clinics and rehabilitation programs that may not otherwise be accessible. If necessary, patients can be seen rapidly by other medical specialists such as oncologists, chest physicians, and palliative care physicians. Patients may finally benefit psychologically from a closer relationship with their surgeon and oncological nurses. All of those benefits are difficult to measure scientifically and accurately, but they are often important to the patient and his or her relatives.

For the surgeon, a potential benefit is the possibility of evaluating the advantages and disadvantages of specific operative procedures and their long-term results. Indeed, any surgeon who simply performs pulmonary resections and never follows patients cannot learn from his or her successes and most importantly from his or her errors. Another important aspect of postresection follow-up is that it provides the surgeon with opportunities to teach the house staff, including residents and nurses, about disease processes, operations, complications, and results.

SUMMARY

The validation of surveillance programs for patients with prior pulmonary resection for lung cancer is an extremely important issue, but unfortunately, the current literature does not provide recommendations based on science. Additionally, there is still much controversy with regards to frequency of follow-ups and who should do them. Taking into account these limitations, most people agree that follow-up is important and that it should be more intense during the first 2 postoperative years. Although the choice of imaging studies that should be done is still undetermined, CT seems better than standard radiographs, and a French study is currently underway comparing minimal follow-up programs to ones that include a chest CT.[42]

REFERENCES

1. Jemal A, Siegal R, Xu J, et al. Cancer statistics, 2010. CA Cancer J Clin 2012;60:277–300.
2. Mountain CF. Revisions in the international system for staging lung cancer. Chest 1997;111:1710–7.
3. Sawada S, Suehisa H, Yamashita M, et al. Current status of postoperative follow-up for lung cancer in Japan: questionnaire survey by the Setouchi Lung Cancer Study Group-A09101. Gen Thorac Cardiovasc Surg 2012;60:104–11.
4. Handy JR, Child AI, Grunkemeier GL, et al. Hospital readmission after pulmonary resection: prevalence, patterns, and predisposing characteristics. Ann Thorac Surg 2001;72:1855–60.
5. Grillo HC, Shepard J, Mathisen DJ, et al. Postpneumonectomy syndrome: diagnosis, management, and results. Ann Thorac Surg 1992;54:638–51.

6. Nezu K, Kushibe K, Tojo T, et al. Recovery and limitations of exercise capacity after lung resection for lung cancer. Chest 1998;113:1511–6.
7. Korst RJ, Ginsberg RJ, Ailawadi M, et al. Lobectomy improves ventilatory function in selected patients when severe COPD. Ann Thorac Surg 1998;66: 898–902.
8. Deslauriers J, Ugalde P, Miro S, et al. Long-term physiologic consequences of pneumonectomy. Semin Thorac Cardiovasc Surg 2011;23:196–202.
9. Merskey H. Classification of chronic pain: description of chronic pain syndrome and definition of pain terms. Pain 1986;3:S138–9.
10. Katz J, Jackson M, Kavanagh B, et al. Acute pain after thoracic surgery predicts long-term post-thoracotomy pain. Clin J Pain 1996;12:50–5.
11. Katz J, Calrke H, Seltzer Z. Preventive analgesia: quo vadimus. Anesth Analg 2011;113:1242–53.
12. Siegal T, Haim N. Cisplatin-induced peripheral neuropathy. Frequent off-therapy deterioration, demyelinating syndromes, and muscles cramps. Cancer 1990;66:1117–23.
13. Martini N, Melamed MR. Multiple primary cancers. J Thorac Cardiovasc Surg 1975;70:606–11.
14. Lou F, Huang J, Sima CS, et al. Patterns of recurrence and second primary lung cancer in early-stage lung cancer survivors followed with routine computed tomography surveillance. J Thorac Cardiovasc Surg 2013;145:75–82.
15. Douillard JY, Rosell R, De Lena M, et al. Adjuvant vinorelbine plus cisplatin versus observation in patients with completely resected stage IB-IIIA non-small-cell lung cancer (Adjuvant Navelbine International Trialist Association [ANITA]): a randomized controlled trial. Lancet Oncol 2006;7:719–27.
16. Lamont JP, Kakuda JT, Smith D, et al. Systematic postoperative radiologic follow-up in patients with non-small cell lung cancer for detecting second primary lung cancer in stage IA. Arch Surg 2002;137: 935–9.
17. Levi F, Randimbison L, Te VC, et al. Second primary cancers in patients with lung carcinoma. Cancer 1999;86:186–90.
18. Colice GL, Rubins J, Unger M. Follow-up and surveillance of the lung cancer patient following curative-intent therapy. Chest 2003;123:272S–83S.
19. Westeel V, Choma D, Clément F, et al. Relevance of an intensive postoperative follow-up after surgery of non-small cell lung cancer. Ann Thorac Surg 2000; 70:1185–90.
20. Walsh GL, O'Connor M, Willis KM, et al. Is follow-up of lung cancer patients after resection medically indicated and cost-effective? Ann Thorac Surg 1995;60:1563–72.
21. Younes RN, Gross JL, Deheinzelin D. Follow-up in lung cancer. How often and for what purpose? Chest 1999;115:1494–9.
22. Gilbert S, Reid KR, Lam MY, et al. Who should follow-up lung cancer patients after operation? Ann Thorac Surg 2000;69:1696–700.
23. Calman L, Beaver K, Hind D, et al. Survival benefits from follow-up of patients with lung cancer. A systematic review and meta-analysis. J Thorac Oncol 2011;6:1993–2004.
24. Moore S, Corner J, Haviland J, et al. Nurse led follow-up and conventional medical follow-up in management of patients with lung cancer: randomized trial. BMJ 2002;325:1145–52.
25. Virgo KS, Naunheim KS, Coplin MA, et al. Lung cancer patient follow-up. Motivation of thoracic surgeons. Chest 1998;114:1519–34.
26. Cox K, Wilson E, Heath L, et al. Preferences for follow-up treatment for lung cancer. Assessing the nurse-led option. Cancer Nurs 2006;29:176–87.
27. Kent MS, Korn P, Port JL, et al. Cost effectiveness of chest computed tomography after lung cancer resection: a decision analysis model. Ann Thorac Surg 2005;80:1215–23.
28. Association of Community Cancer Centers. Oncology management guidelines, version 3.0. Rockville (MD): Association of Community Cancer Centers; 2000.
29. Rubins J, Unger M, Colice GL. Follow-up and surveillance of the lung cancer patient following curative intent therapy. ACCP evidence-based clinical practice guideline (2nd edition). Chest 2007;132: 355S–67S.
30. Crino L, Weder W, van Meerbeeck J, et al. Early stage and locally advanced (non-metastatic) non-small-cell lung cancer: ESMO clinical practice guidelines for diagnosis, treatment and follow-up. Ann Oncol 2010;21(Suppl 5):v103–15.
31. Ettinger DS, Akerley W, Borghaei H, et al. NCCN clinical practice guidelines in oncology (NCCN guidelines): non-small cell lung cancer 2013. Version 1. 2013. Available at: http://www.nccn.org/professionals/physician_gls/pdf/nsclc.pdf. Accessed January 6, 2013.
32. Fontana RS, Sanderson DR, Woolner LB, et al. Lung cancer screening: the Mayo program. J Occup Med 1986;28:746–50.
33. Deslauriers J. Should screening for lung cancer be revisited? J Thorac Cardiovasc Surg 2001;121: 1031–2.
34. Eddy DM. Screening for lung cancer. Ann Intern Med 1989;111:232–7.
35. Varella-Garcia M, Schulte AP, Wolf HJ, et al. Chromosomal aneusomy in sputum, as detected by fluorescence in situ hybridization (FISH) predicts lung cancer incidence. Cancer Prev Res 2010;3: 447–53.
36. Carpagnano GE, Palladino GP, Gramiccioni C, et al. New bimolecular methodologies in diagnosis of lung cancer. Recenti Prog Med 2008;99:417–21.

37. Weigel TL, Kosco PJ, Dacic S, et al. Postoperative fluorescence bronchoscopic surveillance in non-small cell lung cancer patients. Ann Thorac Surg 2001;71:967–70.
38. Yokoi K, Miyazawa N, Arai T. Brain metastasis in resected lung cancer: value of intensive follow-up with computed tomography. Ann Thorac Surg 1996;61: 546–51.
39. Hellwig D, Groschel A, Graeter TP, et al. Diagnostic performance and prognostic impact of FDG-PET in suspected recurrence of surgically treated non-small cell lung cancer. Eur J Nucl Med Mol Imaging 2006;33:13–21.
40. Kanzaki R, Higashiyama M, Maeda J, et al. Clinical value of F18-fluorodeoxyglucose positron emission tomography-computed tomography in patients with non-small cell lung cancer after potentially curative surgery: experience with 241 patients. Interact Cardiovasc Thorac Surg 2010; 10:1009–14.
41. Richardson GE, Tucker MA, Venzon DJ, et al. Smoking cessation after successful treatment of small cell lung cancer is associated with fewer smoking-related second primary cancers. Ann Intern Med 1993;119:383–90.
42. Westeel V, Lebitasy MP, Mercier M, et al. Protocole IFCT-0302: Essai randomise de deux schémas de surveillance dans les cancers bronchiques non à petites cellules complètement réséqués. Rev Mal Respir 2007;24:645–52.

Quality of Life After Pulmonary Resections

Robert J. Cerfolio, MD*, Ayesha S. Bryant, MD, MSPH

KEYWORDS

• Quality of life (QOL) • Pulmonary resection • Morbidity

KEY POINTS

- One of the limitations of the assessment of the quality of life (QOL) is that the topic is inherently subjective.
- Pneumonectomy leads to a worse QOL than lobectomy, and older patients do worse than younger patients.
- Preoperative QOL is an important predictor of postoperative QOL.
- The QOL of patients after all types of medical treatment should continue to be assessed more frequently by patients before surgery.

DATA

Table 1 summarizes recent studies that have evaluated quality of life (QOL) after pulmonary resection.[1,2] QOL is a subjective measure and thus inherent to bias and confounders. It has been evaluated in several studies; however, the instruments, methodology, and metrics used for analysis vary. Attempts to use predictors of operative morbidity (eg, pulmonary function tests, age, comorbidities) have been shown to have poor correlation with QOL.[3,4] For example, Brunelli and colleagues in 2007[5] showed there was little correlation between QOL measurements and the physiologic tests and QOL. Brunelli administered pulmonary function tests (forced expiratory volume in 1 second [FEV_1], carbon monoxide lung diffusion capacity [DLCO]), exercise test, along with QOL assessments (Short Form-36 [SF-36] survey) to 156 patients who underwent pulmonary resection at 1 and 3 months after resection (12 patients had a pneumonectomy and the rest underwent a lobectomy). In addition, he found that the functional variables did not correlate with QOL.

Some investigators have proposed algorithms instead of physiologic data to objectify and predict QOL better after pulmonary resection. For example, Pompili and coworkers[6] performed a prospective observational study on 172 consecutive patients who underwent a lobectomy or pneumonectomy to identify predictors of clinically relevant decline of physical and emotional components of QOL following lung resection. QOL was assessed using SF-36 survey preoperatively and 3 months postoperatively. The authors found 48 patients (28%) had a large decline in the physical component scores (PCS) and 26 (15%) patients had a decline in the mental component scores (MCS). Patients with a better preoperative physical functioning ($P = .0008$) and bodily pain ($P = .048$) scores and those with worse mental health ($P = .0007$) scores were those at higher risk of a relevant physical deterioration. Patients with a lower predicted postoperative forced expiratory volume in 1 second ($ppoFEV_1$; $P = .04$), higher preoperative scores of social functioning ($P = .02$), and mental health ($P = .06$) were those at higher risk of a relevant emotional deterioration. They found

Disclosure: The principle investigator of this study (Robert Cerfolio) has lectured for Intuitive (Sunnyvale, CA).
Division of Cardiothoracic Surgery, University of Alabama at Birmingham, 703 19th Street South, ZRB 739, Birmingham, AL 35294, USA
* Corresponding author.
E-mail address: rcerfolio@uab.edu

Thorac Surg Clin 23 (2013) 437–442
http://dx.doi.org/10.1016/j.thorsurg.2013.05.004
1547-4127/13/$ – see front matter

Table 1
Recent studies evaluating QOL following pulmonary resection

Author	No. of Patients	Cohorts Studied	Tool Used to Assess QOL	Frequency of Survey	Results
Balduyck,[17] 2007	100	Lobectomy, pneumonectomy	EORTC Q-30, LC13	Preoperative, postoperative 1, 3, 6, 12 mo	Both resections associated with an initial decreased QOL in first month postoperatively. Lobectomy patients reported better physical scores and less pain than patients who had pneumonectomy.
Brunelli et al,[5] 2007	156	Lobectomy, pneumonectomy	SF-36, physiologic variables	Preoperative, postoperative 1, 3 mo	Physical component score decreased temporarily 1 mo postoperatively; recovered at 3 mo. Mental QOL score was unaffected. There was no correlation with functional physiologic variables.
Burfeind, 2008	422	Lobectomy (stratified by age, >70 y)	EORTC QLQ-C30, LC-13	Preoperative, postoperative 3, 6 and 12 mo	No significant differences in QOL in older and younger patients. Patients showed a decrease in overall QOL 3 mo postoperatively, but returned to baseline at 6 and 12 mo
Kenny et al,[14] 2008	173	Lobectomy			
Schulte et al,[15] 2009	131	Lobectomy, bilobectomy (stratified by age)		Preoperative, up to 2 y postoperative	Younger patients returned to preoperative QOL faster than elderly patients.
Pompili et al,[16] 2010	252	Lobectomy	SF-36	Preoperative, postoperative 3 mo	Evaluated QOL in patients with COPD. There were no significant differences in physical or mental OQL scores in this cohort.
Leo et al,[10] 2010	41	Pneumonectomy	EORTC QLQ-C30 and LC13	Preoperative, postoperative 1, 3, 5 mo	QOL was impaired in 25% of patients at 6 mo postoperatively. Postoperative QOL was presected by baseline global health scores.
Deslauriers et al,[8] 2011	100	Pneumonectomy	No QOL survey		Most patients were able to adjust to living a "near-normal life" following pneumonectomy
Cerfolio, 2012	111	Pneumonectomy		Postoperative 6 mo to 5 y (median 3.4 y)	PCS component of QOL 1 y after pneumonectomy significantly lower than average population, mental QOL was higher than that of patients with other chronic illnesses
Pompili, 2012	172	Lung resection		Preoperative, 3 mo postoperative	
Moller & Sartipy,[2] 2012	213	Lung resection	SF-36	Preoperative, 6 mo postoperative	The extent of resection, age, and adjuvant therapy were significantly associated with decline in QOL.
Sartipy, 2009	117	Pneumonectomy and lobectomy	SF-36	Postoperative 6 mo	Pneumonectomy resulted in a greater negative impact on the physical component of QOL, than lobectomy at 6 mo postoperatively. The mental component score was not affected by extent of surgical resection.

that patients with a better preoperative physical functioning score and bodily pain scores and worse mental health scores were at higher risk of a relevant physical deterioration after surgery.[6] Patients with a lower $ppoFEV_1$, higher preoperative scores of social functioning, and higher preoperative scores of mental health were at higher risk of a relevant emotional deterioration. Based on their findings, the authors derived logistical regression equations to predict the risk of decline in physical or mental components of QOL after surgery:

$$\frac{\ln R}{1+R} = -11.6 + 0.19XPF\,(\textit{physical functioning}) + 0.05XBP\,(\textit{bodily pain}) - 0.05XMH\,(\textit{mental health})$$

The risk of physical decline computed by:

$$\frac{\ln R1}{1+R1} = -8.06 - 0.03XppoFEV1 + 0.11XSF + 0.55XMH\,(\textit{mental health})$$

Validated tools commonly used to measure QOL include SF-36, a shortened version (SF-12), Health-Related Quality of Life (HRQOL), European Organization for Research and Treatment of Cancer Quality of Life Questionnaire (EORTC QLQ-C30/LC13). Most of these tools have questions to assess MCS and PCS separately.

Given the subjective nature of QOL assessment as well as the different tools and methodology used in studies, a meta-analysis is difficult to perform. **Table 1** summarizes recent studies that have evaluated QOL after pulmonary resection. Most studies about QOL after pulmonary resection concern patients who have undergone pneumonectomy and not lobectomy.

PNEUMONECTOMY

QOL studies show that patients have a poor QOL following pneumonectomy. A recent study by the authors in 2012 evaluating 111 patients using the SF-12 showed that 1 year after pneumonectomy, the overall QOL was significantly lower than the QOL of the average population, yet their mean mental component scores were higher than those of patients with chronic diseases. This difference persisted even in patients who had both a pneumonectomy and a chronic illness, such as diabetes, heart disease, or a patient receiving neo-adjuvant therapy.[7] The univariate analysis of patient characteristics showed that the mental QOL differed significantly by gender (women had a higher mental component score than men, $P<.001$), indication for surgery (patients who underwent resection for malignancy had a higher mental score, $P<.001$), and disease recurrence (patients who had a recurrence had lower mental scores). There was no significant difference observed based on age, preoperative pulmonary function tests, neo-adjuvant therapy, final pathologic stage, smoking status, or co-morbidity. On multivariate analysis, none of these factors remained significantly associated with the mental QOL score.

Univariate analysis showed that physical QOL significantly differed by age (older patients had a lower physical component score, $P = .01$), $FEV_1\%$ score (patients with a higher $FEV_1\%$ had a higher physical component score, $P<.001$), and indication for surgery (patients undergoing surgery for malignancy had a higher physical score, $P = .05$). There were no significant differences observed based on gender, DLCO%, neo-adjuvant therapy, final pathologic stage, smoking status, comorbidity, or recurrence. On multivariate analysis, only age remained significantly associated with physical component score ($P = .02$).

Deslauriers and coworkers in 2011[8] evaluated the QOL of 100 patients 5 or more years after pneumonectomy using only physiologic markers to assess operative risks and estimate QOL. They showed that most patients were able to adjust to living a "near-normal life" following pneumonectomy. Their conclusions were based on the evaluation of physiologic parameters, which included $FEV_1\%$, DLCO%, $Vo_{2\ max}$, 6-minute walk test, chest roentgenogram, ipsilateral diaphragmatic motion, phrenic nerve conduction, and echocardiography. They concluded that most patients can adjust to living with only one lung and are thus able to live a near-normal life. The primary limitation of his study was that his findings provided unique physiologic information but QOL was not directly assessed or correlated with the functional variables.

Menna and colleagues in 2012 evaluated the QOL of 71 patients after pneumonectomy for up to 5 years postoperatively.[9] Twenty-six patients underwent right pneumonectomy (2 of them underwent intrapericardial pneumonectomy), 31 underwent left pneumonectomy (3 of them underwent intrapericardial pneumonectomy), 3 underwent extended pneumonectomy, 3 underwent extrapleural pneumonectomy, and 5 patients had a complete pneumonectomy. Three patients were not included in the study for early postoperative deaths (4.3%). All patients underwent complete preoperative assessment at 1 year after surgery. QOL was assessed by a questionnaire. They found that the 1-year and 5-year survival rates were 93% (N = 63) and 20% (N = 14), respectively. Mean values of FEV_1 decreased from 2.59 ± 0.75 L to 1.8 ± 0.72 L ($P<.001$). One year after surgery, all patients showed moderate tricuspid valve insufficiency; pulmonary artery systemic pressure was significantly higher, and right ventricular free wall thickness was moderately increased. An increased negative effect was recorded in the QQL scores with $P<.001$. Three clinical and surgical parameters were identified as risk or protective factors for the survival outcome. Postoperative mortality was 4.3% and 5-year survival was 20%.

Leo and colleagues in 2010[10] evaluated the QOL in 41 patients who underwent a pneumonectomy. They used the EORTC QLC-30 survey that was administered preoperatively and at 1, 3, and 6 months postoperatively. Poor QOL at 6 months was defined as global health values 10% or more below baseline values. The impact of several clinical variables was tested to discover predictors of poor postoperative QOL. They found that 6 months after pneumonectomy, global health showed a minimal impairment in the whole population (baseline 60.4 ± 26.5, at 6 months 56.3 ± 24.2, $P = .15$). Ten patients (24.4%) were identified as having poor QOL at 6 months. Age of 70 years or greater was identified as a significant risk factor for poor 6-month QOL using multivariate analysis (odds ratio, 1.13; 95% confidence interval, 1–1.26). The baseline global health score was the strongest predictor of postoperative global health QOL (odds ratio, 0.16; 95% confidence interval, 0.02–0.46; $P = .0086$). The overall QOL after pneumonectomy was impaired in 25% of surviving patients at 6 months after surgery; thus, this aspect of recovery should be routinely discussed with patients before pneumonectomy. Patients aged 70 years or more and those with low preoperative QOL seem to be at risk for unsatisfactory QOL after surgery. QOL after pneumonectomy was impaired in 25% of surviving patients at 6 months after surgery; thus, this aspect of recovery should be routinely discussed with patients before pneumonectomy. Older patients (those 70 years or more) and those with low preoperative QOL were at risk for unsatisfactory QOL after surgery.

Many studies have shown a decrease in QOL scores immediately postoperatively, but a return to baseline QOL about 6 to 12 months postoperatively.[11–13] Kenny and coworkers in 2008 evaluated the QOL in patients with stage I or II non-small cell lung carcinoma (NSCLC) who underwent pulmonary resection up to 2 years postoperatively.[14] The authors measured QOL using HRQOL questionnaires before surgery, at discharge, 1 month after surgery, and then every 4 months for 2 years. HRQOL was measured with a generic cancer QOL questionnaire (EORTC-QLQ-C30) and a lung cancer–specific questionnaire (EORTC QLQ-LC13). In their cohort, resection substantially reduced HRQOL across all dimensions except emotional functioning. HRQOL improved in the 2 years after surgery for patients without disease recurrence, although approximately half continued to experience symptoms and functional limitations. For those with recurrence within 2 years, there was some early postoperative recovery in HRQOL, with subsequent deterioration across most dimensions. Surgery had a substantial impact on HRQOL, and although many disease-free survivors experienced recovery, some lived with long-term HRQOL impairment. HRQOL generally worsened with disease recurrence. The authors also observed a substantially reduced QOL in all dimensions except mental score, even as far as 2 years after surgery.[14]

LOBECTOMY/BI-LOBECTOMY

Schulte and colleagues in 2009[15] evaluated 159 patients with NSCLC that underwent surgical resection. QOL and clinical data were assessed before resection and for up to 24 months after surgery by applying the EORTC core questionnaire and the lung-specific questionnaire, the EORTC lung-specific module. QOL was calculated, and QOL following bilobectomy/lobectomy was compared with QOL after pneumonectomy. They found the overall 5-year survival rate was 42%. Mean survival of the pneumonectomy group was slightly lower than that of the bilobectomy/lobectomy group, although the difference was not statistically significant ($P = .058$). The rate of complications was not significantly different between the 2 groups. Most QOL indicators remained near baseline for up to 24 months, with the exception of physical function ($P<.001$), pain ($P = .034$), and dyspnea ($P<.001$), which remained significantly impaired. QOL was significantly better after bilobectomy/lobectomy than after pneumonectomy. However, differences were statistically significant only with regard to physical function (at 3 months), social function (at 3 and 6 months), role function (at 3, 6, and 12 months), global health (at 3 and 6 months), and pain (at 6 months). Patients who underwent lung resection for NSCLC failed to make a complete recovery after 24 months. Patients who underwent pneumonectomy had significantly worse QOL values and a decreased tendency to recover compared with patients who underwent bilobectomy/lobectomy.

Many patients who present for lung resection also have comorbidities such as chronic obstructive pulmonary disease (COPD). Some studies have evaluated the changes in QOL after resection in these cohorts. For example, Pompili and coworkers in 2010[16] evaluated 220 patients who underwent lobectomy for lung cancer. Preoperative and postoperative (3 months) QOL were assessed in all patients via the SF-36 health survey. Compared with non-COPD patients, those with COPD had a 3-fold higher rate of cardiopulmonary morbidity (14 cases vs 5 cases, 28% vs 10%, $P = .04$), lower reduction in FEV_1 (6% vs 13%, $P = .0002$), but lower residual postoperative FEV_1 values (62% vs 74%, $P<.0001$). Postoperative DLCO (69% vs 65%, $P = .1$) and $Vo_{2\ max}$ (15.3 mL kg^{-1}) min^{-1} vs 14.3 mL kg^{-1} min^{-1}; $P = .4$) values were similar between the groups. The authors concluded that there were no significant differences between the groups in any of the preoperative and postoperative physical and mental QOL scores.

PREDICTING CHANGES IN QOL

One of the most significant predictors of changes in QOL is the extent of resection. Patients who underwent pneumonectomy tended to report the greatest decline in QOL (in particular physical domain) as compared with those who had lesser resections.[7,16] Other factors associated with postoperative QOL are shown in **Table 2** and these include age,[2,10] preoperative chronic pain,[6] lower preoperative mental score, and low preoperative DLCO.[12] The surgical approach (video-assisted thoracoscopic surgery, robotic vs open thoracotomy)[2,12] and in the authors' experience, preoperative body mass index seems to impact QOL postoperatively (R.J. Cerfolio, unpublished observations, 2013).

There are conflicting reports about age being a risk factor for QOL. Salati and colleagues (in 2009) showed that age does not seem to impact QOL after lung resection. They evaluated QOL in 218 patients, 85 of whom were elderly (70 years or older), who had completed preoperative and postoperative (3 months) the SF-36v2 health survey. QOL scales were compared between elderly and younger patients. Furthermore, limited to the elderly group, the authors compared the preoperative with the postoperative SF-36v2 measures and the PCS and MCS scores between high-risk patients and low-risk counterparts. The postoperative SF-36 PCS (50.3 vs 50, $P = .7$) and MCS (50.6 vs 49, $P = .2$) and all SF-36 domains did not differ between elderly and younger patients. Within the elderly, the QOL returns to the preoperative values 3 months after the operation. The authors did not find any significant differences between elderly higher risk patients and their lower risk counterparts postoperatively. The information that residual QOL in elderly patients will be similar to the one experienced by younger and fitter individuals may help them in their decision to proceed with surgery.

SUMMARY

One of the limitations of the assessment of the QOL is that the topic is inherently subjective. Therefore, all analyses are limited by this fact. Lack of standardization and multiple metrics for QOL lead to various interpretation of the literature. However it seems clear that pneumonectomy leads to a worse QOL than lobectomy;

Table 2
Factors associated with postoperative QOL in patients who undergo pulmonary resection

Factors	
Preoperative QOL/pain	Patients with better preoperative PCS, MCS, and no bodily pain preoperatively were associated with a better QOL postoperatively
Extent of resection	Pneumonectomy has been shown to decrease QOL significantly more than patients who undergo lobectomy Patients with pneumonectomy had a significantly lower postoperative physical QOL compared with mental QOL[2]
Age	Older age associated with worse postoperative QOL (Leo[10] cited >70 y, Cerfolio[2])
Preoperative PFTs	A DLCO <45% associated with worse overall QOL, as for low $ppoFEV_1$[6] associated with risk of mental declines postoperatively[6] Patients with low $ppoFEV_1$ had a greater perceived risk of postoperative emotional decline[6]
Approach	Patients who had a video-assisted thoracoscopic surgery or robotic resection had a better postoperative physical functioning score, compared with thoracotomy[10] (Cerfolio)
Social support system	Parenthetic data (Cerfolio)

older patients do worse than younger patients, and the preoperative QOL is an important predictor of postoperative QOL. The QOL of patients after all types of medical therapy will continue to be assessed more frequently by patients and by third-party payers. Therefore, more validated tools that better objectify this parameter are needed.

REFERENCES

1. Cykert S, Kissling G, Hansen CJ. Patient preferences regarding possible outcomes of lung resection. What outcomes should preoperative evaluations target? Chest 2000;117:1551–9.
2. Moller A, Sartipy U. Associations between changes in quality of life and survival after lung cancer surgery. J Thorac Oncol 2012;1:183–7.
3. Brunelli A, Charloux A, Bolliger CT, et al. ERS/ESTS clinical guidelines on fitness for radical therapy in lung cancer patients (surgery and chemo-radio therapy). Eur Respir J 2009;34:17–41.
4. Koller M, Kussman J, Lorenz W, et al. Symptom reporting in cancer patients: the role of negative affect and experienced social stigma. Cancer 1996;77:983–95.
5. Brunelli A, Socci L, Refai M, et al. Quality of life before and after major lung resection for lung cancer: a prospective follow-up analysis. Ann Thorac Surg 2007;84:410–6.
6. Pompili C, Brunelli A, Xiume F, et al. Predictors of postoperative decline in quality of life after major lung resections. Eur J Cardiothorac Surg 2011;39:732–7.
7. Bryant AS, Cerfolio RJ, Minnich DJ. Survival and quality of life at least 1 year after pneumonectomy. J Thorac Cardiovasc Surg 2012;144:1139–43.
8. Deslauriers J, Ugalde P, Miro S, et al. Long-term physiological consequences of pneumonectomy. Semin Thorac Cardiovasc Surg 2011;23:196–202.
9. Menna C, Ciccone AM, Ibrahim M, et al. Pneumonectomy: quality of life and long-term results. Minerva Chir 2012;67(3):219–26.
10. Leo F, Scanagatta P, Vannucci F, et al. Impaired quality of life after pneumonectomy: who is at risk? J Thorac Cardiovasc Surg 2010;139:49–52.
11. Win T, Sharples L, Wells FC, et al. Effect of lung cancer surgery on quality of life. Thorax 2005;60: 234–8.
12. Handy JR Jr, Asaph JW, Skokan L, et al. What happens to patients undergoing lung cancer surgery? Outcomes and quality of life before and after surgery. Chest 2002;122:21–30.
13. Dales RE, Belanger R, Shamji FM, et al. Quality of life following thoracotomy for lung cancer. J Clin Epidemiol 1994;47:1443–9.
14. Kenny PM, King MT, Viney RC, et al. Quality of life and survival in the 2 years after surgery for non small-cell lung cancer. J Clin Oncol 2008;26(2): 233–41.
15. Schulte T, Schniewind B, Dohrmann P, et al. The extent of lung parenchyma resection significantly impacts long-term quality of life in patients with non-small cell lung cancer. Chest 2009;135:322–9.
16. Pompili C, Brunelli A, Refai M, et al. Does chronic obstructive pulmonary disease affect postoperative quality of life in patients undergoing lobectomy for lung cancer? A case-matched study. Eur J Cardiothorac Surg 2010;37:525–30.
17. Balduyck B, Hendriks J, Lauwers P, et al. Quality of life evolution after lung cancer surgery: a prospective study in 100 patients. Lung Cancer 2007; 56(3):423–31.

Palliative Care Principles for Thoracic Surgery

Bill Nelems, MD, FRCSC, MEd

KEYWORDS

• Thoracic surgery • Oncology • Pain and symptom control • Palliation • Palliative care

KEY POINTS

- Thoracic surgical practice, heavily oncological in nature, is two-thirds populated with patients who do not survive their illnesses—embedding this practice in palliative medicine.
- Palliative care medicine, now a distinct specialty of its own, was late in forming, launched initially in the United Kingdom in 1967.
- At an international level, palliative care services are woefully inadequate: 5 billion of the world's 7 billion people have minimal or no access to opiods for pain control. Global awareness and advocacy are imperative.
- Research informs that the early identification of patient needs for palliative care services not only improves the quality of care but also saves money.
- A significant part of thoracic surgery practice is specifically aimed at procedures designed to alleviate symptoms and relieve suffering, procedures that are entirely palliative in nature.

Thoracic surgeons have always had an open window into the world of palliative care: 80% of patients referred to a thoracic surgeon have malignant diseases of the chest, and 80% of those patients die of the disease not able to be cured, not even with the support of the multibillion dollar pharmaceutical and radiation industries available.[1]

This worldview says more about the virulence and complexity of lung and esophagus cancer than it does about failure to cure. Nevertheless, whether tasked with the diagnostics of advanced stage cancer, undertaking surgical procedures that are inherently palliative in nature, or undertaking potentially curative surgeries of the chest, from a historical perspective, thoracic surgeons have had a front row seat into the developing world of palliative medicine.

It is surprising that among the various subspecialties of medicine, palliative care is one the most recent to have evolved. It was not until 1967, when Dame Cicely Saunders launched the first hospice unit in the United Kingdom, that this new discipline emerged.[2] In the years since then, there has been an explosion of research, public policy enactments, and World Health Organization directives, culminating in a fascinating Quality of Death Index, published in 2010 by the Economist Intelligence Unit, commissioned by the Lien Foundation in Singapore.[3]

Because of Dr Saunders' founding work, the United Kingdom leads the world in terms of research, funding, and policy. Australia and New Zealand enacted legislation for palliative care integration into their health care systems in 1988 and 1990, respectively, soon after Britain's actions.[4,5] It is not unanticipated then that these 3 countries should lead the Quality of Death Index, a summation of the basic health environment, availability, costs, and quality provided for end-of-life care. Canada and the United States are ranked coequally at 9th on the index. This Quality of Death Index is measured in only 40 countries where data are consistently available. Palliative services are low in the bottom 4 on this list: China, Brazil, Uganda, and India. Recognizing that no data

Department of Surgery, University of British Columbia, 2178 Pandosy Street, Kelowna, BC, V1W 1S8, Canada
E-mail address: billnelems@fastmail.fm

Thorac Surg Clin 23 (2013) 443–446
http://dx.doi.org/10.1016/j.thorsurg.2013.04.006

were available from the remaining 146 countries in the world, palliative services worldwide are woefully inadequate.

The World Health Organization describes palliative care as "an approach that improves the quality of life of patients and their families facing the problems associated with life-threatening illness. This is done through the prevention and relief of suffering by means of early identification and impeccable assessment and treatment of pain and other problems—physical, psychosocial, and spiritual."[6]

It is no surprise then to find advocates for palliative care assemble under the banners of pain and symptom control or of psychosocial, spiritual, or existential advocacy.

The embodiment of both paradigms of care can be concurrently adopted. "Pain management opens the gate to bringing in all the rest that we know—the social, spiritual, cultural issues that are there," say Merriman and Harding.[7] "With pain control, people can start to think again."

Cultural and historical differences explain why there is such diversity in the ways that people approach death and dying and, therefore, the way they enact laws and practice palliative medicine.

Even talking about death and dying is taboo in China, Japan, and India, making it virtually impossible for those countries to legislate policies. In a great many countries, the availability of opioids for the control of pain is restricted for fear of abuse and criminal access to these drugs.[3] In India, fewer that 1% of the public can access narcotic drugs.[3] Despite the World Health Organization's pain ladder for treatment, 5 billion of the world's 7 billion people live in countries with insufficient or no access to medications for the control of severe or moderate pain.[8]

In other parts of the world, in particular Africa, there is a strong sense of community support for the dying, augmented perhaps by the disease endemics that shorten life expectancy. In North America, there is a tendency to medicalize palliative care because of the availability of analgesic drugs, prompted also by the for-profit motives of pharmaceutical companies.[3]

Clarity surrounding any discussion about palliative care blurs in the modern era as topics, such as assisted suicide and euthanasia, enter the debate. Values and attitudes along with historical and religious beliefs vary from one jurisdiction to another, guaranteeing that no worldwide consensus about palliative care is established. This is different from practice guidelines for the treatment of lung cancer informed by scientific evidence.

As the population ages and chronic diseases proliferate, the need for palliative services will skyrocket. Between 50% and 70% of adults older than 70 suffer from chronic pain alone.[9] Although the funding of palliative care services even in first world countries is becoming a challenge, research shows that early intervention in the palliative care cycle can improve quality of care and decrease costs.

Patients receiving early palliative care consultations in intensive care settings had experienced shorter hospital stays, incurring lower costs with no decrease in their overall hospital mortality.[10] By identifying issues quickly on admission to hospital, their initial resolution facilitated early discharge.

A direct quote from the Economist Intelligence Unit report sums up the state of affairs succinctly: "The Governments and providers are in a race against time—however quickly they can beef up their end-of-life care infrastructure, they may still not be able to meet the even faster pace at which their citizens are reaching an age or condition where they need those services. So although calls echo around the world for end-of-life care to become enshrined in national and international policy as a human right, the reality is that even if it achieves that status, for much of the world's population, such a commitment will exist on paper only."[3]

Returning to the theme of palliative care in thoracic surgery, special notice is taken of those operations and procedures designed to relieve suffering and to improve quality of life.

The historical role of bypass procedures for advanced-stage esophageal cancer has given way to stenting, a technology that itself has undergone significant improvement over time. Esophageal stents have proved helpful in managing patients with dysphagia and tracheoesophageal fistulae.[11] A multicenter prospective randomized trial compared the self-expanding metal stent with the newer and self-expanding plastic stents in palliating malignant dysphagia. Both were effective in their palliation of symptoms, although the more-expensive metal stent migrated less frequently than its plastic alternative, with better dysphagia scores.[12]

The successful placement of second self-expanding stents has been reported in dealing with tumor overgrowth of previous stents.[13]

Both Nd:YAG laser débridement, and photodynamic therapy (PDT) have been evaluated in cases of bulky endoluminal tumor.[14] Both offered equivalent relief from esophageal obstruction, the PDT treatment leading to greater tumor ablation. Both treatments have been useful in control of bleeding from esophageal tumor erosion.[15]

Single-dose brachytherapy proved less useful than stenting in relieving dysphagia,[16] and the successful use of stents in the treatment of perforations of the esophagus in both malignant and benign disease has been reported.[17]

The similar use of stenting, YAG laser, and PDT treatments also applies to obstructing lesions of the tracheobronchial tree, where airflow obstruction, bleeding, and obstructive pneumonia pose significant clinical dilemmas.[11]

Mathisen and Grillo[18] report the successful coring out of bulky tumor in 51 of 56 patients. Airway stenting provides prompt and durable palliation in unresectable patients with central airway obstruction. Frequently, multiple stents and multiple procedures are necessary to maintain a satisfactory airway.[19]

Rigid bronchoscopy remains an invaluable tool for the control of massive hemoptysis.[20] Once the site of bleeding has been established and airway control stabilized, bronchial artery embolization, despite known complications, has proved effective in the control of bleeding.[21] Palliative lobectomy remains an option in cases of uncontrolled bleeding.[21]

Surgery plays a role in the management of bulky, infected, skin-eroded chest wall tumors. Extensive resection followed by rotation or by free tissue grafts has proved helpful.[22]

Pearson and MacGregor[23] were the first to describe the use of talc pleurodesis as an effective treatment in the management of malignant pleural effusions. A later randomized trial showed the pleurodesis technique more effective than the talc slurry technique.[24]

The advent of the PleurX catheter (CareFusion Corporation) has proved effective in treating malignant effusion patients in whom the lung is trapped and incapable of full re-expansion.[25] A randomized trial was undertaken comparing PleurX catheter insertion to doxycycline pleurodesis. The PleurX catheter group had a shorter median hospital stay (1.0 day vs 6.5 days) and had fewer recurrences.[26] No study could be found comparing PleurX to talc.

Malignant pericardial effusions, sometimes presenting as acute emergencies, can effectively be treated by surgical drainage, the techniques varying from left minithoracotomy to subxiphoid incision or videoscopic means. A limited pericardial window usually suffices. The use of talc as an irritant has been described.[27]

SUMMARY

The enduring challenge of palliative care, for both thoracic surgeons and the now established palliative care specialty, is to ask research-based questions, to seek answers to those questions, to teach, to learn, and to advocate. It is hoped that this article inspires the curious and informs those anxious to collaborate for a better tomorrow.

REFERENCES

1. Kachuri L, De P, Ellison LF, et al. Cancer incidence, mortality and survival trends in Canada, 1970-2007. Chronic Dis Inj Can 2013;33(2):69–80.
2. Obituary: Dame cicely Saunders. BMJ 2005;331. Available at: http://dx.doi.org/10.1136/bmj.331.7510.238. Accessed April 17, 2013.
3. Economist Intelligence Unit. The quality of death. Ranking end-of-life care across the world. Economist 2010. Available at: www.eiu.com/sponsor/lienfoundation/qualityofdeath. Accessed April 17, 2013.
4. Medical Treatment Act 1988—Australia. Available at: http://www.austlii.edu.au/au/legis/vic/consol_act/mta1988168/. Accessed April 17, 2013.
5. New Zealand Bill of Rights Act 1990. Available at: http://www.legislation.govt.nz/act/public/1990/0109/latest/DLM224792.html. Accessed April 17, 2013.
6. World Health Organization definition of Palliative Care. Available at: http://www.who.int/cancer/palliative/definition/en/. Accessed April 17, 2013.
7. Merriman A, Harding R. Pain Control in the African Context: the Ugandan introduction of affordable morphine to relieve suffering at the end of life. Philos Ethics Humanit Med 2010;5:10. http://dx.doi.org/10.1186/1747-5341-5-10.
8. World Health Organization Briefing note, "Access to Controlled Medications Programme," September, 2008. Available at: http://www.hrw.org/node/86033. Accessed April 17, 2013.
9. Gianni W, Madaio RA, Di Cioccio L, et al. Prevalence of pain in elderly hospitalized patients. Arch Gerontol Geriatr 2010;51(3):273–6. http://dx.doi.org/10.1016/j.archger.2009.11.016.
10. Byock I. Improving palliative care in intensive care units: identifying strategies and interventions that work. Crit Care Med 2006;34(11):S302–5. http://dx.doi.org/10.1097/01.CCM.0000237347.94229.23.
11. Klapper JA, Tong BC. The role of thoracic surgery in palliative care: a review. J Palliat Care Med 2012;2:7. Available at: http://dx.doi.org/10.4172/2165-7386.1000133. Accessed April 17, 2013.
12. Eickhoff A, Hartmann D, Kiesslich R, et al. A multicenter, prospective randomized trial comparing two types of self-expanding stents in the palliation of malignant dysphagia: SEMS (Ultraflex Stent) versus SEPS (Polyflex Stent). JFZ Gastroenterol 2008;46:425. http://dx.doi.org/10.1055/s-0028-1089800.

13. Conio M, Blanchi S, Filiberti R, et al. Self-expanding plastic stent to palliate symptomatic tissue in/overgrowth after self-expanding metal stent placement for esophageal cancer. Dis Esophagus 2010;23(7): 590–6. http://dx.doi.org/10.1111/j.1442-2050.2010.01068.x.
14. Lightdale CJ, Heier SK, Marcon NE, et al. Photodynamic therapy with porfimer sodium versus thermal ablation therapy with Nd:YAG laser for palliation of esophageal cancer: a multicenter randomized trial. Gastrointest Endosc 1995;42:507–12.
15. Suzuki H, Miho O, Watanabe Y, et al. Endoscopic laser therapy in the curative and palliative treatment of upper gastrointestinal cancer. World J Surg 1989; 13:158–64.
16. Homs MY, Essink-Bot ML, Borsboom GJ, et al, Dutch SIREC Study Group. Quality of life after palliative treatment for oesophageal carcinoma—a prospective comparison between stent placement and single dose brachytherapy. Eur J Cancer 2004;40: 1862–71.
17. Gomez-Esquivel R, Raju GS. Endoscopic closure of acute esophageal perforations. Curr Gastroenterol Rep 2013;15(5):321. http://dx.doi.org/10.1007/s11894-013-0321-9.
18. Mathisen DJ, Grillo HC. Endoscopic relief of malignant airway obstruction. Ann Thorac Surg 1989;48: 469–73.
19. Wood DE, Liu YH, Vallières E, et al. Airway stenting for malignant and benign tracheobronchial stenosis. Ann Thorac Surg 2003;76(1):167–72 [discussion: 173–4].
20. Karmy-Jones R, Cuschieri J, Vallières E. Role of bronchoscopy in massive hemoptysis. Chest Surg Clin N Am 2001;11(4):873–906.
21. Hurt K, Bilton D. Haemoptysis: diagnosis and treatment. Acute Med 2012;11(1):39–45.
22. Losken A, Thourani VH, Carlson GW, et al. A reconstructive algorithm for plastic surgery following extensive chest wall resection. Br J Plast Surg 2004;57(4):295–302.
23. Pearson FG, MacGregor DC. Talc poudrage for malignant pleural effusion. J Thorac Cardiovasc Surg 1966;51(5):732–8.
24. Dresler CM, Olak J, Herndon JE 2nd, et al. Phase III intergroup study of talc poudrage vs talc slurry sclerosis for malignant pleural effusion. Chest 2005;127: 909–15.
25. Olden AM, Holloway R. Treatment of malignant pleural effusion: PleuRx catheter or talc pleurodesis? A cost-effectiveness analysis. J Palliat Med 2010;13(1): 59–65. http://dx.doi.org/10.1089/jpm.2009.0220.
26. Putnam JB Jr, Light RW, Rodriguez RM, et al. A randomized comparison of indwelling pleural catheter and doxycycline pleurodesis in the management of malignant pleural effusions. Cancer 1999;86:1992–9.
27. Fibla JJ, Molins L, Mier JM, et al. Pericardial window by videothoracoscope in the treatment of pericardial effusion and tamponade. Cir Esp 2008;83(3):145–8.

Index

Note: Page numbers of article titles are in **boldface** type.

Thorac Surg Clin 23 (2013) 447–452
http://dx.doi.org/10.1016/S1547-4127(13)00105-9
1547-4127/13/$ – see front matter

Q

R

S

T

Printed and bound by CPI Group (UK) Ltd, Croydon, CR0 4YY

03/10/2024

01040370-0007